T0348644

Anesthesia at the Edge of Life

Editors

RANJIT DESHPANDE
STANLEY H. ROSENBAUM

ANESTHESIOLOGY CLINICS

www.anesthesiology.theclinics.com

Consulting Editor
LEE A. FLEISHER

March 2020 • Volume 38 • Number 1

ELSEVIER

1600 John F. Kennedy Boulevard • Suite 1800 • Philadelphia, Pennsylvania, 19103-2899

http://www.theclinics.com

ANESTHESIOLOGY CLINICS Volume 38, Number 1
March 2020 ISSN 1932-2275, ISBN-13: 978-0-323-69621-0

Editor: Colleen Dietzler
Developmental Editor: Kristen Helm

Anesthesiology Clinics (ISSN 1932-2275) is published quarterly by Elsevier Inc., 360 Park Avenue South, New York, NY 10010-1710. Months of issue are March, June, September, and December. Periodicals postage paid at New York, NY and at additional mailing offices. Subscription prices are $100.00 per year (US student/resident), $364.00 per year (US individuals), $446.00 per year (Canadian individuals), $728.00 per year (US institutions), $920.00 per year (Canadian institutions), $100.00 per year (Canadian student/resident), $225.00 per year (foreign student/resident), $474.00 per year (foreign individuals), and $920.00 per year (foreign institutions). To receive student and resident rate, orders must be accompanied by name of affiliated institution, date of term, and the *signature* of program/residency coordinator on institutions letterhead. Orders will be billed at individual rate until proof of status is received. Foreign air speed delivery is included in all *Clinics'* subscription prices. All prices are subject to change without notice. POSTMASTER: Send address changes to *Anesthesiology Clinics,* Elsevier Health Sciences Division, Subscription Customer Service, 3251 Riverport Lane, Maryland Heights, MO 63043. Customer Service (orders, claims, online, change of address): Elsevier Health Sciences Division, Subscription Customer Service, 3251 Riverport Lane, Maryland Heights, MO 63043. **Tel:1-800-654-2452 (U.S. and Canada); 314-447-8871 (outside U.S. and Canada). Fax: 314-447-8029. E-mail: journalscustomerservice-usa@elsevier.com (for print support); journalsonlinesupport-usa@elsevier.com (for online support).**

Reprints. For copies of 100 or more of articles in this publication, please contact the Commercial Reprints Department, Elsevier Inc., 360 Park Avenue South, New York, NY 10010-1710. Tel.: 212-633-3874; Fax: 212-633-3820; E-mail: reprints@elsevier.com.

Anesthesiology Clinics, is also published in Spanish by McGraw-Hill Inter-americana Editores S. A., P.O. Box 5-237, 06500 Mexico D. F., Mexico.

Anesthesiology Clinics, is covered in *MEDLINE/PubMed (Index Medicus), Current Contents/Clinical Medicine, Excerpta Medica, ISI/BIOMED,* and *Chemical Abstracts.*

Contributors

CONSULTING EDITOR

LEE A. FLEISHER, MD, FACC
Robert D. Dripps Professor and Chair of Anesthesiology and Critical Care, Professor of Medicine, Perelman School of Medicine, University of Pennsylvania, Philadelphia, Pennsylvania, USA

EDITORS

RANJIT DESHPANDE, MBBS
Department of Anesthesiology, Director, Transplant Anesthesiology, Yale School of Medicine, Anesthesiology, New Haven, Connecticut, USA

STANLEY H. ROSENBAUM, MA, MD
Professor of Anesthesiology, Internal Medicine, and Surgery, Chief, Section of Perioperative and Adult Anesthesia, Director, Critical Care Fellowship, Vice Chairman for Academic Affairs, Department of Anesthesiology, Yale School of Medicine, New Haven, Connecticut, USA

AUTHORS

CHRISTINE ACHO, DO
Resident, Department of Anesthesiology, Pain Management and Perioperative Medicine, Henry Ford Hospital, Detroit, Michigan, USA

MEREDITH A. ALBRECHT, MD, PhD
Associate Professor, Department of Anesthesiology, Medical College of Wisconsin, Milwaukee, Wisconsin, USA

AYMEN AWAD ALIAN, MBBCh
Associate Professor, Department of Anesthesiology, Yale School of Medicine, New Haven, Connecticut, USA

LOVKESH ARORA, MD
Clinical Associate Professor, Department of Anesthesia, University of Iowa Hospitals and Clinics, Iowa City, Iowa, USA

RAFI AVITSIAN, MD, FASA
Professor, Department of General Anesthesiology, Cleveland Clinic Foundation, Cleveland, Ohio, USA

AMIT BARDIA, MBBS
Department of Anesthesiology, Yale School of Medicine, New Haven, Connecticut, USA

NIBRAS BUGHRARA, MD
Director of Anesthesia Critical Care Division, Director of Critical Care Echocardiography Program, Assistant Professor, Departments of Anesthesiology and Surgery, Albany Medical College, Albany, New York, USA

STEPHANIE CHA, MD
Assistant Professor of Anesthesiology and Critical Care Medicine, Divisions of Cardiothoracic Anesthesiology and Critical Care, Johns Hopkins School of Medicine, Baltimore, Maryland, USA

NIKHIL CHAWLA, MBBS
Assistant Professor, Department of Anesthesiology, Yale School of Medicine, Yale University, New Haven, Connecticut, USA

ANOOP CHHINA, MD
Anesthesiologist and Surgical Critical Care Intensivist, Department of Anesthesiology, Pain Management and Perioperative Medicine, Henry Ford Hospital, Detroit, Michigan, USA

JOSE L. DIAZ-GOMEZ, MD
Section Chief, Cardiothoracic, Circulatory Support, and Transplant Critical Care, Director, Critical Care Echocardiography and Point of Care Ultrasonography, Associate Chief, Staff Professional Development, Education, and Clinical Research, Senior Faculty, Baylor College of Medicine, Division of Cardiovascular Anesthesia and Critical Care Medicine, Critical Care Medicine Services, Texas Heart Institute, Baylor St Luke's Medical Center, Houston, Texas, USA

HERODOTOS ELLINAS, MD
Associate Professor, Department of Anesthesiology, Medical College of Wisconsin, Milwaukee, Wisconsin, USA

KRISTEN L. FARDELMANN, MD
Assistant Professor, Department of Anesthesiology, Yale School of Medicine, New Haven, Connecticut, USA

ALEXANDER C. FORT, MD
Assistant Professor of Clinical Anesthesiology, Department of Anesthesiology, Perioperative Medicine and Pain Management, University of Miami Miller School of Medicine, University of Miami, Miami, Florida, USA

DRAGOS GALUSCA, MD
Anesthesiologist, Division Head of Surgical Critical Care, Department of Anesthesiology, Pain Management and Perioperative Medicine, Henry Ford Hospital, Detroit, Michigan, USA

CALVIN C. KUAN, MD, FAAP
Department of Anesthesiology, Perioperative and Pain Medicine, Stanford University School of Medicine, Stanford, California, USA

ASAD LATIF, MD, MPH
Department of Anesthesiology and Critical Care Medicine, Johns Hopkins School of Medicine, Armstrong Institute for Patient Safety and Quality, Johns Hopkins Medicine, Baltimore, Maryland, USA

SEUNG LEE, MD
Department of Anesthesiology and Critical Care Medicine, Johns Hopkins School of Medicine, Baltimore, Maryland, USA

SINEAD McCARTHY, MB BCh BAO, FCAI
Abdominal Organ Transplantation Anesthesia Fellowship Program, Department of Anesthesia and Pain Management, Toronto General Hospital, University Health Network, Toronto, Ontario, Canada

STUART A. McCLUSKEY, MD, PhD, FRCPC
Department of Anesthesia and Pain Management, Toronto General Hospital, University Health Network, University of Toronto, Toronto, Ontario, Canada

SARA NIKRAVAN, MD
Director of Perioperative Echocardiography and Point of Care Ultrasound, Divisions of Cardiothoracic Anesthesiology and Critical Care Medicine, Department of Anesthesiology, Virginia Mason Medical Center, Seattle, Washington, USA

AZUKA ONYE, MD
Department of Anesthesiology and Critical Care Medicine, Johns Hopkins School of Medicine, Baltimore, Maryland, USA

DASUN PERAMUNAGE, MD
Anesthesiology Resident, CA-3, Department of Anesthesiology, Virginia Mason Medical Center, Seattle, Washington, USA

ALIAKSEI PUSTAVOITAU, MD, MHS, FCCM
Assistant Professor of Anesthesiology and Critical Care Medicine, Division of Adult Critical Care Medicine, Director of Perioperative Ultrasound Program, Medical Director of Respiratory Care Services, Co-director of Liver Transplant Anesthesia Fellowship, Johns Hopkins School of Medicine, Baltimore, Maryland, USA

SHILPA RAO, MD
Assistant Professor, Department of Anesthesiology, Yale School of Medicine, Yale New Haven Hospital, New Haven, Connecticut, USA

RADWAN SAFA, MD
Assistant Professor, Departments of Anesthesiology and Surgery, Albany Medical College, Albany, New York, USA

JAGROOP S. SARAN, MD
Abdominal Organ Transplantation Anesthesia Fellowship Program, Department of Anesthesia and Pain Management, Toronto General Hospital, University Health Network, University of Toronto, Toronto, Ontario, Canada

SURANGAMA SHARMA, MD
Clinical Assistant Professor, Department of Anesthesia, University of Iowa Hospitals and Clinics, Iowa City, Iowa, USA

SUSANNA J. SHAW, MD
Department of Anesthesiology, Perioperative and Pain Medicine, Stanford University School of Medicine, Stanford, California, USA

AIDAN SPRING, LRCP&SI, MB BCh BAO, FCAI
Abdominal Organ Transplantation Anesthesia Fellowship Program, Department of Anesthesia and Pain Management, Toronto General Hospital, University Health Network, University of Toronto, Toronto, Ontario, Canada

WENDY SUHRE, MD
Assistant Professor, Department of Anesthesiology and Pain Medicine, University of Washington School of Medicine, Seattle, Washington, USA

MAYANKA TICKOO, MD, MS
Pulmonary and Critical Care Medicine, Department of Internal Medicine, Yale School of Medicine, New Haven, Connecticut, USA

GAIL A. VAN NORMAN, MD
Professor, Anesthesiology and Pain Medicine, Adjunct Professor, Bioethics, University of Washington, Seattle, Washington, USA

RICHARD A. ZACK-GUASP, MD
Assistant Professor of Clinical Anesthesiology, Department of Anesthesiology, Bruce W. Carter Medical Center, Department of Veteran's Health Administration, Miami, Florida, USA

Contents

Perioperative risk of morbidity and mortality for neonates is significantly higher than that for older children and adults. At particular risk are neonates born prematurely, neonates with major or severe congenital heart disease, and neonates with pulmonary hypertension. Presently no consensus exists regarding the safest anesthetic regimen for neonates. Regional anesthesia appears to be safe, but does not reduce the overall risk of postoperative apnea. Former preterm infants require postoperative observation for apnea. The anesthesiologist caring for the neonate for major surgery should be knowledgeable of the unique physiology of the neonate and maintain the highest level of vigilance throughout.

Mechanical circulatory support devices are increasingly being used for patients presenting with heart failure. The primary goal of these devices is to maintain perfusion to all organs. Intra-aortic balloon pump and extracorporeal membrane oxygenators are temporary devices that are usually reserved for patients presenting with acute heart failure. A left ventricular assist device may be implanted either as a bridge to heart transplant or to cardiac recovery, or for destination therapy in refractory heart failure. Familiarization with these devices is key to patient management in the perioperative period, especially for patients presenting for noncardiac surgeries.

The incidence of liver failure continues to increase, and it is associated with increased perioperative morbidity and mortality. Liver failure is associated with multiorgan dysfunction, including central nervous, cardiac, respiratory, gastrointestinal, renal, and hematological systems. Preoperative identification, optimization, and tailored anesthetic management are essential for optimum outcomes in patients with liver disease undergoing surgery. The coagulopathy of liver failure is a balanced coagulopathy better assessed by thromboelastography than conventional testing, and it is not directly associated with bleeding risk.

Video content accompanies this article at www.anesthesiology.
theclinics.com.

Point-of-care ultrasound is capable of identifying the precise causes of
hemodynamic failure in patients with septic shock. Patients in shock
demonstrate complex alterations in their circulation, including changes
in loading conditions (preload and afterload), right and left ventricular
function, and development of obstructive physiology, and some of
them have a burden of underlying cardiac disease. Knowledge of underlying hemodynamic derangements in such situations allows targeted interventions, that is, fluids, vasoactive, and inotropic medications, to
optimize patient's perfusion. One example of competing goals involves
a patient with hypertrophic "thick" left ventricle (LV), which is easily identified using point-of-care ultrasound (POCUS). Such patients usually have
diastolic dysfunction and commonly require higher filling pressures
(mainly grade II and III diastolic dysfunction) to maintain adequate cardiac
output. They are vulnerable to the effects of hypovolemia with the potential for dynamic LV outflow tract (LVOT) obstruction. The use of inotrope is
harmful under these circumstances and could lead to worsening of the
obstructive physiology because of systolic anterior motion of the mitral
valve leaflet and mitral regurgitation with rapid progression toward a cardiac arrest. Recognizing the increasingly important role of POCUS in the
perioperative arena, in this review, we highlight how POCUS allows anesthesiologists to recognize and manage hemodynamic derangements in
patients with sepsis and septic shock. We provide a systematic approach
to the evaluation of this patient population using qualitative assessment
of myocardial performance, fluid responsiveness, and fluid tolerance.
Our approach is based on a limited number of ultrasound views: subcostal, inferior vena cava (IVC), and lung views are obtained in rapid succes-
sion. A combination of findings in these views is grouped into distinct
hemodynamic phenotypes, each of them requiring their own approach
to management.

Trauma anesthesiology is a unique and growing subspecialty. With the
growing number of adult and pediatric trauma centers in the United
States, a thorough understanding of the early management of severely
injured patients with trauma is an important aspect of anesthesia.
Trauma anesthesiology requires the ability to adapt to different work
environments, including the trauma bay, the operating room, and
even the intensive care unit, where a patient room may require conversion to an operating suite for emergencies. This article provides a review of the anesthetic management for patients with extensive
trauma, focusing on physiology, pharmacology, and bedside
management.

countries can help fill this gap, particularly during crises, but it is critical to provide care responsibly and ethically. Most unmet surgical need is in low-income and middle-income countries where limited infrastructural, human, and material resources pose significant challenges. Anesthesia providers must recognize these difficulties as they apply to the local context and plan accordingly. This article outlines some of the unique issues and provides a framework of considerations for safe and responsible anesthesia delivery in resource-limited areas.

End-of-life vital organ transplantation involves singular ethical issues, because survival of the donor is impossible, and organ retrieval is ideally as close to the death of the donor as possible to minimize organ ischemic time. Historical efforts to define death have been met with confusion and discord. Fifty years on, the Harvard criteria for brain death continue to be problematic and now face significant legislative efforts to limit their authority.

ANESTHESIOLOGY CLINICS

THE CLINICS ARE AVAILABLE ONLINE!
Access your subscription at:
www.theclinics.com

Foreword

Anesthesia at the Edge of Life

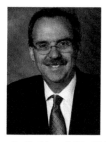

Lee A. Fleisher, MD, FACC
Consulting Editor

Anesthesiology has been lauded for being a leader in patient safety with an amazing record of markedly reducing deaths directly attributable to the delivery of surgical anesthesia. These advancements have led surgeons and other proceduralists to perform procedures on increasingly ill individuals. Many of these individuals would have died without a procedure several decades ago, but increasingly, the skill of anesthesiologists in the operating room and intensive care units has led to surviving these physiologic insults. In this issue of the *Anesthesiology Clinics*, innovations in perioperative management of extreme conditions and the ethical issues, including resource-limited areas, are discussed.

In order to assemble a series of articles for Anesthesia at the Edge of Life, I enlisted an editor with much experience in the area and an editor of several previous issues of the *Clinics*, Stanley H. Rosenbaum, MA, MD. Dr Rosenbaum is Professor of Anesthesiology, Internal Medicine, and Surgery. He is Vice-Chair for Academic Affairs and Section Chief of Perioperative and Adult Anesthesia. In addition, he taught me how to provide anesthesia care for patients at the edge of life. He is joined by his colleague, Ranjit Deshpande, MBBS. Dr Deshpande is Assistant Professor of Anesthesiology and Director of Transplant Anesthesiology at Yale School of Medicine. Together, they have assembled an all-star group of authors to educate in this area.

Lee A. Fleisher, MD, FACC
Perelman School of Medicine
University of Pennsylvania
3400 Spruce Street, Dulles 680
Philadelphia, PA 19104, USA

E-mail address:
lee.fleisher@uphs.upenn.edu

https://doi.org/10.1016/j.anclin.2019.12.002
1932-2275/20/© 2019 Published by Elsevier Inc.
anesthesiology.theclinics.com

Preface

Anesthesia at the Edge of Life

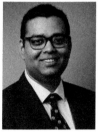
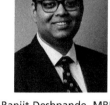

Ranjit Deshpande, MBBS   Stanley H. Rosenbaum, MA, MD
Editors

The evolution and advance of medical science in the contemporary era have greatly improved the quality of care for the sickest patients in the perioperative arena. In this issue, dealing with these critically ill patients at the edge of life and death, we focus on a series of different situations the clinician might encounter.

This issue of *Anesthesiology Clinics* is meant to update the anesthesia provider who cares for extremely sick patients needing emergency surgery in a well-resourced or resource-limited area. We start with neonatal anesthesia, where in-hospital mortality for noncardiac surgery is 5 times higher for preterm neonates than full-term neonates. We also review organ failure, neurosurgical emergencies, high-risk obstetrics, septic shock, trauma, endocrine emergencies, malignant hyperthermia, electroconvulsive therapy, obesity, and anesthesia in resource-limited areas.

The articles on septic shock focus on the use of ultrasound to help manage shock; they are sure to engage our readers with the novel and valuable uses of this technology. Our final article brings forward the sensitive ethical issues of organ donation.

Anesthesiology Clin 38 (2020) xv–xvi
https://doi.org/10.1016/j.anclin.2019.12.001
1932-2275/20/© 2019 Published by Elsevier Inc.

anesthesiology.theclinics.com

We thank the authors who have made this a success and hope that the readers enjoy the issue while they learn just as we have.

Ranjit Deshpande, MBBS
Department of Anesthesiology
Yale School of Medicine
333 Cedar Street
New Haven, CT 06520-8051, USA

Stanley H. Rosenbaum, MA, MD
Department of Anesthesiology
Internal Medicine, and Surgery
Section of Perioperative and Adult Anesthesia
Critical Care Fellowship
Department of Anesthesiology
Yale School of Medicine
333 Cedar Street
New Haven, CT 06520-8051, USA

E-mail addresses:
ranjit.deshpande@yale.edu (R. Deshpande)
stanley.rosenbaum@yale.edu (S.H. Rosenbaum)

Anesthesia for Major Surgery in the Neonate

Calvin C. Kuan, MD*, Susanna J. Shaw, MD

KEYWORDS

- Pediatric anesthesia • Neonatal anesthesia • Neonate • Preterm infant
- Pediatric surgery • Neonatal surgery

KEY POINTS

- Neonates and preterm neonates are at significantly higher risk for perioperative complications compared with older children and adults.
- Children with major or severe congenital heart disease and pulmonary hypertension require specialized perioperative care.
- Former premature infants require postoperative monitoring because of an increased risk of apnea and bradycardia.

INTRODUCTION

Children are not just little adults

This often-spoken aphorism could not be more relevant than in the care of our youngest, smallest, and most fragile patients. The anesthesiologist caring for the neonate must have an intimate understanding of anatomy, physiology, and pharmacology and how anesthesia impacts these newborns who are transitioning to life outside the womb. A neonate is defined as a newborn up to 28 days of life, regardless of gestational age (GA). This article is intended to assist the anesthesiologist tasked to care for the neonate but will also be applicable to preterm infants and infants.

EVOLUTION/HISTORY OF ANESTHESIA FOR THE NEONATE

A newborn undergoing major surgery before the 1980s would have likely received an anesthetic consisting solely of nitrous oxide and muscle relaxant. Historically, this "Liverpool technique" of light general anesthesia devoid of opiates was the standard of care.[1] The prevailing thought at the time was that neonates were not able to feel pain because they lacked a mature sensory nervous system. Analgesia for neonates

Department of Anesthesiology, Perioperative and Pain Medicine, Stanford University School of Medicine, 300 Pasteur Drive, H3582, Stanford, CA 94305, USA
* Corresponding author.
E-mail address: ckuan@stanford.edu

Anesthesiology Clin 38 (2020) 1–18
https://doi.org/10.1016/j.anclin.2019.10.001
anesthesiology.theclinics.com

undergoing any procedure was considered unnecessary or even contraindicated because of concerns for hemodynamic instability. In the 1980s, Robinson and Gregory[2] demonstrated that fentanyl could be safely administered to neonates for ligation of patent ductus arteriosus (PDA), and Anand and colleagues[3] published their seminal study showing that the addition of fentanyl to the anesthetic regimen of nitrous oxide and D-tubocurarine diminished the stress response and decreased postoperative complications. These studies changed the mindset allowing for the use of a wider spectrum of anesthetics for neonates.

RISK OF PERIOPERATIVE CARDIAC ARREST FOR THE NEONATE

Beecher and Todd[4] were some of the first to recognize that anesthesia mortality was "disproportionately high in the first decade of life." Over the years, other groups have examined the risk of anesthesia in children grouping neonates with infants less than 1 year of age.[5,6] One study[7] that did break down the patients into smaller age subcategories found that neonates and infants were at the highest risk of cardiac arrest from any cause compared with older children. With the advent of pulse oximetry in the 1980s and technological advancements in ventilation, and pharmacology, the overall mortality for anesthesia has dropped significantly globally. Even so, the mortality in neonates and premature infants continues to be significantly greater than that for older children or adults.[8]

More recent studies have attempted to delve deeper into this question by examining risks of minor and major complications in addition to cardiac arrest in neonates and specific subgroups that may be at higher risk.

THE NEONATE BORN PREMATURELY

GA has been identified as an independent risk factor.[9,10] The in-hospital mortality for noncardiac surgery is 5 times higher for preterm neonates than full-term neonates (10.5% vs 2%).[11]

THE NEONATE WITH CONGENITAL HEART DISEASE

Analyzing data from the Pediatric Perioperative Cardiac Arrest Registry, Ramamoorthy and colleagues[12] found that children younger than 2 years of age were more likely to have cardiac arrest, and that children with congenital heart disease (CHD) are more likely to have a cardiac arrest during noncardiac surgery than during cardiac surgery and the interventional cardiac catheterization laboratory combined. This study also determined that the causes of cardiac arrest in patients with CHD were not different when they occurred in the general operating room (OR) versus the cardiac OR. The investigators suggested that the reason for this is that the underlying cardiac lesion and condition may be more important than the type of surgery. A separate study[13] found that the highest incidence of mortality within 24 hours and 30 days after anesthesia occurred in neonates, and that patients undergoing cardiac surgery had a much higher mortality compared with patients who had noncardiac surgery.

It is important to note that not all congenital cardiac conditions pose the same risk. The American College of Surgeons National Surgical Quality Improvement Program classifies CHD into 3 categories (**Table 1**). Patients with minor CHD are generally considered appropriate for care by any pediatric anesthesiologist in an ambulatory setting, whereas patients with major or severe CHD require a pediatric anesthesiologist with expertise caring for these complex patients in a tertiary setting.[14]

Table 1	
Risk stratification for congenital heart disease for noncardiac surgery	
Classification	**Definition and Criteria**
Minor CHD	• Cardiac condition with or without medication and maintenance (eg, atrial septal defect, small to moderate ventricular septal defect with no symptoms) • Repair of congenital heart defect with normal cardiovascular function and no medication
Major CHD	• Repair of congenital heart defect with residual hemodynamic abnormality with or without medications (eg, tetralogy of Fallot with wide open pulmonary insufficiency; hypoplastic left heart syndrome, including stage 1 repair)
Severe CHD	• Uncorrected cyanotic heart disease • Patients with any documented PH • Patients with ventricular dysfunction requiring medications • Listed for heart transplant

From Faraoni D, Zurakowski D, Vo D, et al. Post-operative outcomes in children with and without congenital heart disease undergoing noncardiac surgery. Journal of the American College of Cardiology 2016;67(7):795; with permission.

THE NEONATE WITH PULMONARY HYPERTENSION

Children with pulmonary hypertension (PH) have been consistently described as having among the highest risk of major complications, including cardiac arrest and death with any anesthetic, with the risk increasing in proportion to severity of the PH.[13] The cause of the PH does not appear to affect the risk. Bernier and colleagues[15] found that patients receiving PH-targeted pharmacologic therapy (eg, prostacyclin analogue or inhaled nitric oxide) appear to have a lower incidence of minor intraoperative events than those not on medication. This study also found that 4.7% of these patients experienced a cardiac arrest up to 7 days postoperatively, even when admitted to an intensive care unit (ICU) postoperatively. Because the risk for patients with PH in the postoperative period appears to be at least as dangerous as the intraoperative period, continued vigilance is advised during the emergence period, and an elevated level of postoperative care should be considered even for minor procedures.

RISK STRATIFICATION

Recent research into perioperative mortality has taken into consideration the interaction of patient comorbidities with the intrinsic risk of the surgical procedure (**Table 2**). Nasr and colleagues[16] identified the following 5 major comorbid conditions that impact outcome:

- Weight of patient less than 5 kg
- American Society of Anesthesiologists (ASA) status III or higher
- Preoperative sepsis
- Inotropic support
- Ventilator dependence

When these 5 conditions were analyzed in the context of surgical procedures divided into low- to high-risk quartiles, they found that the risk of 30-day mortality was 0% when patients with no comorbidities underwent a low-risk procedure and 4.74% when patients with all 5 comorbidities had low-risk procedures. The risk of 30-day mortality was 0.07% when patients with no comorbidities had high-risk procedures, whereas the risk increased to 46.7% when patients with all 5 comorbidities had high-risk procedures. Of particular relevance is that the authors found that being a neonate in and of itself did not increase risk significantly. One possible explanation for this is that the arbitrary distinction of age was less meaningful than the weight of the patient.

Table 2	
Risk factors associated with perioperative complications in neonates	
Risk Factor	**Source**
Prematurity	Lillehei et al,[11] 2012
CHD	
Serious respiratory condition	
NEC	
Neonatal sepsis	
Prematurity	Michelet et al,[9] 2017
CHD	
BPD	
NEC	
Preoperative ICU status	
Intraoperative fluid bolus administration	
Weight <5 kg	Nasr et al,[16] 2019
ASA III or greater	
Preoperative sepsis	
Inotropic support	
Ventilator dependence	

Abbreviations: BPD, bronchopulmonary dysplasia; NEC, necrotizing enterocolitis.

RISK OF NEUROTOXICITY WITH GENERAL ANESTHESIA

All commonly used anesthetic agents have been associated with neurotoxicity across a spectrum of animal species, including nonhuman primates, and there is no consensus whether these findings are translatable to humans.[17] Taken collectively, the clinical studies in humans have been inconclusive because of the myriad of variables that are difficult to control.[18] The sole prospective, randomized, controlled study of infants has provided the strongest and most reassuring evidence to date, that a single, short exposure (ie, <1 hour) to general anesthesia does not affect neurodevelopmental outcomes at 5 years.[19] This lack of association between anesthetic exposure and negative neurocognitive outcome is consistent with other major cohort studies.[20,21] The data regarding effects on the neonate after repeated or longer exposures to general anesthesia are less clear. Adding to the uncertainty are factors that are much more difficult to control, including the underlying disease process (eg, cyanotic heart disease), hypotension, and altered cerebral blood flow.[8] Based on the Food and Drug Administration's (FDA) latest warning, procedures requiring general anesthesia should be postponed for children younger than 3 years. Most conditions requiring major surgery in the neonate are urgent and cannot be delayed. Therefore, it may be prudent to minimize exposure by attempting to schedule multiple procedures under a single anesthetic when medically feasible.

ANATOMY AND PHYSIOLOGY OF THE NEONATE

One of the more challenging aspects of delivering anesthetic care to the neonate is their unique physiology. The following is a brief discussion by relevant systems of the challenges often faced when caring for a neonate.

Airway: Cuffed Versus Uncuffed Endotracheal Tubes

Historically, there was concern that cuffed endotracheal tubes (ETT) caused tracheal damage; however, current evidence supports the use of cuffed tubes even in the neonatal population. Cuffed tubes have not been found to result in more postoperative stridor or increased need for reintubation. Furthermore, cuffed tubes are associated with fewer leaks, higher tidal volumes, and less hoarseness/sore throat than uncuffed tubes.[22,23] One study of infants <3 kg intubated in the OR found no difference between the cuffed versus uncuffed tubes in regard to duration of intubation, tube changes, unplanned extubations, ventilator leaks, atelectasis, plugging of the tube, pneumonia, or postextubation stridor.[24]

Recalling Poiseuille's law describing flow through a cylinder in which the radius is raised to the fourth power, even a 0.5- mm-diameter change can have significant implications for work of breathing, especially when small tubes are used (**Fig. 1**). Thomas and colleagues[25] simulated differences in work of breathing between an uncuffed 3.5 ETT and a 3.0 ETT. They found that although work of breathing was higher with a cuffed tube (by approximately 10%), this difference was neutralized by the application of pressure support and automatic tube compensation. Given the risk of worsening lung compliance during major surgery in the neonate, a cuffed ETT provides the safest way to ventilate without having to upsize the tube.

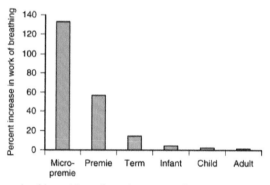

Fig. 1. Change in work of breathing after placement of an appropriately sized ETT. (*From* Spaeth JP, Lam JE. The Extremely premature infant (micropremie) and common neonatal emergencies. In: Coté CJ, Lerman J, Anderson BJ, editors. A Practice of Anesthesia for Infants and Children, 6th edition. Philadelphia: Elsevier; 2019; with permission.)

Respiratory Physiology

Biochemical and Reflex Respiratory Control

The respiratory control systems, including the brainstem respiratory rhythmogenesis areas and the central and peripheral chemoreceptors, are still immature in the term neonate. These patients, particularly preterm neonates, are susceptible to apnea at baseline, and this is exacerbated in the postoperative setting. Preterm infants can have life-threatening postoperative apneic episodes up to 60 weeks' postconceptional age (**Fig. 2**).[26] The neonate also has a notably different response to hypoxia. Whereas an older child compensates with a protective phase of increased ventilation in response to a hypoxic mixture, the neonate has only a brief period of hyperpnea followed by significant bradypnea, which can contribute to the rapid development of hypoxemia and lead to apnea. Although term infants appear to have the same ventilatory response curve as adults (with hypercapnea causing increased minute ventilation), this response is blunted in preterm infants. In addition, neonates also have an exaggerated apneic response to both afferent laryngeal stimulation and excessive inflation of the lung (ie, Hering Breuer Inflation reflex).

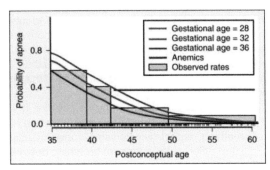

Fig. 2. Predicted probability of apnea for all patients by GA and weeks of postconceptual age. (*From* Gregory GA, Brett CM. Neonatology for Anesthesiologists. In: Davis PJ, Cladis FP, editors. Smith's Anesthesia for Infants and Children, 9th edition. Philadelphia: Elsevier; 2017; with permission.)

Lung anatomy

Neonates have anatomic differences that primarily aggregate to increase their work of breathing and decrease their apneic time compared with older children and adults. In addition to smaller airways, neonates, particularly preterm infants, are at increased risk of having laryngomalacia, tracheomalacia, tracheal stenosis, and subglottic stenosis, which can further decrease airway size and gas conductance. The chest wall in infants is highly compliant with a horizontally aligned rib structure (rather than the angled rib structure of older children and adults). This anatomic difference decreases chest wall elasticity and increases work of breathing as well as risk of airway collapse and atelectasis. All of this contributes to closing volumes that are greater than functional residual capacity (FRC). As a result, neonates can experience terminal airway closure during normal breathing. Finally, the diaphragm in neonates contains less type 1 fibers (endurance fibers) so they are more likely to quickly fatigue.

To maintain FRC, infants have high respiratory rates and short expiratory time (creating auto–positive end expiratory pressure [PEEP]). They also maintain partial laryngeal adduction in expiration to increase expiratory airway resistance. The effects of general anesthesia eliminate the natural mechanisms the neonate has in place to maintain an open airway and prevent atelectasis. When an infant becomes apneic, FRC is lost and hypoxemia rapidly develops. This phenomenon is exacerbated by the infant's increased oxygen consumption (Vo_2). These factors together highlight the importance of preoxygenation.

Mechanical ventilation

In the neonatal intensive care unit (NICU), lung-protective strategies are used to avoid volutrauma, barotrauma, and atelectotrauma by using PEEP and recruitment maneuvers. Volume-targeted ventilation (VTV) methods are preferred over pressure-limited ventilation (PLV). A recent Cochrane review of the literature found that infants ventilated using VTV modes had reduced rates of death or bronchopulmonary dysplasia (BPD), pneumothoraces, hypocarbia, severe cranial ultrasound pathologic conditions, and duration of ventilation compared with infants ventilated using PLV modes.[27] Mild permissive hypercapnea is advised and can help prevent BPD.[28] For many years, it had been accepted that hyperoxia was associated with retinopathy of prematurity

(ROP) and BPD of the premature lung. Although some investigations have indicated that mortality in extremely premature infants is increased when the targeted oxygen saturation is 85% to 89% versus 91% to 95%,[29] new investigations have suggested no difference in mortality, BPD, ROP, or neurodevelopment in extremely preterm neonates when a more liberal SpO$_2$ (85%–95%) is permitted.[30]

Cardiovascular Physiology

Maintenance of cardiac output

The neonatal heart is extremely dependent on heart rate to maintain adequate cardiac output. Consider the formula for cardiac output (CO) (CO = heart rate [HR] x stroke volume [SV]), where stroke volume is determined by a combination of preload, afterload, and contractility. Hypovolemia will certainly result in decreased cardiac output, but because fetal myocardial cells are disorganized and the ventricles are poorly compliant, increasing preload in a euvolemic neonate will not necessarily augment stroke volume. Moreover, a rapid fluid bolus may cause increased ventricular wall tension and decreased coronary perfusion, putting the neonatal heart at risk for overdistension and heart failure.

To best optimize cardiac output during anesthesia in the neonate, it is essential to maintain heart rate in the normal range with a normal sinus cardiac rhythm. Although β-agonists can be used to increase contractility, they should be used judiciously because the neonatal myocardium is vulnerable to cardiotoxicity from circulating epinephrine. Calcium may be a useful inotrope to improve contractility in the neonate. Unlike the adult myocardium, which uses sarcoplasmic reticulum calcium stores, neonatal cardiac cells rely on both extracellular and nuclear calcium for contraction.

Maintenance of blood pressure

Neonatologists use a mean arterial blood pressure equivalent to the GA in weeks as an adequate minimal value. Among pediatric anesthesiologists, there is a wide variety in practice as when to treat hypotension. Most use a systolic blood pressure of 40 to 50 mm Hg or a decrease of 20% to 30% from baseline as the threshold. These numbers are significantly lower than the fifth percentile as defined in various normative studies, suggesting that most anesthesiologists accept lower values in a neonate under anesthesia.[31] Without an established nominal value as a guide, treatment should follow 3 paradigms: (1) "normative," according to population derived data; (2) "physiologic," based on the point at which low blood pressure is detrimental to organ perfusion; and (3) "operational," the point at which the anesthesiologist should intervene.[32] The physiologic point at which blood pressure no longer supports adequate tissue perfusion is largely theoretic, and efforts to associate hypotension with decrease in perfusion of vital organs have not always shown correlation. Olbrecht and colleagues[33] measured cerebral oxygenation during anesthesia in the neonate using near-infrared spectroscopy (NIRS) and noted that many periods of low arterial pressure were not necessarily associated with low cerebral oxygenation.

Fluid, Glucose, and Electrolytes

Sodium and fluids

Electrolyte needs were initially calculated based on their presence in human breast milk, which amounts to a hypotonic solution (0.2% saline equivalent). More recent clinical observations have questioned whether hypotonic solutions are appropriate, and the current recommendation is that patients from 28 days to 18 years receive isotonic fluids.[34] Although these guidelines exclude neonates, there is some evidence that this population is also at risk for hyponatremia when given hypotonic solutions.[35]

Glucose

Neonates need 4 to 8 mg/kg/min of glucose to sustain brain development and prevent hypoglycemia, even short episodes of which can cause neurological injury in the neonate. Generally, a normal intraoperative serum glucose level is maintained by neonates undergoing major surgery (notable exceptions are when a preoperative glucose infusion is interrupted or in neonates less than 48 hours old). Although there is no consensus on the threshold to treat hypoglycemia, ensuring that serum glucose level is great than 50 mg/dL is suggested while under anesthesia.[36] There is evidence that moderate hyperglycemia is not detrimental in the same way it is in adults and may in fact be protective in neonates.[37] Although neonates need dextrose supplementation during surgery, the rate may be lower than their normal maintenance requirement. A recent review of available literature, examining dextrose-containing fluids in pediatric populations, suggests that 1% to 2.5% dextrose-containing isotonic fluids for intraoperative maintenance in neonates and infants may be adequate to provide the appropriate homeostasis.[38] Current standard practice advises administration of 5% to 10% dextrose-containing fluids.[36] The most prudent practice would be to monitor glucose levels at frequent intervals.

Hematology and Coagulation

Although there is an increasing body of evidence meant to guide transfusion parameters in the neonate, consensus is still lacking, and there is considerable variation in transfusion practices. Guidelines have been published guiding transfusion in patients less than 4 months that recommend transfusion for hematocrit less than 20% in an otherwise healthy infant, less than 30% in an infant on supplemental oxygen, and less than 35% in an infant on noninvasive or invasive positive pressure and when there is acute blood loss of 10% of the blood volume.[39] In the preterm infant, and especially the micropremies, even a very small amount of blood loss can represent a huge portion of the blood volume (**Table 3**). A study by Goobie and colleagues[40] found an independent association between preoperative anemia (defined as a hematocrit <40%) and in-hospital mortality in neonates 0 to 30 days old. A 2016 review suggests for infants greater than 1000 g and without other risk factors (eg, cyanotic CHD) that the threshold should be greater than 35% (or >30% for patients at physiologic nadir).[41]

Although the neonatal clotting system is described as immature, a healthy term neonate is not at particular risk for clotting or bleeding.[42] Platelet counts are similar to normal adult values in term neonates but are lower in premature infants. Prolonged prothrombin times and activated partial thromboplastin times may not indicate a bleeding diathesis. Age-appropriate reference ranges should be used and clinical context considered to prevent overtreating.[42] Newborn infants are deficient in vitamin K and are at risk for vitamin K deficiency bleeding (VKDB). A single intramuscular dose (1 mg) of vitamin K is effective in preventing classic VKDB in the term infant. Although preterm infants are at risk for potential vitamin K deficiency secondary to immature hepatic and hemostatic function, delayed feeding and, therefore, delayed colonization of the gut with vitamin K_2–producing microflora, VKDB has not been well described in the preterm infant. Although neonatal intensive care practices may vary, most NICU patients empirically receive ongoing vitamin K supplementation through either parenteral or enteral nutrition during their hospital stay.[43] If a neonate has not received a prophylactic dose of vitamin K at birth, a dose before major surgery is advisable. There are no data regarding the administration of additional doses in term or preterm infants before invasive procedures.

Table 3
Circulating blood volume in micropremies, premies, full-term neonates, infants, and children

	Blood Volume (mL/kg)	Weight (kg)	Total Blood Volume (mL)	25-mL Blood Loss Proportion of Total Blood Volume (%)
Micropremie	110	1	110	23
Premie	100	1.75	175	14
Full-term neonate	90	3	270	9
Infant	80	10	800	3
Child	70	20	1400	2

From Spaeth JP, Lam JE. The Extremely premature infant (micropremie) and common neonatal emergencies. In: Coté CJ, Lerman J, Anderson BJ, editors. A Practice of Anesthesia for Infants and Children, 6th edition. Philadelphia: Elsevier; 2019; with permission.

Pharmacology

Pharmacokinetics and pharmacodynamics in neonates differ from infants, older children, and adults and are rapidly changing in the first few months after birth. Post-conceptional age rather than postnatal age determines the level of maturation. Absorption, distribution, and clearance are all altered in this period.

Absorption

Gastroenteric absorption is decreased because of delayed gastric emptying in neonates. Transdermal absorption of topical medications (ie, steroids or EMLA cream) is increased because of large surface area and increased skin perfusion. The epidural space in the neonate has increased vascularity and smaller absorptive surface for local anesthetics compared with older children.[44] The absorption half-time of epidural levobupivacaine decreases from birth until 6 months postnatal age and also has reduced clearance by the cytochrome P450 enzyme, CYP3A4, causing a delay to maximal plasma concentration.[45]

Distribution

The neonate has a greater extracellular and total-body water space compared with older children. In addition, adipose stores have a higher ratio of water to lipid. As a result, plasma levels of hydrophilic drugs, such as morphine, have a reduced volume of distribution in neonates, and the initial dose (in milligram per kilograms) should be less than that administered to an adult.[44]

Neonates also have a higher free fraction of protein-bound drugs, both because of a decrease in circulating plasma proteins (eg, albumin and α_1-acid glycoprotein) and because of the presence of exogenous substances (eg, bilirubin and free fatty acids) that displace drugs bound to albumin-binding sites. The epidural dose of bupivacaine will have an increased unbound and therefore active fraction of the drug, decreasing the recommended bolus dose in neonates.[44]

Clearance

Phase I reactions by the cytochrome P-450 isoenzymes activate at birth (except CYP3A7, which is present in the fetal liver) and continue to develop over the first few days to weeks in a term neonate. Over the first weeks of life, infants will have variable responses to certain medications. For example, CYP3A4 is required for clearance of levobupivacaine or midazolam and starts to appear sometime in the first week of life. Ropivacaine is cleared by CYP1A2, which is the last enzyme to appear.

Sulfate conjugation is mature in the term neonate, but other phase II reactions, such as glucuronidation, are not. Glucuronidation is responsible for the clearance of several drugs, including acetaminophen, morphine, and propofol (although propofol is also metabolized by cytochrome P450 enzymes) (**Fig. 3**). Failure to appreciate immaturity of uridine diphosphate-glucuronosyltransferase resulted in the cardiovascular collapse of neonates given chloramphenicol in the late 1950s. **Table 4** provides further information regarding commonly used drugs in anesthesia and use in neonate.

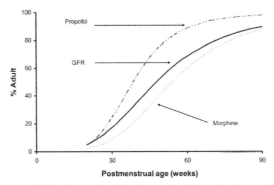

Fig. 3. Clearance curve. GFR, glomerular filtration rate. (*From* Anderson BJ, Allegaert K. The pharmacology of anaesthetics in the neonate. Best Pract Res Clin Anaesthesiol 2010;24(3):425; with permission.)

Pain

The immature brain is especially susceptible to alterations in somatosensory pathways that can have long-term effects on pain pathways and future sensitivity to pain.[53]

Regional anesthetics

The use of regional anesthesia in neonates continues to be an area of focus to optimize pain control and decrease exposure to potentially neurotoxic drugs. The Pediatric Regional Anesthesia Network recently published data from 100,000 patients, of which 1% were neonates. There were no adverse events reported in the neonatal population.[54] Pharmacokinetic studies also show an acceptable safety profile when local anesthetics are dosed properly. Suresh and De Oliveira[55] demonstrated low-plasma bupivacaine levels after single-shot transversus abdominis plane blocks with 0.125% bupivacaine 1 mL/kg in neonates. Safe levels of bupivacaine and ropivacaine have also been demonstrated with continuous infusions at 0.2 mg/kg/h.[56]

CONSIDERATIONS FOR ANESTHETIC MANAGEMENT
Location: Operating Room Versus Intensive Care Unit

Certain surgical procedures are routinely performed at the patient's bedside in the NICU (eg, PDA ligation). Occasionally a patient, particularly an ex-preterm very low-birth-weight infant, may be too unstable for transport, or may be receiving therapies that would make transport challenging (eg, extracorporeal membrane oxygenation, or high-frequency oscillatory ventilation). In these cases, the decision of the location for surgical procedures should be made after a discussion between the anesthesiologist, surgeon, and primary medical team.

Table 4 Commonly used drugs	
Drug	**Consideration in Neonate**
Inhaled anesthetics	• MAC less in neonates than infants • More rapid wash-in in neonates than older children • Higher rate of cardiovascular instability during mask induction than in older children
Morphine	• Decreased clearance in preterm infants • Morphine clearance correlates with GA • Neonates less sensitive to morphine-6-glucuronide (metabolite-causing respiratory depression)
Fentanyl	• Commonly used in the OR • No significant maturational change • Even small doses can cause chest wall rigidity
Remifentanil	• Pharmacokinetics similar to older children • Chest wall rigidity also seen
Acetaminophen	• Can decrease opioid need in neonate[46] • Higher volume of distribution causes lower peak concentration • Decreased clearance can result in accumulation
Ketorolac	• No increase in CT output or creatinine with 48 h of treatment after cardiac surgery[47] • Bleeding events reported after multiple doses in infants with risk factor of age <21 d or GA <37 wk[48]
Codeine	• Contraindicated in neonates and children • The European Medicines Agency, Health Canada, and American Academy of Pediatrics recommend restricted use in patients younger than 12 y • FDA has a black box warning against use in patients undergoing tonsillectomy and adenoidectomy[49]
Dexmedetomidine	• Safe in preterm and term children as sedation • Preterm children may have decreased plasma clearance • Recent evidence that it is less neurotoxic and maybe neuroprotective[50]
NMBD	• Increased sensitivity at neuromuscular junction due to reduced release of Ach due to immature motor nerves[51] • Prolonged effect
Succinylcholine	• Dose response studies suggest dose of 3 mg/kg in infants due to high volume of distribution[51] • Cholinergic effects of second dose can lead to bradycardia and arrest
Sugammadex	• No specific data in neonate • Case reports describing efficacy in neonates[52]

Abbreviations: Ach, acetylcholine; CT, chest tube; MAC, mean alveolar concentration; NMBD, neuromuscular blockade.

Preoperative evaluation and preparation

Operating room: Temperature Prevention of hypothermia in the tiny infant is critical. Therefore, the following actions should be considered:

- Increased ambient temperature in the OR
- Use of radiant warmer (eg, "French fry lights"), forced-air warming device, circulating water mattress, or intravenous (IV) fluid warmer
- Humidified and heated circuit
- Plastic wrap on the patient

Preparation in the neonatal intensive care unit for transport to the operating room
Airway and ventilator A blender to deliver a variable Fio_2 may be necessary for patients with cyanotic mixing heart lesions and for preterm infants to avoid hyperoxia. For intubated patients, discuss with the neonatologist whether the patient is stable for transport with hand ventilation, or if the patient should be transported on the ICU ventilator. Very low-birth-weight babies may need to remain in their isolette to avoid hypothermia. For patients on PEEP greater than 5 cm H_2O, keeping the patient on the ICU ventilator or adding a PEEP valve for hand ventilation should be considered.

Lines and tubing Neonatal units may use slip tip connectors for IV catheters to avoid pressure sores. Changing the slip tip connectors to Luer lock connectors would minimize risk of inadvertent disconnections during surgery. PICC lines in neonates tend to be long and of small caliber, which provide high resistance to rapid fluid administration. If the patient is receiving total parenteral nutrition (TPN) through a central venous line, one way to free up the line is to convert the TPN to an equivalent dextrose and sodium–containing fluid, but without other electrolytes. Not having TPN actively infusing will permit the line to be used without risk of administering a bolus of potassium or calcium that might precipitate with medications.

Umbilical arterial and venous lines Umbilical arterial catheters should be positioned with the distal end above the diaphragm between the sixth and tenth vertebrae. Umbilical venous catheters should be positioned with the distal end in the inferior vena cava just outside the right atrium.[57]

Fluids and nutrition Preventing hypoglycemia is critical, particularly the preterm neonate. Neonates who are receiving continuous tube feeds are at particular risk of developing hypoglycemia when the feeds are discontinued. Patients receiving TPN should have an equivalent infusion of dextrose continued in the OR. Other groups of patients at higher risk of hypoglycemia are infants of diabetic mothers, small-for-gestational-age or large-for-gestational-age infants, and preterm infants.

Anticipation and planning Depending on the condition of the patient and the nature of the surgical procedure, the following should be considered:

- Inhaled nitric oxide
- ICU ventilator for more precise ventilation or alternative modes of ventilation
- Echocardiography with appropriately sized probes
- NIRS monitoring
- Ordering red blood cells (RBC) to be washed to minimize potassium load
- Ordering platelets to be volume reduced to minimize volume

Intraoperative care
Monitoring of patient In addition to standard ASA monitors, special attention must be paid to monitoring core temperature. Direct arterial pressure and central venous pressure monitoring are likely warranted for a neonate undergoing major surgery. PICC lines may be used for central venous pressure monitoring in adults[58]; however, they are less reliable for monitoring central venous pressure in infants. In the authors' experience, if the PICC line distal tip is in a central vein, and pressure can be transduced with a reasonable venous waveform, then the pressure may be followed at least for trends. Peripherally positioned venous lines are not accurate for monitoring central venous pressure.[59] NIRS monitoring should be considered for procedures that might

result in alterations in cerebral blood flow (eg, cardiac surgery, risk of major blood loss, thoracic surgery).[60]

Positioning of patient Surgeons may want to position the patient further down on the operating table closer to equipment or to have better access to the patient, especially when the patient is very small. The anesthesiologist should ensure that the patient's head is within arm's reach to allow for emergency airway management throughout the entire procedure. Ensuring that the patient is closer to the anesthesiologist will also permit the IV tubing to be shorter, which will decrease the flush volume as well as time for changes in infusion rate to reach the patient.

Lines/access Prevention of intravascular entrainment of air and paradoxic air embolus is essential in all children, but especially in preterm infants who may still have a PDA or other intracardiac connection (eg, patent foramen ovale). All IV lines, connections, stopcocks, and access ports must be meticulously examined for air bubbles. In addition, care must be taken to ensure that air bubbles are not injected when administering medication by syringe by aspirating before injecting and using a "plunger highest" technique: holding the plunger upright while injecting so air bubbles will float up.

Careful fluid management, particularly avoiding fluid overload, is imperative for smaller neonates. For example, the maintenance hourly fluid rate for a 2-kg child is approximately 8 mL per hour. If the dead space in the IV tubing is 5 mL, the hourly rate would be exceeded after just 2 medication doses. For very low-weight patients, the authors recommend attaching only "dead-end" IV tubing (ie, not connected to a bag of IV fluid). Alternatively, IV sets that include a reservoir between the fluid bag and the tubing (eg, buretrol) can be used. Because buretrols can also be left open unintentionally, the authors recommend filling the reservoir with no more than 10 mL/kg of fluid at a time. Additional precautions may include attaching smaller bags of IV fluid (eg, 50 mL instead of 1000 mL), shortening the length of tubing for all lines, and batching the administration of medications together to minimize flush volume.

Airway/ventilation Because the distance from vocal cords to carina is short (around 5 cm),[61] the risk of accidental mainstem intubation or extubation is significant especially with procedures that require manipulation of the head or airway.[62] This risk is elevated in premature infants who are intubated with shorter ETTs. It is the practice of the authors' institution to obtain a chest radiograph to confirm position of the ETT for infants undergoing cardiothoracic or major abdominal surgery.

There are limited options for lung isolation in the neonate. Patients must be around 30 kg to fit the smallest double lumen tube. Patients should be older than 6 months of age for bronchial blockers.[63] Therefore, the preferred method for lung isolation in the neonate is endobronchial intubation with a single-lumen tracheal tube. If the chosen tube does not insert easily into the desired bronchus, downsizing should be considered.

Blood product administration Risks of transfusion include hyperkalemia, hypocalcemia, volume overload, and dilution of coagulation factors. Strategies to reduce risks include the following:

- Communication with transfusion services to
  - Order the freshest blood products
  - Wash RBC to lower potassium load

○ Reduce the amount of plasma in a unit of platelets bringing the total volume from more than 200 cc to less than 50 cc
- Preemptively administer diuretics (eg, furosemide) to decrease intravascular volume and total body potassium
- Administer calcium with transfusion
- Monitor central venous pressure for evidence of hypervolemia
- Record baseline electrocardiogram and monitor tracing for signs of hyperkalemia

Postoperative Care

The risk of postoperative apnea in the both the term and especially the pre-term infant must be taken into consideration when determining postoperative disposition. A meta-analysis by Cote and colleagues[64] could not provide definitive data on when risk was acceptable and concluded that preterm infants up to 56 weeks postmenstrual age could be susceptible. In term neonates aged 44 to 46 weeks, discharge appears safe after 4 hours of uneventful postoperative monitoring.

The General Anesthesia compared to Spinal Anesthesia study concluded that there was no evidence that regional anesthesia reduced the overall risk of postoperative apnea, and that because the failure rate of regional anesthesia is up to 20%, general anesthesia must always be available.[65]

Because there is no consensus regarding what postmenstrual age (PMA) is required to minimize the risk of a postoperative apneic event, each institution must determine their own criteria. The policy at the authors' institution is to admit (to a monitored bed for a minimum of 12 hours after anesthesia and continued for at least 12 hours after any apneic event) any patient meeting any of the following criteria:

- Born before 37 weeks' GA *AND* current age is less than 52 weeks' PMA
- All infants less than 44 weeks' PMA irrespective of GA
- Born before 37 weeks' GA *AND* currently less than 60 weeks' PMA *AND* have concurrent pertinent medical issues as defined by the anesthesiologist (eg, ongoing apneic events, significant anemia)

SUMMARY

The perioperative risk of morbidity and mortality for neonates is significantly higher than that for older children and adults.[8] Patients at particular risk include neonates born prematurely, with major or severe CHD, and with PH. There is presently no consensus regarding the safest anesthetic regimen for neonates. The anesthesiologist caring for the neonate should be knowledgeable of the unique physiology of the neonate and maintain the highest level of vigilance throughout the case.

DISCLOSURE

The authors have nothing to disclose.

REFERENCES

1. Kuratani N. The cutting edge of neonatal anesthesia: the tide of history is changing. J Anesth 2015;29:1–3.
2. Robinson S, Gregory GA. Fentanyl-air-oxygen anesthesia for ligation of patent ductus arteriosus in preterm infants. Anesth Analg 1981;60:331–4.
3. Anand KJS, Sippell WG, Aynsley-Green A. Randomised trial of fentanyl anaesthesia in preterm babies undergoing surgery: effects on the stress response. Lancet 1987;1:243–8.

4. Beecher HK, Todd DP. A study of the deaths associated with anesthesia and surgery. Ann Surg 1954;100(1):2–34.
5. Bhananker SM, Ramamoorthy C, Geiduschek JM, et al. Anesthesia-related cardiac arrest in children: update from the Pediatric Cardiac Arrest Registry. Anesth Analg 2007;105(2):344–50.
6. Morray JP, Geiduschek JM, Ramamoorthy C, et al. Anesthesia-related cardiac arrest in children: initial findings of the Pediatric Perioperative Cardiac Arrest (POCA) Registry. Anesthesiology 2000;93(1):6–14.
7. Flick R, Sprung J, Harrison TE, et al. Perioperative cardiac arrests in children between 1988 and 2005 at a tertiary referral center. Anesthesiology 2007;106: 226–37.
8. Houck CS, Vinson AE. Anaesthetic considerations for surgery in newborns. Arch Dis Child Fetal Neonatal Ed 2017;102:F359–63.
9. Michelet D, Brasher C, Ben Kaddour H, et al. Postoperative complications following neonatal and infant surgery: common events and predictive factors. Anaesth Crit Care Med 2017;36:163–9.
10. Weinberg AC, Huang L, Jiang H, et al. Perioperative risk factors for major complications in pediatric surgery: a study in surgical risk assessment for children. J Am Coll Surg 2011;212:768–78.
11. Lillehei C, Gauvreau K, Jenkins KJ. Risk adjustment for neonatal surgery: a method for comparison of in-hospital mortality. Pediatrics 2012;130(3):e560–74.
12. Ramamoorthy C, Haberkern CM, Bhananker SM, et al. Anesthesia-related cardiac arrest in children with heart disease: data from the Pediatric Perioperative Cardiac Arrest (POCA) Registry. Anesth Analg 2010;110(5):1376–82.
13. Van de Griend BF, Lister NA, McKenzie IM, et al. Postoperative mortality in children after 101,885 anesthetics at a tertiary pediatric hospital. Anesth Analg 2011; 112(6):1440–7.
14. Taylor D, Habre W. Risk associated with anesthesia for non-cardiac surgery in children with congenital heart disease. Pediatr Anesth 2019;29:426–34.
15. Bernier ML, Jacob AI, Collaco JM, et al. Perioperative events in children with pulmonary hypertension undergoing non-cardiac procedures. Pulm Circ 2017; 8(1):1–10.
16. Nasr V, Staffa SJ, Zurakowski D, et al. Pediatric risk stratification is improved by integrating both patient comorbidities and intrinsic surgical risk. Anesthesiology 2019;130:971–80.
17. Lin EP, Soriano SG, Loepke AW. Anesthetic neurotoxicity. Anesthesiol Clin 2014; 32:133–55.
18. Walkden GJ, Pickering AE, Gill H. Assessing long-term neurodevelopmental outcome following general anesthesia in early childhood: challenges and opportunities. Anesth Analg 2019;128(4):681–94.
19. McCann ME, de Graaff JC, Dorris L, et al. Neurodevelopmental ouitcome at 5 years of age after general anesthesia or awake-regional anesthesia in infancy (GAS): an international, multicenter, randomized, controlled equivalence trial. Lancet 2019;393:664–77.
20. Wilder RT, Flick RP, Sprung J, et al. Early exposure to anesthesia and learning disabilities in a population-based birth cohort. Anesthesiology 2009;110(4): 796–804.
21. Sun LS, Li G, Miller TK, et al. Association between a single general anesthesia exposure before age 36 months and neurocognitive outcomes in later childhood. JAMA 2016;315(21):2312–20.

22. Chambers NA, Ramgolam A, Sommerfield D, et al. Cuffed vs. uncuffed tracheal tubes in children: a randomised controlled trial comparing leak, tidal volume and complications. Anaesthesia 2017;73:160–8.
23. Cole F. Pediatric formulas for the anesthesiologist. AMA J Dis Child 1957;94:672–3.
24. Thomas RE, Rao SC, Minutillo C, et al. Cuffed endotracheal tubes in infants less than 3 kg: a retrospective cohort study. Paediatr Anaesth 2018;28(3):204–9.
25. Thomas J, Weiss M, Cannizzaro V, et al. Work of breathing for cuffed and uncuffed pediatric endotracheal tubes in an in vitro lung model setting. Paediatr Anaesth 2018;28(9):780–7.
26. Kurth CD, Spitzer AR, Broennle AM, et al. Postoperative apnea in preterm infants. Anesthesiology 1987;66:483–8.
27. Klingenberg C, Wheeler KI, McCallion N, et al. Volume-targeted versus pressure-limited ventilation in neonates. Cochrane Database Syst Rev 2017;10:CD003666.
28. Thome UH, Ambalavanan N. Permissive hypercapnia to decrease lung injury in ventilated preterm neonates. Semin Fetal Neonatal Med 2009;14(1):21–7.
29. BOOST II United Kingdom Collaborative Group, BOOST II Australia Collaborative Group, BOOST II New Zealand Collaborative Group, Stenson BJ, Tarnow-Mordi WO, Darlow BA, et al. Oxygen saturation and outcomes in preterm infants. N Engl J Med 2013;368:2094–104.
30. Manja V, Lakshminrusimha S, Cook DJ. Oxygen saturation target range for extremely preterm infants: a systematic review and metaanalysis. JAMA Pediatr 2015;169:332–40.
31. Nafiu OO, Voepel-Lewis T, Morris M, et al. How do pediatric anesthesiologists define intraoperative hypotension? Pediatr Anaesth 2009;19:1048–53.
32. Cayabyab R, McLean CW, Seri I. Definition of hypotension and assessment of hemodynamics in the preterm neonate. J Perinatol 2009;29:S58–62.
33. Olbrecht VA, Skowno J, Marchesini V, et al. An international, multicenter, observational study of cerebral oxygenation during infant and neonatal anesthesia. Anesthesiology 2018;128(1):85–96.
34. Feld LG, Neuspiel DR, Foster BA, et al. Clinical Practice Guideline: maintenance intravenous fluids in children. Subcommittee on fluid and electrolyte therapy. Pediatrics 2018;142(6):2018–3083.
35. Edjo Nkilly G, Michelet D, Hilly J, et al. Postoperative decrease in plasma sodium concentration after infusion of hypotonic intravenous solutions in neonatal surgery. Br J Anaesth 2014;112(3):540–5.
36. Gregory G, Brett C. Neonatology for anesthesia. In: Cladis FP, Davis PJ, editors. Smith's anesthesia for infants and children. 9th edition. Philadelphia: Elsevir Moby; 2017. p. 513–70.
37. de Ferranti S, Gauvreau K, Hickey PR, et al. Intraoperative hyperglycemia during infant cardiac surgery is not associated with adverse neurodevelopmental outcomes at 1, 4, and 8 years. Anesthesiology 2004;100(6):1345–52.
38. Datta PK, Aravindan A. Glucose for children during surgery: pros, cons, and protocols: a postgraduate educational review. Anesth Essays Res 2017;11(3):539–43.
39. Roseff SD, Luban NLC, Manno CS. Guidelines for assessing appropriateness of pediatric transfusion. Transfusion 2002;42(11):1398–413.
40. Goobie SM, Faraoni D, Zurakowski D, et al. Association of preoperative anemia with postoperative mortality in neonates. JAMA Pediatr 2016;170(9):855–62.
41. Colombatti R, Sainati L, Trevisanuto D. Anemia and transfusion in the neonate. Semin Fetal Neonatal Med 2016;21(1):2–9.

42. Revel-Vilk S. The conundrum of neonatal coagulopathy. Hematology Am Soc Hematol Educ Program 2012;12:450–4.

43. Offringa M, Ovelman C, Soll R, et al. Prophylactic vitamin K for the prevention of vitamin K deficiency bleeding in preterm neonates. Cochrane Database Syst Rev 2018;2018(2):CD008342.

44. Anderson BJ, Allegaert K. The pharmacology of anaesthetics in the neonate. Clin Aneaesthesiol 2010;24(3):419–31.

45. Chalkiadis GA, Anderson BJ. Age and size are the major covariates for prediction of levobupivacaine clearance in children. Paediatr Anaesth 2006;16:275–82.

46. Ceelie I, de Wildt SN, van Dijk M, et al. Effect of intravenous paracetamol on postoperative morphine requirements in neonates and infants undergoing major noncardiac surgery: a randomized controlled trial. JAMA 2013;309(2):149–54.

47. Gupta A, Daggett C, Drant S, et al. Prospective randomized trial of ketorolac after congenital heart surgery. J Cadiothorac Vasc Anesth 2004;18(4):454–7.

48. Aldrink JH, Ma M, Wang W, et al. Safety of ketorolac in surgical neonates and infants 0 to 3 months old. J Pediatr Surg 2011;46(6):1081–5.

49. Tobias J, Weiss M, Cannizzaro V, et al. Codeine: time to say "no." Section on anesthesiology and pain medicine, committee on drugs. Pediatrics 2016;10(4):138.

50. Shan Y, Yang F, Tang Z, et al. Dexmedetomidine ameliorates the neurotoxicity of sevoflurane on the immature brain through th BMP/SMAD signaling pathway. Front Neurosci 2018;12(964).

51. Meakin G. Neuromuscular blocking drugs in infants and children. Cont Educ Anaesth Crit Care Pain 2007;7:143–4.

52. Langley RJ, McFadzean J, McCormack J. The presumed central nervous system effects of rocuronium in a neonate and its reversal with sugammadex. Paediatr Anaesth 2016;26(1):109–11.

53. Ririe DG. How long does incisional pain last: early life vulnerability could make it last a lifetime. Anesthesiology 2015;122:1189–91.

54. Walker BJ, Long JB, Sathyamoorthy M, et al. Complications in pediatric regional anesthesia: an analysis of more than 100,000 blocks from the pediatric regional anesthesia network. Anesthesiology 2018;129(4):721–32.

55. Suresh S, De Oliveira GS Jr. Blood bupivacaine concentrations after transversus abdominis plane block in neonates: a prospective observational study. Anesth Analg 2016;122(3):814–7.

56. Calder A, Bell GT, Anderson M, et al. Pharmacokinetic profiles of epidural bupivacaine and ropivacaine following single-shot and continuous epidural use in young infants. Paediatr Anaesth 2012;22(5):430–7.

57. Bayley G. Special considerations in the premature and ex-premature infant. Anaesth Intensive Care Med 2014;15(3):107–10.

58. Latham HE, Rawson ST, Dwyer TT, et al. Peripherally inserted central catheters are equivalent to centrally inserted catheters in intensive care unit patients for central venous pressure monitoring. J Clin Monit Comput 2012;26(2):85–90.

59. Leipoldt CC, McKay WP, Clunie M, et al. Peripheral venous pressure predicts central venous pressure poorly in pediatric patients. Can J Anaesth 2006;53(12):1207–12.

60. Vutskits L. Cerebral blood flow in the neonate. Paediatr Anaesth 2014;24:22–9.

61. Lee K, Yan C. Tracheal length of infants under three months old. Ann Otol Rhinol Laryngol 2001;110:268–70.

62. Wagner KM, Raskin JS, Carling NP, et al. Unplanned intraoperative extubations in pediatric neurosurgery: analysis of case series to increase patient safety. World Neurosurg 2018;115:E1–6.

63. Letal M, Theam M. Paediatric lung isolation. BJA Educ 2017;17(2):57–62.
64. Cote CJ, Zaslavsky A, Downes JJ, et al. Postoperative apnea in former preterm infants after inguinal herniorrhaphy: a combined analysis. Anesthesiology 1995; 82:809–22.
65. Davidson AJ, Morton NS, Arnup SJ, et al. Apnea after awake-regional and general anesthesia in infants: the General Anesthesia compared to Spinal Anesthesia Gas study. Anesthesiology 2015;123(1):38–54.

Anesthesia at the Edge of Life: Mechanical Circulatory Support

Mayanka Tickoo, MD, MS[a], Amit Bardia, MBBS[b],*

KEYWORDS

- Anesthesia • Mechanical circulatory support • ECMO • LVAD • IABP

KEY POINTS

- Intra-aortic balloon pumps (IABPs extracorporeal membrane oxygenators (ECMOs), and left ventricular assist devices (LVADs) are commonly used mechanical circulatory support devices, placed in patients with compromised cardiac function.
- IABP is a device placed in the thoracic aorta consisting of a polyethylene balloon that inflates during diastole and deflates during systole, augmenting left ventricular stroke volume.
- ECMO can have a venovenous (VV) or a venoarterial (VA) configuration depending on its indication for use: pulmonary or cardiopulmonary support.
- An implantable LVAD usually consists of an inflow cannula placed at the apex of the heart, a pump, and an outflow cannula placed in the ascending aorta.
- Maintaining adequate right ventricular support is key to the management of patients with LVADs.

Mechanical circulatory support (MCS) devices are used for patients with cardiogenic compromise. The choice of mechanical circulatory device depends on the patient's clinical condition, including acuity, severity, and cause of the decompensation. Commonly used MCS devices include intra-aortic balloon pump (IABP), extracorporeal membrane oxygenators (ECMOs), and left ventricular assist devices (LVADs). With the advances in technology, the indications, management, and outcomes of patient with these devices are constantly evolving. In general, the use of these devices has increased over the last couple of decades. An understanding of their working principles and their effects on hemodynamics is essential for the management of these patients in the perioperative period. This article provides a brief synopsis of the MCS devices and key anesthetic considerations of patients with these devices presenting for noncardiac surgeries.

[a] Pulmonary and Critical Care Medicine, Department of Internal Medicine, Yale School of Medicine, 333 Cedar Street, New Haven, CT 06510, USA; [b] Department of Anesthesiology, Yale School of Medicine, 20 York Street, New Haven, CT 06510, USA
* Corresponding author.
E-mail address: amit.bardia@yale.edu

Anesthesiology Clin 38 (2020) 19–33
https://doi.org/10.1016/j.anclin.2019.11.002
anesthesiology.theclinics.com
1932-2275/20/© 2019 Elsevier Inc. All rights reserved.

INTRA-AORTIC BALLOON PUMP
Background

IABP is one of the most commonly used mechanical assist devices in patients with cardiogenic shock unresponsive to medical management, severe acute mitral regurgitation such as papillary muscle rupture, severe aortic stenosis, and acute ventricular septal defect.[1,2] It is also used in patients with cardiogenic shock to downtitrate pharmaceutical support, especially in patients with refractory ventricular arrhythmias triggered by high doses of inotropic agents.[3]

The device consists of a polyethylene balloon mounted on a flexible catheter usually inserted from the femoral artery, which is positioned in the descending thoracic aorta and terminates 1 to 2 cm below the origin of the left subclavian artery.[4] Its proximal end terminates before the origin of the renal arteries. This system is connected to a console that houses helium, which is used to inflate the balloon. Other insertion sites, such as the axillary artery, are less common.

Intra-aortic Balloon Pump: Effect on Hemodynamics

The IABP inflates during diastole and deflates during systole. IABP is used for its salutary effect on the myocardial energy balance because it augments myocardial blood flow and decreases the cardiac workload. Coronary perfusion pressure (CPP) is the difference between diastolic blood pressure and left ventricular end-diastolic pressure (LVEDP). Inflation of the balloon during diastole augments the diastolic blood pressure and in turn improves the CPP, enhancing coronary blood flow. During systole, the balloon deflates, decreasing the pressure in the descending aorta, which in turn decreases the cardiac afterload (**Fig. 1**).

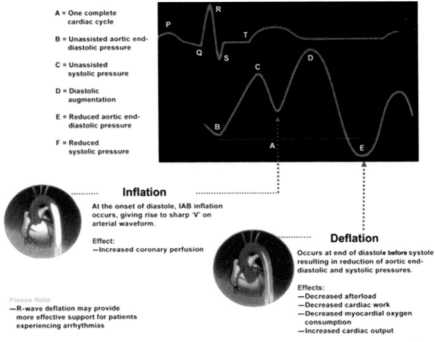

Fig. 1. Hemodynamic changes associated with IABP. IAB, intra-aortic balloon. (*From* Sodhi N, Lasala JM. Mechanical Circulatory Support in Acute Decompensated Heart Failure and Shock. Interv Cardiol Clin 2017;6(3):389; with permission.)

Timing

Optimal operation of the IABP requires inflation of the balloon during the period of aortic valve closure (marked by the dicrotic notch in the arterial pressure waveform) and deflation before the opening of the aortic valve (marked by the end of downslope in the arterial pressure waveform). Improper timing of balloon inflation and deflation may have negative consequences, as described in **Table 1**.

Trigger

To ensure proper timing of the balloon inflation/deflation (counterpulsation) with respect to the cardiac cycle, the device can be programmed to use the following sources:

1. ECG (electrocardiogram): the R wave indicates the beginning of the cardiac cycle.
2. Arterial pressure waveform: the upstroke of the pressure waveform indicates aortic valve opening.
3. Internal waveform: this is used when there is no cardiac output, such as cardiopulmonary bypass or cardiac arrest.

In addition, the balloon pump may be programmed to special modes such as A pacing, V pacing, and atrial fibrillation modes for proper trigger identification for specific clinical scenarios.

Anesthetic Considerations

Only emergent surgeries should be performed in patients with IABP. Before transport, proper positioning of the IABP should be ensured based on the patient's recent chest radiograph (**Fig. 2**). Similarly, utmost care must be taken that the position of the IABP does not change during transport/patient positioning. In patients with femoral arterial cannulation, the hips should not be flexed to avoid injury to the femoral artery. Anticoagulation with heparin is usually not required in patients with IABP, especially if the

Table 1
Improper timing of intra-aortic balloon pump inflation and deflation

Event	Event Definition	Hemodynamic Consequence
Early inflation	Inflation while aortic valve is still open (before the dicrotic notch)	Increase in cardiac afterload leading to myocardial oxygen demand Premature closure of aortic valve leading to increase in LVEDP
Late deflation	Deflation after aortic valve opens (during the upslope of the arterial pressure waveform)	Cardiac ejection against an inflated balloon leads to an increase in cardiac afterload leading to myocardial oxygen demand
Early deflation	Deflation while the aortic valve is still closed (during the downslope of the arterial pressure waveform)	Early deflation leading to decrease in diastolic pressures leading to suboptimal diastolic augmentation and hence suboptimal coronary perfusion
Late inflation	Inflation after the aortic valve closes (after the dicrotic notch)	Late inflation leading to suboptimal diastolic augmentation and hence suboptimal coronary perfusion

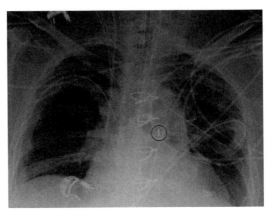

Fig. 2. Chest radiograph of a patient showing appropriate positioning of the IABP. The red circle indicates the IABP terminating in proximal descending aorta just caudal to the aortic knuckle.

device is programmed to provide counterpulsation on every beat (1:1 mode). However, an active type and screen should be available because bleeding from the arterial insertion site is common.

As with other mechanical circulatory devices, the mean arterial pressure (MAP) goal is usually greater than 65 mm Hg or as dictated by the clinical scenario. If there is inappropriate triggering caused by ECG interference from electrocautery, the trigger may be switched from ECG to arterial pressure waveform. Common alarms and troubleshooting are described in **Table 2**.

Management of Cardiopulmonary Arrest in Patients with Intra-aortic Balloon Pumps

In the event of cardiac arrest, standard cardiopulmonary resuscitation (CPR) and post-arrest care should be performed as per the American Heart Association (AHA) guidelines.[5] During asystole, in the absence of ECG waveform and arterial pressure signal, the IABP shows a trigger loss alarm and stops counterpulsation. The internal trigger could then be selected for asynchronous counterpulsation. The trigger must be changed back to the original appropriate trigger once return of spontaneous circulation is achieved.

Table 2
Common alarms and troubleshooting in patients with intra-aortic balloon pumps

Serial Number	Alarm	Action
1	Loss of trigger	Ensure proper ECG tracing and/or pressure tracing
2	Loss of pressure trace	Ensure arterial line is patent, pressure bag is appropriately inflated, and transducer connection is appropriate
3	Rapid gas loss	Ensure connections to the helium disk and the connecting tube is intact. Ensure catheter tubing is not kinked
4	Blood in line	Indicates rupture of balloon, which may become nidus for thrombi. Immediate plans for heparinization and IABP removal should be initiated

EXTRACORPOREAL MEMBRANE OXYGENATION

ECMO is a modified form of cardiopulmonary bypass that can provide temporary (days to months) support for respiratory and cardiovascular failure and that is making a resurgence in adult critical care. Although this form of extracorporeal support has been widely used in the pediatric population, it had not found wide acceptance in adult critically ill patients because of the lack of evidence for improved outcomes and a high rate of complications until recently. However, ECMO is rapidly becoming an acceptable rescue modality for a wide variety of patients in multiple clinical settings and therefore necessities a degree of familiarization for practicing anesthesiologists. With an increase in both the number of centers performing ECMO nationally as well as the total number of patients supported on ECMO annually, it is becoming a rapidly used mode of cardiorespiratory support.[6]

Extracorporeal Membrane Oxygenation: Types and Hemodynamics Principles

In patients on ECMO support, venous blood is drained through an outflow cannula, passed through a membrane oxygenator that can add oxygen as well as remove carbon dioxide, and then pumped back into the patient in the arterial or venous circulation depending on the configuration of extracorporeal support used. Although the basics of design are similar to a cardiac bypass circuit used during cardiac surgery, improvements in technology have allowed this modified form of support to be brought outside the operating room. There are 2 basic configurations of ECMO: venovenous (VV) and venoarterial (VA), although sometimes hybrid configurations can also be used. Depending on the clinical indication, ECMO can be configured to provide oxygen, achieve CO_2 clearance, as well as support perfusion.[7]

VENOVENOUS EXTRACORPOREAL MEMBRANE OXYGENATION

The VV configuration is used in acute respiratory failure with preserved circulatory response, especially when conventional mechanical ventilation is either insufficient to maintain desired oxygenation goals or is proving to be injurious to the patient. There are 2 cannulation strategies used in VV ECMO: single bicaval cannula (double-lumen cannula placed in the right internal jugular [IJ] vein) or 2 separate venous cannulas (femoral-femoral/IJ-femoral). The 2-cannula strategy involves placement of the outflow cannula into the femoral vein and, following gas exchange, using the inflow cannula to return blood to the patient's contralateral femoral vein (femoral-femoral) or IJ (femoral-IJ) vein. The bicaval approach consists of placement of a concentric double-lumen cannula with the outflow (external) cannula drawing blood out and the inner cannula (tip directed toward the tricuspid valve) returning oxygenated blood to the right ventricle (**Fig. 3**). The VV support system then depends on the intrinsic cardiac activity to maintain the patient's systemic hemodynamics and supply oxygenated blood to the body. The bicaval approach is preferred because it requires single-vein cannulation, which allows for the possibility of ambulation and rehabilitation while the patient is on ECMO.

In addition, with the 2 -approach, because of issues with the position of the inflow and outflow cannulas, occasionally the venous inflow cannula may entrain oxygenated blood exiting the venous outflow cannula. As a result, a certain amount of oxygenated blood volume loops around the VV ECMO circuit and does not mix with the systemic circulation. Consequently, the predominant systemic circulating blood volume

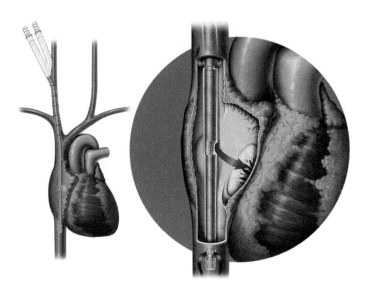

Fig. 3. Avalon bicaval dual-lumen cannula in correct position. (*Courtesy of* Getinge, Wayne, NJ.)

continues to be poorly oxygenated. This phenomenon is known as recirculation. Management steps include echocardiographic confirmation of cannula position by the institutional imaging team and, possibly, adjustment of the cannulas under echocardiographic guidance. Attempts should be made to optimize the ventilatory settings in the interim.

VENOARTERIAL EXTRACORPOREAL MEMBRANE OXYGENATION

The VA configuration is used for cardiovascular support. ECMO for cardiovascular support is used in refractory cardiogenic shock as a bridge to recovery, placement of destination ventricular assist devices, or heart transplant. Common indications for VA ECMO include after myocardial infarction cardiogenic shock, fulminant myocarditis, and postcardiotomy, or following primary heart transplant graft failure.[8,9] Previously thought of contraindications including postpartum status and right ventricular (RV) failure (following pulmonary embolism or pulmonary hypertension) are now being considered as viable situations for ECMO support in appropriate patients.[9,10] Hemodynamic support is maintained by a combination of pump flow plus native cardiac output. Access for VA ECMO can be established via central as well as peripheral cannulation (**Fig. 4**). In central cannulation, the drainage cannula is usually placed directly into the right atrium and the return cannula in the proximal ascending aorta. This strategy is most commonly used in the operating room for patients undergoing cardiac surgery who require extracorporeal support. The peripheral cannulation for VA ECMO involves placement of the drainage cannula in a central vein (IJ or femoral advanced into superior vena cava). In this mode of peripheral cannulation, blood from the ECMO circuit flows in a retrograde fashion into the descending aorta. The direction of this blood flow is reverse to the native cardiac output. This process in turn increases the cardiac afterload, impeding left ventricular (LV) emptying. It is important to ensure proper LV ejection because, in the absence of LV ejection, blood clots may form in the LV cavity and may form a nidus for thromboembolic complications. In addition, in

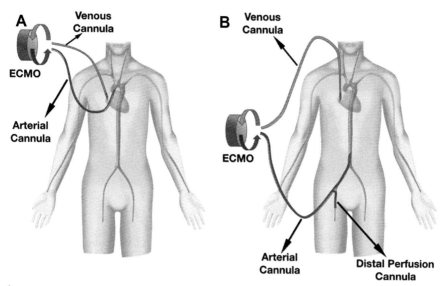

Fig. 4. Commonly used VA ECMO cannulation strategies. (*A*) Central cannulation. (*B*) Peripheral cannulation. (*Adapted from* Le Gall A, Follin A, Cholley B, et al. Veno-arterial-ECMO in the intensive care unit: From technical aspects to clinical practice. Anaesth Crit Care Pain Med 2018;37(3):261; with permission.)

the absence of LV ejection, accumulation of blood in the left ventricle may cause distention of the LV cavity. This distention increases the LV end-diastolic pressure and hence decreases the CPP, impairing myocardial blood flow. Appropriate LV ejection can be monitored by visualizing a dicrotic notch in the pressure tracing from an arterial line placed in the right upper extremity. The choice of obtaining arterial access in the right upper extremity is extremely important because the right brachiocephalic artery is the first arterial take-off from the aortic arch and closely reflects native cardiac function. Low-dose inotropic support or an IABP may be used to ensure LV emptying.

In patients with peripheral VA ECMO cannulation, the point where blood ejected from the native circulation meets the retrograde flow from the peripheral ECMO is known as the mixing point (**Fig. 5**). If the cardiac function improves but the pulmonary function continues to be impaired, poorly oxygenated blood will be ejected by the heart. If the mixing point is at the descending aorta, the heart (via the coronaries) and the brain (via the carotids) will be perfused by this poorly oxygenated blood. This phenomenon is known as north south syndrome or harlequin syndrome.[11] Arterial blood gases drawn from the right-sided arterial access will show poor PaO_2 concentration reflecting native cardiac output. Management steps include optimizing mechanical ventilatory settings to improve oxygenation, titrating down inotropic support (while still ensuring LV ejection), and in severe cases switching to VV ECMO (or hybrid) configurations.

In patients with arterial femoral cannulas, distal ischemic complications are often noted because of the large size of the ECMO cannula and associated limited perfusion of the specific extremity. Use of small-bore retrograde cannulas to establish distal flow to the lower extremity can help avoid this complication. Ensuring good Doppler flow of the pedal arteries is important to rule out leg ischemia, especially in patients with lactic acidosis on peripheral VA ECMO.

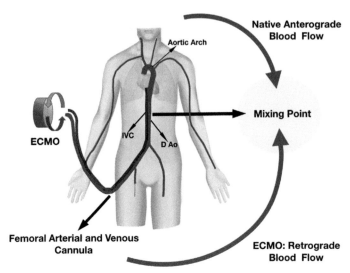

Fig. 5. Pathophysiology of north south syndrome or harlequin syndrome seen with peripheral VA ECMO. D Ao, descending aorta; IVC, inferior vena cava. (*Adapted from* Le Gall A, Follin A, Cholley B, et al. Veno-arterial-ECMO in the intensive care unit: From technical aspects to clinical practice. Anaesth Crit Care Pain Med 2018;37(3):261; with permission.)

MANAGEMENT CONSIDERATIONS IN EXTRACORPOREAL MEMBRANE OXYGENATION

For cardiovascular support in VA ECMO, the pump rotation determines the flow being delivered to the patient. After initial cannulation, pump rotation is gradually increased to determine the maximum flow through the circuit depending on the individual patient's intrinsic vascular as well as cannula resistance. The flow is then decreased to the lowest limit necessary to meet the patient's requirements, which can be variable depending on the cause of cardiovascular failure (eg, cardiogenic vs septic shock). ECMO circuits are by their intrinsic nature prone to clot formation and, therefore, patients on circuit require systemic anticoagulation. The recommended agent is unfractionated heparin administered as a continuous infusion with close follow-up of anticoagulation parameters such as activated clotting time (ACT; goal 1.5 times normal), measurement of factor Xa level or partial thromboplastin time (tends to be less accurate). Patients on ECMO can develop thrombocytopenia as circulating platelets bind to the surface of the ECMO circuit and become activated, causing increased platelet plug formation, which also increases the risk of microthrombus and macrothrombus formation, cell injury, and hemolysis. These processes can ultimately mimic a diffuse intravascular coagulation–like consumptive coagulopathy, which can be detrimental to the patient. Excessive clot formation often requires a change in the ECMO circuit, as well as appropriate blood product transfusion to maintain platelet goal greater than 80,000/μL and normal fibrinogen and antithrombin III levels.[12]

Whether the patient is on VA or VV ECMO, the recommendation for ventilator management is to maintain the ventilator on lung-rest settings to minimize ventilator-associated lung injury. This recommendation often includes a low respiratory rate, low inspiratory pressure, appropriate positive end-expiratory pressure to allow lung recruitment, and low fraction of inspired oxygen to minimize hyperoxia-induced lung injury.

Anesthetic Considerations

Similar to patients with IABPs, only emergent surgeries should be performed on patients with ECMOs. Bleeding in the setting of systemic anticoagulation, thrombocytopenia, and poor platelet function is one of the most dreaded complications of ECMO. An active type and screen and appropriate blood products should be available before the surgical procedure. Care should be taken to minimize invasive procedures, including venipuncture, insertion of catheters such as Foley/central venous catheters, as well as suctioning of endotracheal tubes/tracheostomies.

Appropriate ACT levels should be ensured perioperatively. Suspension of systemic anticoagulation, if needed, should be individualized on a case-by-case basis after a multidisciplinary discussion with the institutional team that routinely manages patients with ECMOs.

Blood stream infections are challenging to manage because, often, exchange of ECMO cannulas is not possible because of the patient's clinical condition. Infections are commonly encountered in patients with ECMOs. Special attention to antisepsis should be undertaken while obtaining new vascular access or accessing vascular ports/lines. Proper perioperative antibiotic prophylaxis should be administered before the surgery.

Configuration-specific complications (north south syndrome, recirculation) should be recognized and managed as described previously. Right upper extremity arterial line access should be ensured in patients with peripheral (femoral) VA ECMO. Similarly, arterial line waveform should be closely monitored to ensure presence of dicrotic notch as a surrogate for LV opening in patients with peripheral VA ECMO. Usual MAP goal is usually greater than 65-70 mm Hg unless dictated by a particular clinical scenario.

Patients requiring ECMO support often develop renal failure requiring appropriate use of diuretics or renal replacement therapy needing close vigilance and management of serum electrolytes and drug dose adjustments. Similarly, lipophilic drugs such as fentanyl need much higher doses because a sizable amount of administered drug is adsorbed by the ECMO membrane.[13]

Utmost care should be undertaken during patient positioning and transport to ensure prevention of dislodgment/migration of ECMO cannulas. Resumption of anticoagulation after the surgical procedure should be made on a case-by-case basis after a multidisciplinary discussion.

Management of Cardiopulmonary Arrest in Patients with Extracorporeal Membrane Oxygenators

Management of cardiac arrest in patients with ECMOs depends on the type of ECMO configuration and the destination plans for the patient. In patients with VV ECMO, CPR and postarrest care should be performed as per the AHA guidelines.[5] In patients with VA ECMO, management of malignant rhythm depends on the destination plans for the patient. If the VA ECMO is used as a salvage therapy with ultimate plans for LVAD implantation or decannulation, malignant rhythms should be defibrillated. As with standard CPR, every effort to correct the underlying cause should always be made.

LEFT VENTRICULAR ASSIST DEVICES
Background

LVADs are placed in patients with advanced heart failure as a bridge to transplant or as destination therapy. The use of LVADs in patients with end-stage heart failure has been shown to be superior to medical therapy alone.[14] An LVAD consists of an inflow cannula, which is usually positioned in the LV cavity; a pump; and an outflow cannula, which is commonly placed in the ascending aorta.[15] First-generation devices have mostly been phased out and second-generation and third-generation devices are being used in current practice. Second-generation devices are nonpulsatile and use axial-flow pumps.

SECOND-GENERATION DEVICES

The HeartMate II (HM II) is a second-generation LVAD, consisting of an axial-flow pump that is electrically powered by a percutaneous lead that connects the pump to an external system controller and power source[16] (**Fig. 6**). When the rotor spins on its axis, blood is drawn continuously from the LV apex through the pump and is propelled into the ascending aorta.[17] The parameters that are shown by the device include speed (revolutions per minute [RPM]), power (watts), pulsatility index (PI), and flow (liters per minute). Its speed can be adjusted by the clinical care team. Although the pump speed can range from 6000 to 15,000 RPM, typical speeds between 8000 and 10,000 RPM are used in the clinical setting.[18] The flow is a calculated number based on pump speed and power. It is not exactly the same as cardiac output and only provides a rough estimate of the cardiac output.[19] The display speed usually matches the actual speed within 100 RPM under normal conditions. PI is a dimensionless number and represents the flow pulse through the device. With the increase in LV pressure during native LV contraction, flow through the pump increases compared with LV diastole. The PI represents the difference in flow during systole and diastole, and is calculated by the formula:

$$PI = \frac{Q_{max} - Q_{min}}{Q_{Avg}}$$

Where Q_{max} is the maximum flow during systole, Q_{min} is the minimum flow during diastole, and Q_{Avg} is the average flow during cardiac cycle.[20]

The device usually checks the change in PI from the previous 15-second average. Its usual range for HM II is between 3 and 4.

THIRD-GENERATION DEVICES

These devices are continuous-flow centrifugal pumps that are designed with a focus on smaller size and a low risk of hemolysis or thrombosis. The HeartWare and the

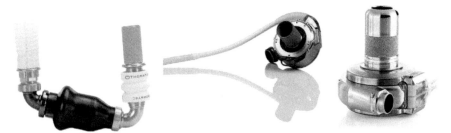

Fig. 6. Commercially available LVAD devices: HeartMate II, HeartMate III, and Heartware HVAD. (*Adapted from* Dalia AA, Cronin B, Stone ME, et al. Anesthetic Management of Patients With Continuous-Flow Left Ventricular Assist Devices Undergoing Noncardiac Surgery: An Update for Anesthesiologists. J Cardiothorac Vasc Anesth 2018;32(2):1002; *Courtesy of* Abbott, Abbott Park, IL; Reproduced with permission of Medtronic, Inc; with permission.)

HeartMate III (HM III) are the 2 commercially available third-generation LVAD devices.

The HeartWare HVAD system consists of a centrifugal-flow pump, an external controller, and an external power source. The pumping mechanism consists of an impeller with a hybrid suspension system that uses passive magnetic and hydrodynamic thrust bearings to create a contact-free rotation of the impeller.[21] This pump is highly compact and is the integrated inflow cannula, allowing its placement in the pericardial space (see **Fig. 6**). The adjustable speed for this device ranges from 1800 to 4000 RPM. The flow estimate is computed based on the electrical current, impeller speed, and a fixed viscosity value. Blood viscosity is determined by several factors, including the patient's hematocrit, which may affect the flow estimation. The device also consists of a cyclical controlled speed change function, because of which the impeller rotational speed decreases to less than the set speed by 200 RPM for 2 seconds, then increases 400 RPM (200 RPM more than the set speed) for 1 second, and then returns to the set point when the HVAD speeds are set between 2000 and 3800 RPM.[21] This function allows for decrease in areas of blood stasis.

The HM III is based on an intrapericardial centrifugal-flow pump with a full magnetically levitated rotor (see **Fig. 6**). This design is designed to eliminate the need for mechanical bearings or hydrodynamic blood bearings. Although the pump speed can range from 4800 to 6200 RPM, typically speeds between 5200 and 5800 RPM are used in the clinical setting.[22] The device also creates an artificial pulse by alternating the pump rotor speed 30 times per minute to increase pulsatile flow, which also allows for regular washing of flow pathways within the pump.[23] Like the HM II, the HM III flow readings are based on the power and speed. These readings usually maintain a linear relationship at a given speed. However, increase in power caused by factors not related to increased flow (eg, thrombus) may lead to artificially high flow readings.

Left Ventricular Assist Device Physiology and Effect on Hemodynamics

The LVAD is primarily designed to support the functioning of the left ventricle. However, because most of the congestive heart failure pathophysiology is biventricular, LVAD insertion often unmasks RV dysfunction. Ensuring adequate RV function to match up with the LV and LVAD output is key to patient management and often requires the addition of inotropes and RV afterload–reducing agent such as inhaled NO. Central venous pressure (CVP) monitoring may be helpful in these patients because an increase in CVP with low flows, low PI, and/or low MAPs may indicate RV compromise. In contrast, hypovolemia is usually associated with low CVPs along with low flows, low PI, and/or low MAPs.

In addition, patients with LVADs are prone to ventricular arrhythmias.[24] Because the LV (and LVAD) functioning depends on adequate RV output, ensuring an optimal cardiac rhythm is of vital importance. Ventricular tachycardia may lead to poor RV output and hence poor LV preload, which may lead to decrease in LV volume caused by continued emptying of the LV cavity by the LVAD. As a result, the interatrial septum may get suctioned by the inflow cannula of the LVAD. This occurrence is called a suction event. Suction events lead to ventricular irritability and may cause ventricular arrhythmias. In addition, they draw the septal wall away from the midline, further compromising RV function. In order to minimize such events, the HeartMate devices are programmed to undergo a decrease in their speed to a predetermined lower speed when the PI decreases suddenly (>45%). The LVAD returns to the original speed once the PI is restored, which allows a decrease in emptying of the LV cavity because of lower speed, allowing restoration of the LV volume. This event is registered in the LVAD event log as a PI event. The Heartware similarly has a suction-detection algorithm that monitors the estimated flow waveforms for a sudden decrease in instantaneous flow.[21] The algorithm establishes a baseline estimated flow based on the average minimum estimated flow, which is recalculated every 2 seconds. The suction trigger value is established at 40% less than the estimated flow baseline. If the flow remains lower than this baseline, the device alarms. The alarm stops once the estimated flow baseline surpasses the threshold limit for 20 seconds.

Another important determinant of the amount of blood flow across the device at a particular speed is the differential pressure across the pump. The difference between preload (LV pressure) and afterload (aortic pressure) governs blood flow through the pump. Because the flow is not pulsatile, the afterload is measured as MAP (and not as systolic and diastolic components). In general, the goal MAP for patients with LVAD is usually between 70 and 90 mm Hg.[25] Lower MAPs despite adequate flows may lead to decreased end-organ perfusion, whereas high MAPs may decrease flows because of increased afterload and are also associated with cerebrovascular accidents.[26]

Anesthetic Considerations

Preoperative work-up

The center's LVAD team should be contacted because they provide invaluable expertise in device management.[27] Depending on the center, it could include LVAD nurse, heart failure cardiologist, cardiothoracic surgeon, perfusionists, and so forth. The LVAD should be connected to a power source and have batteries available for backup.

When evaluating a patient with an LVAD, key considerations include enquiring about the type of LVAD, baseline display parameters (flow, speed, power and so forth), how long ago the device was placed, any recent issues from the device, as well as anticoagulation status. A recent echocardiogram may provide vital information about the patient's RV function. Recent hospitalizations, inotrope requirement, increased jugular venous pressure, and/or pedal edema may also signal RV dysfunction. Deranged RV function increases the perioperative risk. Securing a preinduction arterial access and having inotropes for hemodynamic support available is recommended by the authors in such cases. Because of the absence of a strong pulsatile flow with continuous-flow devices, a pulse for arterial line placement may not be palpable. Ultrasonography-guided arterial line placement is often used for the same reason.

Patients with LVADs are generally on anticoagulants to prevent device thrombosis. If possible, baseline hematocrit levels and anticoagulation tests should be obtained before the surgery. At present there are no clear guidelines on perioperative anticoagulation management.[28] The center's heart failure team/cardiothoracic surgeon may help in deciding the best anticoagulation management plan depending on the type/urgency of the surgery. Anticoagulants are usually not reversed/held if risk of bleeding is low. If the risk of bleeding is higher, Coumadin (and/or antiplatelet therapy) is held and anticoagulation is bridged to heparin infusion. The infusion is held in the perioperative period and restarted as soon as deemed safe by the perioperative clinical team. Patients with LVADs are prone to bleeding complications because they are usually on anticoagulation, have impaired platelet aggregation, and have vascular angiodysplasia.[29] Having a current type and screen (or type and crossmatch as appropriate) for these patients is of paramount importance. It is also important to discuss the patient's LVAD status (destination therapy or bridge to transplant) with the cardiology team because multiple blood transfusions in patients with LVADs can lead to development of circulating antibodies, complicating the organ match process.

In addition, patients with LVADs often have automatic implantable cardioverter-defibrillators (AICDs). Standard perioperative guidelines for cardiac implantable electronic device management should be followed for patients with AICDs.[30]

Intraoperative management

Standard American Society of Anesthesiologists (ASA) monitors should be used for intraoperative monitoring. However, there are several monitor-related caveats for patients with LVADs. The pulse oximeter signals are often imprecise if the pulse pressure is low because the device uses pulse to differentiate between arterial and venous waveforms. Similarly, noninvasive blood pressure readings may not be accurate in patients with LVADs.[31,32] Although invasive arterial line continues to be the gold standard, measurement of blood pressure with Doppler ultrasonography is a more reliable alternative.[31] Other noninvasive devices, such as the Terumo device and Mobil-O-Graph devices, have been reported to have higher levels of accuracy compared with noninvasive devices.[32,33] Depending on the invasiveness of the surgical procedure, a central venous line may be considered for CVP monitoring and use of inopressor support. As mentioned earlier, inotropic support should readily be available for patients to support the right ventricle. Similarly, other insults, such as hypercarbia, hypoxia, and volume overloading, should be avoided to maintain adequate RV function. Intraoperative echocardiography may be helpful in estimating changes in RV function and guiding fluid therapy, especially in surgeries involving massive fluid shifts.

Another important consideration is to precisely note the location of the driveline, especially in abdominal surgeries. Proper localization may prevent iatrogenic driveline injury and possible driveline infections.

Postoperative management

Postoperative care should be performed in a setting with health care providers familiar with the devices. As mentioned earlier, hypoxia and hypercarbia should be avoided to prevent iatrogenic RV injury. Adequate postoperative nausea and vomiting prophylaxis should be provided because vomiting/dry heaving increases intrathoracic pressure and RV afterload. AICD devices should again be reprogrammed to their initial preoperative settings.

Anticoagulation should be resumed after a multidisciplinary discussion with the patient's cardiologist and the surgeon, to balance the risk of bleeding and thromboembolic events.

Management of Cardiopulmonary Arrest in Patients with Left Ventricular Assist Devices

Recently the AHA published guidelines on CPR in patients with LVADs.[34] Per the guidelines, an end-tidal CO_2 of less than 20 mm Hg in an unresponsive, correctly intubated pulseless patient with an LVAD would be a reasonable indicator of poor systemic perfusion and chest compressions should be initiated. LVAD should be assessed for proper function and connections by listening for a hum over the left chest and left upper abdominal quadrant. Standard CPR and postarrest care should be performed, including mild therapeutic hypothermia as per the AHA guidelines.[5]

OTHER MECHANICAL CIRCULATORY SUPPORT DEVICES

Other than these commonly used MCS devices, other devices, such as Impella, RV assist devices, and tandem hearts, are also used for hemodynamic support.

Familiarization with the devices at the relevant institutions may be very useful, especially when patients present for emergent surgical procedures. With advancing technology, the use of these devices is expected to grow. Management of these patients in an interdisciplinary collaborative fashion is imperative for optimal patient outcomes.

ACKNOWLEDGMENTS

None.

CONFLICTS OF INTEREST

The authors have no relevant conflicts of interest.

DISCLOSURE

None.

REFERENCES

1. Gold HK, Leinbach RC, Sanders CA, et al. Intraaortic balloon pumping for ventricular septal defect or mitral regurgitation complicating acute myocardial infarction. Circulation 1973;47:1191–6.
2. Aksoy O, Yousefzai R, Singh D, et al. Cardiogenic shock in the setting of severe aortic stenosis: role of intra-aortic balloon pump support. Heart 2011;97:838–43.
3. Fotopoulos GD, Mason MJ, Walker S, et al. Stabilisation of medically refractory ventricular arrhythmia by intra-aortic balloon counterpulsation. Heart 1999;82: 96–100.
4. Papaioannou TG, Stefanadis C. Basic principles of the intraaortic balloon pump and mechanisms affecting its performance. ASAIO J 2005;51:296–300.
5. AHA CPR Guidelines. Available at: https://eccguidelines.heart.org/index.php/circulation/cpr-ecc-guidelines-2/part-7-adult-advanced-cardiovascular-life-support/. Accessed August 06, 2019.
6. ELSO Registry. Available at: https://www.elso.org/Registry/Statistics.aspx. Accessed August 13, 2019.
7. Kulkarni T, Sharma NS, Diaz-Guzman E. Extracorporeal membrane oxygenation in adults: a practical guide for internists. Cleve Clin J Med 2016;83:373–84.
8. Bardia A, Schonberger RB. Postcardiotomy venoarterial extracorporeal membrane oxygenation (VA ECMO) in adult patients - many questions, few answers, and hard choices. J Cardiothorac Vasc Anesth 2018;32:1183–4.
9. ELSO Guidelines. Available at: https://www.elso.org/Portals/0/IGD/Archive/FileManager/e76ef78eabcusersshyerdocumentselsoguidelinesforadultcardiacfailure1.3.pdf. Accessed August 10, 2019.
10. Guglin M, Zucker MJ, Bazan VM, et al. Venoarterial ECMO for adults: JACC Scientific Expert Panel. J Am Coll Cardiol 2019;73:698–716.
11. Rupprecht L, Lunz D, Philipp A, et al. Pitfalls in percutaneous ECMO cannulation. Heart Lung Vessel 2015;7:320–6.
12. ELSO guidelines. Available at: https://www.elso.org/Portals/0/ELSO Guidelines General All ECLS Version 1_4.pdf. Accessed August 15, 2019.
13. Cheng V, Abdul-Aziz MH, Roberts JA, et al. Optimising drug dosing in patients receiving extracorporeal membrane oxygenation. J Thorac Dis 2018;10:S629–41.
14. Rose EA, Gelijns AC, Moskowitz AJ, et al. Long-term use of a left ventricular assist device for end-stage heart failure. N Engl J Med 2001;345:1435–43.

15. Pratt AK, Shah NS, Boyce SW. Left ventricular assist device management in the ICU. Crit Care Med 2014;42:158–68.
16. Slaughter MS, Rogers JG, Milano CA, et al. Advanced heart failure treated with continuous-flow left ventricular assist device. N Engl J Med 2009;361:2241–51.
17. Miller LW, Pagani FD, Russell SD, et al. Use of a continuous-flow device in patients awaiting heart transplantation. N Engl J Med 2007;357:885–96.
18. Griffith BP, Kormos RL, Borovetz HS, et al. HeartMate II left ventricular assist system: from concept to first clinical use. Ann Thorac Surg 2001;71:S116–20 [discussion: S114–6].
19. Slaughter MS, Bartoli CR, Sobieski MA, et al. Intraoperative evaluation of the HeartMate II flow estimator. J Heart Lung Transplant 2009;28:39–43.
20. Capoccia M. Mechanical circulatory support for advanced heart failure: are we about to witness a new "gold standard"? J Cardiovasc Dev Dis 2016;3 [pii:E35].
21. Larose JA, Tamez D, Ashenuga M, et al. Design concepts and principle of operation of the HeartWare ventricular assist system. ASAIO J 2010;56:285–9.
22. Tchoukina I, Smallfield MC, Shah KB. Device management and flow optimization on left ventricular assist device support. Crit Care Clin 2018;34:453–63.
23. Schmitto JD, Hanke JS, Rojas SV, et al. First implantation in man of a new magnetically levitated left ventricular assist device (HeartMate III). J Heart Lung Transplant 2015;34:858–60.
24. Feldman D, Pamboukian SV, Teuteberg JJ, et al. The 2013 International Society for Heart and Lung Transplantation guidelines for mechanical circulatory support: executive summary. J Heart Lung Transplant 2013;32:157–87.
25. Wilson SR, Givertz MM, Stewart GC, et al. Ventricular assist devices the challenges of outpatient management. J Am Coll Cardiol 2009;54:1647–59.
26. DeVore AD, Stewart GC. The risk of stroke on left ventricular assist device support: steady gains or stalled progress? JACC Heart Fail 2017;5:712–4.
27. Nicolosi AC, Pagel PS. Perioperative considerations in the patient with a left ventricular assist device. Anesthesiology 2003;98:565–70.
28. Chung M. Perioperative management of the patient with a left ventricular assist device for noncardiac surgery. Anesth Analg 2018;126:1839–50.
29. Birks EJ. Stopping LVAD bleeding: a piece of the puzzle. Circ Res 2017;121:902–4.
30. American Society of Anesthesiologists. Practice advisory for the perioperative management of patients with cardiac implantable electronic devices: pacemakers and implantable cardioverter-defibrillators: an updated report by the american society of anesthesiologists task force on perioperative management of patients with cardiac implantable electronic devices. Anesthesiology 2011;114:247–61.
31. Bennett MK, Roberts CA, Dordunoo D, et al. Ideal methodology to assess systemic blood pressure in patients with continuous-flow left ventricular assist devices. J Heart Lung Transplant 2010;29:593–4.
32. Lanier GM, Orlanes K, Hayashi Y, et al. Validity and reliability of a novel slow cuff-deflation system for noninvasive blood pressure monitoring in patients with continuous-flow left ventricular assist device. Circ Heart Fail 2013;6:1005–12.
33. Castagna F, McDonnell BJ, Stohr EJ, et al. Non-invasive measurement of peripheral, central and 24-hour blood pressure in patients with continuous-flow left ventricular assist device. J Heart Lung Transplant 2017;36:694–7.
34. Peberdy MA, Gluck JA, Ornato JP, et al. Cardiopulmonary resuscitation in adults and children with mechanical circulatory support: a scientific statement from the American Heart Association. Circulation 2017;135:e1115–34.

Anesthesia for the Patient with Severe Liver Failure

Aidan Spring, LRCP&SI, MB BCh BAO, FCAI[a], Jagroop S. Saran, MD[a],
Sinead McCarthy, MB BCh BAO, FCAI[a], Stuart A. McCluskey, MD, PhD, FRCPC[b,]*

KEYWORDS

- Anesthesia • End-stage liver disease • Liver failure • Anesthesia considerations

KEY POINTS

- The incidence of liver failure continues to increase, and it is associated with increased perioperative morbidity and mortality.
- Liver failure is associated with multiorgan dysfunction, including central nervous, cardiac, respiratory, gastrointestinal, renal, and hematological systems.
- Preoperative identification, optimization, and tailored anesthetic management are essential for optimum outcomes in patients with liver disease undergoing surgery.
- The coagulopathy of liver failure is a balanced coagulopathy better assessed by thromboelastography than conventional testing, and it is not directly associated with bleeding risk.

INTRODUCTION

Worldwide, liver disease is estimated to be responsible for 2 million deaths each year, the vast majority owing to complications of cirrhosis, viral hepatitis, and hepatocellular carcinoma.[1] The incidence and prevalence of chronic liver disease are not well established and are likely considerably higher best estimates. The cause and burden of liver disease are also known to vary with geographic region, ethnicity, and socioeconomic status.

The liver has many essential functions, including the production of bile, the synthesis of plasma proteins (eg, clotting factors), drug metabolism, and the storage of vitamins, minerals, and glucose, among many others. Historically, the liver was divided

Financial Disclosures: None.
[a] Abdominal Organ Transplantation Anesthesia Fellowship Program, Department of Anesthesia and Pain Management, Toronto General Hospital, University Health Network, University of Toronto, 3 Eaton North, 200 Elizabeth Street, Toronto, Ontario M5G 2C4, Canada;
[b] Department of Anesthesia and Pain Management, Toronto General Hospital, University Health Network, University of Toronto, 3 Eaton North, 200 Elizabeth Street, Toronto, Ontario M5G 2C4, Canada
* Corresponding author.
E-mail address: Stuart.McCluskey@uhn.ca

Anesthesiology Clin 38 (2020) 35–50
https://doi.org/10.1016/j.anclin.2019.10.002
1932-2275/20/Crown Copyright © 2019 Published by Elsevier Inc. All rights reserved.

anesthesiology.theclinics.com

into right and left lobes according to liver topography. The functional and surgical anatomy of the liver is divided into 8 segments according to vascular anatomy and biliary drainage.[2] The vascular anatomy provides a unique blood supply, receiving blood from both the hepatic portal vein and the hepatic arteries. The hepatic portal vein supplies approximately 75% of hepatic blood flow and 50% of the liver's oxygen.[3] A novel flow relationship exists between these 2 blood supplies in that the hepatic artery can produce compensatory flow changes in response to changes in hepatic portal venous inflow. This compensatory blood flow is known as the hepatic arterial buffer response and maintains constant hepatic blood flow or oxygen supply.[3]

Liver disease is a multisystem disorder (**Fig. 1**) and is described as acute or chronic according to time between symptom onset and the inciting event. Acute liver failure is defined by the development of symptoms of severe liver injury with encephalopathy, and impaired synthetic function in a patient without preexisting liver disease, and an illness duration of less than 26 weeks.[4] Anesthesia for patients with acute liver failure occurs mainly in the context of orthotopic liver transplantation and will not be discussed further in this review. Progressive chronic liver disease results in liver fibrosis, and cirrhosis is a term used to describe advanced fibrosis. Cirrhosis is a histologic description characterized by islands of hepatic regeneration surrounded by thin fibrous septa resulting in parenchymal destruction and vascular distortion.[5] Advanced chronic liver disease may remain compensated for many years; the change to

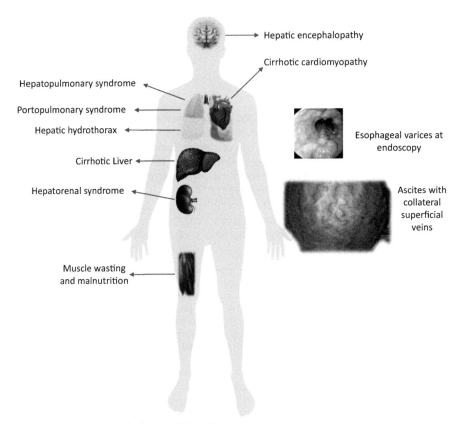

Fig. 1. Complications of advanced liver disease.

decompensated cirrhosis occurs when features such as ascites, variceal bleeding, or encephalopathy develop. Decompensated cirrhosis is associated with increased mortality, and median survival decreases from 12 years to 2 years.[6] Another entity known as acute-on-chronic liver failure has more recently been described.[7] This syndrome is associated with increased short-term mortality and is characterized by acute and severe hepatic disorder in patients with underlying chronic liver disease.

CAUSE OF LIVER DISEASE

The causes of liver disease include infection, toxins, metabolic abnormalities, autoimmune conditions, and vascular abnormalities. In the United States, infection with the hepatitis C virus, alcohol, and increasingly, nonalcoholic fatty liver disease (NAFLD) are the leading causes of cirrhosis.[1,8] The obesity epidemic is strongly associated with the increase in NAFLD. Therapies used to manage obesity and its associated metabolic syndrome are being evaluated.[9]

The pathophysiology of cirrhosis is complex and involves inflammation, fibrogenesis, and angiogenesis. These processes result in hepatic microvascular changes remodeling of hepatic sinusoids and the formation of intrahepatic shunts.[5] Increasing hepatic resistance to portal vein flow causes portal hypertension, a hallmark of cirrhosis. Portal blood flow is enhanced further by splanchnic vasodilation, and this ultimately leads to the development of portal hypertension, ascites, and portosystemic shunts, such as gastric varices. Shunting of compounds such as ammonia directly into the systemic circulation are thought to have a role in the development of hepatic encephalopathy. The complex interaction of the failing liver with other organs can result in hepatorenal syndrome, portopulmonary hypertension, hepatopulmonary syndrome, and cirrhotic cardiomyopathy.[10]

Patients with liver disease present for surgery as part of their liver disease treatment or to manage complications. Surgical procedures may include hepatic resection for hepatocellular carcinoma or the creation of transjugular intrahepatic portosystemic shunts (TIPS) to decompress the portal system in the case of refractory variceal bleeds or massive ascites. However, more concerning are the patients presenting for surgery with advanced liver disease who are unaware of their health status.[8]

RISK STRATIFICATION

A direct relationship between increased perioperative risk and the severity of chronic liver disease has held for some time.[11] Acute hepatitis, particularly alcoholic hepatitis, is regarded as a contraindication to nonemergent surgery because it is associated with unacceptably high mortality.[12] However, assessment of perioperative risk in other patients with liver disease is not straightforward. Certainly, the urgency and nature of the proposed surgery as well as comorbid medical issues need to be considered, but the challenge is to determine whether it is feasible to proceed with a procedure as proposed, to postpone until optimization/liver transplantation, or to defer indefinitely. A variety of clinical scoring systems are used to help make this determination. The two most commonly used are the Child-Turcotte-Pugh (CTP) score and the Model for End-Stage Liver Disease (MELD) score.

The CTP score was developed in the 1960s to predict operative mortality associated with portocaval shunt surgery. It consists of 5 measures: serum albumin, bilirubin, prothrombin time, and the presence of hepatic encephalopathy and ascites. The patient is assigned to group A, B, or C in order of increasing liver disease severity by adding the score for each parameter (**Table 1**). A 2011 single-center retrospective analysis

Table 1
Child-Turcotte-Pugh score

	Points Assigned		
Variable	1	2	3
Serum bilirubin (μmol/L)	<34	34–50	>50
Serum albumin (g/L)	>35	23–35	<28
INR	<1.7	1.7–2.3	>2.3
Ascites	None	Mild	Severe
Encephalopathy[a]	None	Grade I to II	Grade III to IV

[a] West Haven classification of hepatic encephalopathy.

of patients undergoing general surgery found that in-hospital mortality was 63% in CTP group C, 17% in group B, and 10% in group A.[13]

The MELD score was originally developed to predict mortality following TIPS placement and is now used to prioritize patients on the liver transplant list.[14] It includes serum bilirubin, creatinine, and the international normalized ratio (INR). Higher MELD scores have been shown to correlate with increased mortality in nontransplant surgery with a MELD score greater than 15 associated with 54% in-hospital mortality.[13] Another study found that the addition of serum albumin less than 2.5 mg/dL (25 g/L) to a MELD score ≥15 identified a subset of patients at particularly high perioperative risk, that is, greater than 60%.[15] However, when considering retrospective analyses, it should be borne in mind that patients with advanced liver disease (CTP group C or MELD >15) are typically not considered for elective surgery and so disproportionately undergo emergent procedures. Emergent procedures are consistently associated with high mortality in those with advanced liver disease.[13,15] Other factors shown to be associated with adverse outcome include intraoperative blood transfusion[13,15,16] and high American Society of Anesthesiologists (ASA) Physical Status classification score.[11,13,15,17] Laparoscopic approaches may be protective in abdominal surgery.[18] A scoring system has been developed specifically to assess perioperative risk in patients with cirrhosis; essentially age and ASA classification are added to the MELD score.[17] This prediction rule was derived from a Mayo Clinic surgical database and is available as an online calculator.[19] This study also concluded that although ASA classification was best at predicting 7-day mortality, MELD was superior at predicting later mortality. No scoring system provides a clear identification of which elective surgery should proceed safely, and risk scores must be viewed in their clinical context.

ASSESSMENT AND INVESTIGATIONS

As liver disease progresses to cirrhosis, the systemic effects of liver failure become manifest (see **Fig. 1**). A thorough multimodal assessment is required before undertaking elective surgery in these patients relying on history, examination, and focused investigation.

In brief, the history should determine the underlying cause and duration of liver failure, the presence of complications, and treatments used. Knowing whether a patient is currently active on a transplant list can also be very informative. In such cases, it is advisable to consult with the transplant center before any elective procedure. The presence of other medical comorbidities should also be actively sought because conditions such as coronary artery disease and diabetes tend to occur at higher frequency in those with advanced liver disease.[20]

Examination can reveal evidence of decompensated disease, including hepatic encephalopathy and ascites. The presence of hepatic encephalopathy will likely result in delayed emergence from anesthesia and increased susceptibility to anesthetic drugs, such as benzodiazepines and delirium.[21] Evidence of muscle wasting (sarcopenia) often seen in advanced liver cirrhosis has important prognostic implications.[22] Assessment of frailty is a logical progression from this, and measures of sarcopenia are included in many frailty scoring systems. Frailty is an important topic in preoperative risk assessment, and early work suggests that it can be similarly applied to cirrhosis.[23]

A minimum set of blood investigations should include a complete blood count, coagulation profile, liver function tests as well as serum electrolytes and creatinine. Coagulopathy, electrolyte disturbances, and renal dysfunction are commonly encountered in cirrhotic patients and have obvious perioperative implications. The differential diagnosis of deteriorating renal function in cirrhosis is broad and can include sepsis, nephrotoxins, aggressive diuresis causing hypovolemia, and hepatorenal syndrome. Reversible causes of renal dysfunction should be explored and should prompt treatment. Hepatorenal syndrome is a diagnosis of exclusion and is thought to be caused by renal hypoperfusion. Splanchnic vasodilation leads to a state of relative hypovolemia, which is compounded by increased renal vascular resistance owing to activation of the renin angiotensin and sympathetic nervous systems. The reader is directed to a detailed review of the condition, but it suffices to say that the onset of hepatorenal syndrome (particularly type 1) portends a poor prognosis.[24]

Liver function tests commonly include serum aminotransferases, gamma glutamyl transferase, and bilirubin. Despite the name, these tests are poor assays of liver function and can be elevated for other reasons. Nonetheless, they are useful because the serum aminotransferases are markers of hepatocellular damage, and patterns of elevation are suggestive of particular causes of liver injury.[25] Serum albumin is regarded as a marker of hepatic synthetic function, but may have a more complicated cause related to chronic inflammation.[26]

Given the prevalence of electrolyte disturbances and comorbid cardiac issues, a recent electrocardiogram is a minimum requirement, but more focused cardiac assessment may be indicated. A transthoracic echocardiogram (TTE) can evaluate ventricular function and cirrhotic cardiomyopathy, screen for portopulmonary hypertension, and diagnose hepatopulmonary syndrome. Cirrhotic cardiomyopathy is defined as chronic cardiac dysfunction characterized by impaired systolic and diastolic dysfunction with electrophysiologic abnormalities in the absence of known cardiac disease.[27] Worryingly, this condition is typically silent at rest and only manifests with stress. TIPS used to decompress the portal system as a treatment of ascites and variceal bleeding may precipitate heart failure in patients with cirrhotic cardiomyopathy. Chronotropic incompetence is an electrophysiological feature of cirrhotic cardiomyopathy and is defined as the failure of the heart rate to increase in response to metabolic demand.[28] For this reason cardiac stress testing in patients with advanced cirrhosis is typically nondiagnostic for ischemia.

Pulmonary hypertension is defined as an elevation of the mean pulmonary artery pressure ≥ 25 mm Hg. In the presence of portal hypertension, it is known as portopulmonary hypertension, but it is not correlated with cause or severity of cirrhosis. Estimated right ventricular systolic pressures greater than 45 mm Hg or signs of right heart dysfunction should prompt right heart catheterization to establish a formal diagnosis. The presence of portopulmonary hypertension is an indication for liver transplantation, but severe cases are considered exceptionally high risk and are deferred until pulmonary pressures are reduced.[29] Undertaking anesthesia in these patients outside of liver transplantation should not be considered lightly.

Hepatopulmonary syndrome is another pulmonary manifestation of cirrhosis, and the diagnosis is suspected in the presence of shortness of breath relieved by sitting up (platypnea) and desaturation in the lying position (orthodeoxia). It is the result of intrapulmonary shunting of deoxygenated blood, and the diagnosis is established by TTE contrast echocardiography. It is a relatively common condition (up to 20%) in those with cirrhosis, and liver transplantation is the only known treatment. Perioperative hypoxemia should be anticipated, and prolonged mechanical ventilation with the need for rescue therapies should be considered and avoided if possible by accepting reasonable criteria for arterial oxygenation.[30]

The anesthesiologist routinely managing patients with advanced liver failure should be able to appreciate the significance of more focused liver investigations, particularly when contemplating procedures on the hepatobiliary system, such as hepatic resection or TIPS. Liver ultrasound, triphasic computed tomography, and MRI liver may point to the cause of liver failure and likely anesthetic and operative difficulties. For example, a significant hepatic hydrothorax may require thoracentesis before an elective procedure. The presence of portal vein thrombus can make TIPS a more complicated and involved procedure.[31] Similarly, the presence of ectopic biliary varices may make for a more challenging hepatic dissection. Portal vein pressure measurements are more esoteric and probably less clinically useful, although successful lowering of portal pressure during TIPS is crucial, especially if performed emergently for variceal hemorrhage. Anesthesiologists working in interventional radiology suites in liver centers will often hear portal pressure measurements discussed. Portal pressure measurement may be performed directly through the portal vein puncture during TIPS, although more commonly it is determined indirectly by measuring the hepatic venous pressure gradient (HPVG). The HVPG is the difference between balloon wedged hepatic vein pressure and free hepatic vein pressure. A gradient of greater than 10 mm Hg predicts the likelihood of developing decompensation. It may also predict the likelihood of decompensation after liver resection.[32]

PREOPTIMIZATION

Every effort should be made to optimize patients with advanced liver disease when coming to the operating room. Hepatologists can be invaluable in this and should be consulted early. In particular, reversible causes for deterioration in cognition, pulmonary function, and cardiac and renal status should be sought, and prompt treatment should be instituted. Treatment may involve the addition of laxatives and rifaximin to treat hepatic encephalopathy[33] or treating alcohol withdrawal syndrome. It is also important to remember that cirrhosis is a state of relative immunosuppression,[34] and a high index of suspicion for infection should be maintained. Infections such as spontaneous bacterial peritonitis can precipitate deterioration in cognition and organ function. Current medications should also be reviewed in the context of upcoming surgery. Diuretics, sedatives, and anticoagulants may need to be adjusted perioperatively.

Uncontrolled ascites is a contraindication to elective abdominal surgery because it can compromise wound healing culminating in postoperative ascitic leaks[35] and later incisional hernias. Ascites may be controlled using a low-sodium diet and diuresis. Preemptive TIPS before surgery has been described to control refractory ascites and decompress portosystemic shunts to reduce bleeding, but it cannot be recommended as standard of care.[36]

Malnutrition is very common among patients with advanced liver disease. The likely cause is multifactorial, including reduced intake owing to anorexia and ascites, impaired absorption, and increased catabolism. Malnutrition is an independent risk factor for mortality in these patients, and early specialist input to optimize nutrition appears to be beneficial.[37] As mentioned previously, serum albumin is a marker of hepatic synthetic function, and hypoalbuminemia is a predictor of mortality in cirrhotics undergoing surgery. Importantly, the administration of intravenous albumin replacement does not modify this risk.[38] Restriction of dietary protein intake in those at risk of hepatic encephalopathy is not evidence-based practice and may have adverse effects.[39]

Prehabilitation of patients with advanced liver failure, particularly in those awaiting liver transplantation, is being considered.[40] Prehabilitation has been shown to be feasible in this population with 1 study showing improved cardiovascular fitness and reduced insulin resistance.[41] Over the next few years, prehabilitation may become recognized as critical to securing better outcomes for patients with advanced liver disease.

INTRAOPERATIVE MANAGEMENT
Monitoring

Standard anesthesia monitors should be placed as per society guidelines. In patients with severe liver disease, there should be a low threshold to place an invasive arterial catheter to monitor blood pressure and to allow frequent blood sampling to monitor respiratory and acid-base status. Central venous catheter (CVC) placement should be considered when additional venous access is needed or when vasopressor administration anticipated. Type and duration of surgery, anticipated blood loss, hemodynamic swings, and extent of liver disease should also be considered when determining invasive monitoring. CVC placement solely for central venous pressure monitoring is controversial.[42]

Intraoperative transesophageal echocardiography (TEE) may be considered in decompensated liver disease and where significant intraoperative fluid shifts are anticipated. The presence of esophageal varices should be taken into consideration; however, the risk of complications appears to be low. Single-center, retrospective studies from TEE use during liver transplantation place the risk at less than 1%.[43,44]

Anesthetic Medications

Liver disease alters the drug pharmacokinetics by altering protein binding, drug metabolism, and volume of distribution. Drug choice and dose adjustments should be considered for patients with advanced disease as evidenced by portal hypertension, renal dysfunction, or encephalopathy, but anesthetic requirements are generally lower in patients with liver disease.[45,46]

Sedative-Hypnotics

Patients with liver disease have similar clearance rates of induction doses used in routine clinical practice, such as propofol, etomidate, and methohexital, when compared with healthy patients.[47–49] Elimination half-time and free drug levels of benzodiazepines are increased in severe liver disease with the exception of oxazepam and temazepam.

Analgesics

For the most part, analgesics are metabolized in the liver with renal elimination. In liver disease, decreased doses of opioids with increased intervals should be used to prevent drug accumulation. Long-acting opioids, such as morphine and meperidine, should be avoided, but shorter-acting opioids, such as fentanyl and hydromorphone, are well tolerated when used in lower doses and titrated to effect. Acetaminophen is usually well tolerated, but caution should be used in patients with advanced cirrhosis, especially malnourished patients. Nonsteroidal anti-inflammatories should be used, bearing in mind risk of gastrointestinal bleeding and renal function.

Neuromuscular Blockade

The aminosteroid neuromuscular agents, rocuronium and vecuronium, are metabolized in part by the liver, and their duration of action may be prolonged in liver failure. These drugs should be titrated to effect using peripheral nerve stimulators. Benzylisoquinolinium neuromuscular agents, atracurium and cis-atracurium, are not affected in liver disease. Succinylcholine is metabolized by plasma cholinesterase, an enzyme produced by the liver; although the duration of action of succinylcholine is prolonged, it is not clinically significant.

Volatile Anesthetics

Modern halogenated volatile anesthetics are safe to use in cirrhotic patients. Isoflurane and desflurane, but not sevoflurane, are metabolized to trifluoroacetyl chloride, the compound implicated in halothane hepatitis, to a much lesser extent than halothane.

Coagulation

Liver disease affects both procoagulant and anticoagulant components of hemostasis leading to a new "balanced" steady state.[50] As such, conventional tests of coagulation, including INR, prothrombin time, and activated partial thromboplastin time, do not reflect the risks of bleeding and thrombosis. The assumption that patients with liver disease are autoanticoagulated is incorrect.

Viscoelastic testing, such as rotational thromboelastometry (ROTEM) or thromboelastography (TEG), reflects dynamic changes in clot formation and lysis. These tests are superior and potentially provide a clinically relevant picture in patients with liver disease. These tests can also be used to guide specific blood product transfusion (ie, cryoprecipitate, and fresh frozen plasma).[51]

Postoperative Analgesia

Providing effective perioperative analgesia to the patients with advanced liver disease is challenging, balancing the risks of oversedation and uncontrolled bleeding with optimal pain control. A potential coagulopathy made worse with surgery is rightly regarded as a contraindication to neuraxial procedures given the devastating consequences of epidural hematoma.[52] However, neuraxial blockade has been used successfully in patients with cirrhosis as part of enhanced recovery protocols in abdominal surgery.[53] The best available evidence suggests that epidural use is superior in terms of pain control to patient-controlled opioid analgesia, and it is associated with reduced incidence of postoperative respiratory failure.[52]

Other regional anesthetic techniques offer significant benefit without the bleeding risk and should be considered, including subcostal transversus abdominis plane (TAP), erector spinae, and quadratus lumborum blocks.[54] They are performed using real-time ultrasound guidance, and catheters can be placed if required for a more durable effect. Studies have shown that these blocks achieve better pain control and reduce postoperative opioid requirements compared with intravenous opioids alone. The erector spinae and quadratus lumborum blocks are more recently described.

They are ultrasound-guided blocks, and unlike TAP blocks, may offer visceral analgesia in addition to somatic analgesia.[55]

CONSIDERATIONS FOR SPECIFIC PROCEDURES
Cardiac Surgery

With increasingly complex patients, a wider variety of surgical procedures being offered, and an increased prevalence of hepatic disease, there are an increasing number of patients with liver cirrhosis presenting for cardiac surgery.[56] There is little doubt that liver disease or its perioperative management has a negative impact on postoperative mortality[57] and morbidity.[58] Despite this observation, the evaluation of liver function has not been included in many of the most widely used cardiac surgery risk scoring systems, including EuroSCORE II and Society of Thoracic Surgeons risk prediction model.[59,60]

Studies have identified CTP score as well as Na-MELD score as predictors of early postoperative mortality following cardiac surgery.[61,62] The mortalities in these patients range from 9.88% for patients in CTP class A to 69.23% for patients with CTP class C.[56] Using robust risk adjustments, outcome at 5 years postoperatively was strongly associated with CTP: 82.4% for Child A, 47.6% for Child B, and 33.3% for Child C ($P = .001$).[63] A Taiwanese population-based study looking at 10-year survival demonstrated a similar pattern of reduced long-term survival following cardiac surgery in cirrhotic patients. Cirrhotic patients had a higher incidence of readmission primarily with liver and heart failure, with most deaths being due to the progression of the primary liver disease.[64] Although cardiac surgery can be successfully carried out with careful patient selection, mortality with redo procedures has been reported as high as 50%.[62]

Cardiopulmonary bypass can exacerbate a preexisting coagulopathy by inducing platelet dysfunction, fibrinolysis, and/or hypocalcemia.[65] Dhoble and colleagues[66] looked at the outcomes in cirrhotic patients undergoing aortic valve surgery with transcatheter aortic valve replacements (TAVR, n = 156) versus surgical aortic valve replacements (SAVR, n = 189). Interestingly, after propensity matching, there were no significant differences between in-hospital mortality, readmissions, hospitalization costs, and discharges to home within the TAVR and SAVR groups. Postprocedure length of stay (6.3 vs 10.2 days; $P < .001$) and blood transfusion rates (22% vs 58%; $P < .001$) were significantly lower in TAVR patients.

TRAUMA

Multiple studies have identified that patients with cirrhosis and severe liver disease who present with traumatic injuries are at increased risk for morbidity and mortality. Hepatic cirrhosis is a poor prognostic factor in trauma, with as high as a 4-fold increase in mortality independent of their CTP classification.[67] This association appears to be consistent with the most common traumatic injuries, for example, abdominal trauma and traumatic brain injury.[68,69] Mortalities and morbidities were increased even for patients considered to have relatively minor trauma.[70] A 12-year study from Demetriades and colleagues[70] looked at outcomes following trauma laparotomy in cirrhotic patients versus control matched noncirrhotic patients undergoing trauma laparotomy. The mortality in the cirrhotic group was significantly higher than that in the matched noncirrhotic group, even in low Injury Severity Score (ISS) groups (29% vs 5%, ISS <16) with an overall mortality of 45% versus 24% ($P = .021$). Based on this significant increase in mortality, they suggested, regardless of the severity of the injury, these cirrhotic patients should be monitored in a level 1 or 2 intensive care environment in the postoperative period. A more recent systematic review focusing on trauma and orthopedic surgery in the cirrhotic patient showed increased mortality in the cirrhotic versus the noncirrhotic group (12% vs 6%). This association included an increased incidence of complications, such as acute respiratory distress syndrome, trauma coagulopathy, and sepsis.[71] Cirrhotic patients are significantly more likely to suffer severe morbidity (10% vs 4%) and mortality (40%) compared with that of noncirrhotic at 15%.[72]

An analysis of the national trauma databank over an 8-year period from 2002 to 2010 of adult patients with blunt splenic injury revealed that cirrhotic patients had a lower success rate (83% vs 90%, P = .004) of nonoperative management of their injury[73] with an increased rate of splenectomy.[74] Cirrhotic patients were also discovered to have a higher rate of complications per patient, increased length of intensive care and inpatient length of stay, and higher overall mortality (22% vs 6%, $P<.0001$), regardless of their treatment group. Factors contributing to unsuccessful nonoperative management were preexisting coagulopathy and grade 4 to 5 blunt splenic injury. Male sex, hypotension, preexisting coagulopathy, and a Glasgow Coma Score of less than 13 were predictors of mortality.[73]

Traumatic brain injury as an isolated injury demonstrated much the same pattern of increased mortality. An analysis of nearly nine thousand trauma patients showed that hepatic cirrhosis patients had an increased rate of mortality compared to matched non-cirrhotic controls (31% vs 17%, P = .03) and were also less likely to proceed to urgent operative interventions (12% vs 25%, P = .03).[69]

ANESTHESIA FOR TRANSHEPATIC PORTOSYSTEMIC SHUNT AND MINOR PROCEDURES

Transhepatic portosystemic shunt is a percutaneous procedure carried out under sedation or general anesthesia to reduce portal pressure by creating a shunt between the hepatic vein and the intrahepatic portal vein.[75] Performance of a TIPS procedure can be complex, requiring multiple attempts, and general anesthesia may be indicated for patients who cannot tolerate sedation or those who cannot lie flat for several hours. In addition, preprocedural screening for congestive heart failure and pulmonary hypertension is imperative because an increased systemic flow can worsen both of these conditions.

Patients for minor procedures, such as liver biopsies, tunneled intravenous lines, drain insertion, interventional radiology procedures, and paracentesis that requires sedation, are often encephalopathic and require intubation for risk of aspiration. In addition, many cannot tolerate lying flat secondary to massive ascites and pleural effusions. Aside from the complexity of these high-risk patients undergoing sedation or general anesthesia, the anesthesiologist must consider that these procedures mainly occur outside of the operating room environment, primarily in radiology suites. Additional factors, such as unfamiliar equipment, lack of trained help, hostile environmental factors, such as a cold room with an inability to warm the patient, poor access to the patient, and rotating workspace, all contribute to making these procedures more difficult.[76]

Blood typing and screen should be performed in case of a need for blood products. Goals should be a platelet count greater than 50 × 10^9/L and fibrinogen greater than 150 to 200 mg/dL, without attempts to correct the INR. Viscoelastic testing (ie, thromboelastography) may be used to guide therapy, if available. Correction of INR is not recommended because multiple studies have shown INR is a poor correlation for bleeding risk in the cirrhotic patients.[77–82]

ABDOMINAL SURGERY

Gastrointestinal surgery, including both elective and emergency surgery, comprises the bulk of the operations performed on cirrhotic patients. Laparoscopic and open approaches are associated with increased morbidity and mortality. Cholecystectomy is the most frequently performed surgery in cirrhotic patients.[83] A prospective randomized trial demonstrated that an open cholecystectomy was associated with increased morbidity (including bleeding, length of hospital stay, and length of surgery) compared with laparoscopic procedures (30% vs 13%) and a favorable benefit in mortality (0% vs 0%–7%)[84]; however, the difference in morbidity during elective hernia repair was not statistically significant compared with noncirrhotic controls.[85] Abdominal wall hernias develop in 20% of all cirrhotic patients, and elective repair is associated with morbidity (7%–15%) and significant mortality (0%–5%).[85] However, multiple studies acknowledge significantly higher morbidity and mortality in emergency hernia repair compared with elective repair.[85–87] Mortality was 7-fold higher in emergencies (3.8% vs 0.5%; $P<.0001$), and elective repair in these patients may be the optimal course to pursue to avoid increased mortality.[85]

For hepatic resection secondary to hepatocellular carcinoma, preoperative screening can identify those patients with an increased risk of mortality by detecting an increased MELD score. Although previous studies have reported mortality approaching as high as 25%, careful selection and screening have led to improved outcomes and mortality.[88] The MELD score is a strong predictor of both perioperative mortality and long-term survival in patients with cirrhosis undergoing hepatic resection for hepatocellular cancer. In patients with cirrhosis, hepatic resection with an MELD score less than 9 was associated with no perioperative mortality versus 29% for patients with an MELD score greater than 9 ($P<.01$).[89]

CONFLICTS OF INTEREST

None.

REFERENCES

1. Asrani SK, Devarbhavi H, Eaton J, et al. Burden of liver diseases in the world. J Hepatol 2019;70(1):151–71.
2. Juza RM, Pauli EM. Clinical and surgical anatomy of the liver: a review for clinicians. Clin Anat 2014;27(5):764–9.
3. Eipel C, Abshagen K, Vollmar B. Regulation of hepatic blood flow: the hepatic arterial buffer response revisited. World J Gastroenterol 2010;16(48):6046–57.
4. Lee WM, Stravitz RT, Larson AM. Introduction to the revised American Association for the Study of Liver Diseases Position Paper on acute liver failure 2011. Hepatology 2012;55(3):965–7.
5. Tsochatzis EA, Bosch J, Burroughs AK. Liver cirrhosis. Lancet 2014;383(9930):1749–61.
6. D'Amico G, Garcia-Tsao G, Pagliaro L. Natural history and prognostic indicators of survival in cirrhosis: a systematic review of 118 studies. J Hepatol 2006;44(1):217–31.
7. Hernaez R, Sola E, Moreau R, et al. Acute-on-chronic liver failure: an update. Gut 2017;66(3):541–53.
8. Scaglione S, Kliethermes S, Cao G, et al. The epidemiology of cirrhosis in the United States: a population-based study. J Clin Gastroenterol 2015;49(8):690–6.

9. Bril F, Kalavalapalli S, Clark VC, et al. Response to pioglitazone in patients with nonalcoholic steatohepatitis with vs without type 2 diabetes. Clin Gastroenterol Hepatol 2018;16(4):558–66.e2.

10. European Association for the Study of the Liver. Electronic address eee, European Association for the Study of the Liver. EASL clinical practice guidelines for the management of patients with decompensated cirrhosis. J Hepatol 2018; 69(2):406–60.

11. Ziser A, Plevak DJ, Wiesner RH, et al. Morbidity and mortality in cirrhotic patients undergoing anesthesia and surgery. Anesthesiology 1999;90(1):42–53.

12. Powell-Jackson P, Greenway B, Williams R. Adverse effects of exploratory laparotomy in patients with unsuspected liver disease. Br J Surg 1982;69(8):449–51.

13. Neeff H, Mariaskin D, Spangenberg HC, et al. Perioperative mortality after non-hepatic general surgery in patients with liver cirrhosis: an analysis of 138 operations in the 2000s using child and MELD scores. J Gastrointest Surg 2011; 15(1):1–11.

14. Northup PG, Friedman LS, Kamath PS. AGA clinical practice update on surgical risk assessment and perioperative management in cirrhosis: expert review. Clin Gastroenterol Hepatol 2019;17(4):595–606.

15. Telem DA, Schiano T, Goldstone R, et al. Factors that predict outcome of abdominal operations in patients with advanced cirrhosis. Clin Gastroenterol Hepatol 2010;8(5):451–7 [quiz: e458].

16. Garrison RN, Cryer HM, Howard DA, et al. Clarification of risk factors for abdominal operations in patients with hepatic cirrhosis. Ann Surg 1984;199(6):648–55.

17. Teh SH, Nagorney DM, Stevens SR, et al. Risk factors for mortality after surgery in patients with cirrhosis. Gastroenterology 2007;132(4):1261–9.

18. Laurence JM, Tran PD, Richardson AJ, et al. Laparoscopic or open cholecystectomy in cirrhosis: a systematic review of outcomes and meta-analysis of randomized trials. HPB (Oxford) 2012;14(3):153–61.

19. Post-operative mortality risk in patients with cirrhosis. [Online Calculator]. 2019. Post-operative mortality risk in patients with cirrhosis. Available at: https://www.mayoclinic.org/medical-professionals/transplant-medicine/calculators/post-operative-mortality-risk-in-patients-with-cirrhosis/itt-20434721. Accessed June 30, 2019.

20. Jepsen P. Comorbidity in cirrhosis. World J Gastroenterol 2014;20(23):7223–30.

21. Haq MM, Faisal N, Khalil A, et al. Midazolam for sedation during diagnostic or therapeutic upper gastrointestinal endoscopy in cirrhotic patients. Eur J Gastroenterol Hepatol 2012;24(10):1214–8.

22. Kim HY, Jang JW. Sarcopenia in the prognosis of cirrhosis: going beyond the MELD score. World J Gastroenterol 2015;21(25):7637–47.

23. Laube R, Wang H, Park L, et al. Frailty in advanced liver disease. Liver Int 2018; 38(12):2117–28.

24. Mindikoglu AL, Pappas SC. New developments in hepatorenal syndrome. Clin Gastroenterol Hepatol 2018;16(2):162–77.e1.

25. Giannini EG, Testa R, Savarino V. Liver enzyme alteration: a guide for clinicians. CMAJ 2005;172(3):367–79.

26. Redelmeier DA. New thinking about postoperative hypoalbuminemia: a hypothesis of occult protein-losing enteropathy. Open Med 2009;3(4):e215–9.

27. Ruiz-del-Arbol L, Serradilla R. Cirrhotic cardiomyopathy. World J Gastroenterol 2015;21(41):11502–21.

28. Rudzinski W, Waller AH, Prasad A, et al. New index for assessing the chronotropic response in patients with end-stage liver disease who are undergoing dobutamine stress echocardiography. Liver Transpl 2012;18(3):355–60.

29. Safdar Z, Bartolome S, Sussman N. Portopulmonary hypertension: an update. Liver Transpl 2012;18(8):881–91.

30. Fauconnet P, Klopfenstein CE, Schiffer E. Hepatopulmonary syndrome: the anaesthetic considerations. Eur J Anaesthesiol 2013;30(12):721–30.

31. Sharma AK, Kaufman DC. TIPS performed in a patient with complete portal vein thrombosis. Radiol Case Rep 2017;12(2):327–30.

32. Suk KT. Hepatic venous pressure gradient: clinical use in chronic liver disease. Clin Mol Hepatol 2014;20(1):6–14.

33. Swaminathan M, Ellul MA, Cross TJ. Hepatic encephalopathy: current challenges and future prospects. Hepat Med 2018;10:1–11.

34. Albillos A, Lario M, Alvarez-Mon M. Cirrhosis-associated immune dysfunction: distinctive features and clinical relevance. J Hepatol 2014;61(6):1385–96.

35. Rosemurgy AS, Statman RC, Murphy CG, et al. Postoperative ascitic leaks: the ongoing challenge. Surgery 1992;111(6):623–5.

36. Jain D, Mahmood E, V-Bandres M, et al. Preoperative elective transjugular intrahepatic portosystemic shunt for cirrhotic patients undergoing abdominal surgery. Ann Gastroenterol 2018;31(3):330–7.

37. Tsiaousi ET, Hatzitolios AI, Trygonis SK, et al. Malnutrition in end stage liver disease: recommendations and nutritional support. J Gastroenterol Hepatol 2008; 23(4):527–33.

38. Mukhtar A, EL Masry A, Moniem AA, et al. The impact of maintaining normal serum albumin level following living related liver transplantation: does serum albumin level affect the course? A pilot study. Transplant Proc 2007;39(10):3214–8.

39. Amodio P, Bemeur C, Butterworth R, et al. The nutritional management of hepatic encephalopathy in patients with cirrhosis: International Society for Hepatic Encephalopathy and Nitrogen Metabolism Consensus. Hepatology 2013;58(1): 325–36.

40. Morkane CM, Kearney O, Bruce D, et al. An outpatient hospital-based exercise training program for patients with cirrhotic liver disease awaiting transplantation: a feasibility trial. Transplantation 2020;104(1):97–103.

41. Kaibori M, Ishizaki M, Matsui K, et al. Perioperative exercise for chronic liver injury patients with hepatocellular carcinoma undergoing hepatectomy. Am J Surg 2013;206(2):202–9.

42. Marik PE, Baram M, Vahid B. Does central venous pressure predict fluid responsiveness? A systematic review of the literature and the tale of seven mares. Chest 2008;134(1):172–8.

43. Markin NW, Sharma A, Grant W, et al. The safety of transesophageal echocardiography in patients undergoing orthotopic liver transplantation. J Cardiothorac Vasc Anesth 2015;29(3):588–93.

44. Myo Bui CC, Worapot A, Xia W, et al. Gastroesophageal and hemorrhagic complications associated with intraoperative transesophageal echocardiography in patients with model for end-stage liver disease score 25 or higher. J Cardiothorac Vasc Anesth 2015;29(3):594–7.

45. Kang JG, Ko JS, Kim GS, et al. The relationship between inhalational anesthetic requirements and the severity of liver disease in liver transplant recipients according to three phases of liver transplantation. Transplant Proc 2010;42(3): 854–7.

46. Song JC, Sun YM, Zhang MZ, et al. The etomidate requirement is decreased in patients with obstructive jaundice. Anesth Analg 2011;113(5):1028–32.

47. Servin F, Desmonts JM, Haberer JP, et al. Pharmacokinetics and protein binding of propofol in patients with cirrhosis. Anesthesiology 1988;69(6):887–91.

48. van Beem H, Manger FW, van Boxtel C, et al. Etomidate anaesthesia in patients with cirrhosis of the liver: pharmacokinetic data. Anaesthesia 1983; 38(Suppl):61–2.

49. Duvaldestin P, Chauvin M, Lebrault C, et al. Effect of upper abdominal surgery and cirrhosis upon the pharmacokinetics of methohexital. Acta Anaesthesiol Scand 1991;35(2):159–63.

50. Lisman T, Porte RJ. Rebalanced hemostasis in patients with liver disease: evidence and clinical consequences. Blood 2010;116(6):878–85.

51. Verbeek TA, Stine JG, Saner FH, et al. Hypercoagulability in end-stage liver disease: review of epidemiology, etiology, and management. Transplant Direct 2018; 4(11):e403.

52. Choi PT, Beattie WS, Bryson GL, et al. Effects of neuraxial blockade may be difficult to study using large randomized controlled trials: the PeriOperative Epidural Trial (POET) Pilot Study. PLoS One 2009;4(2):e4644.

53. Siniscalchi A, Gamberini L, Bardi T, et al. Role of epidural anesthesia in a fast track liver resection protocol for cirrhotic patients - results after three years of practice. World J Hepatol 2016;8(26):1097–104.

54. Karanicolas P, Cleary S, McHardy P, et al. Medial open transversus abdominis plane (MOTAP) catheters for analgesia following open liver resection: study protocol for a randomized controlled trial. Trials 2014;15:241.

55. Chin KJ, Malhas L, Perlas A. The erector spinae plane block provides visceral abdominal analgesia in bariatric surgery: a report of 3 cases. Reg Anesth Pain Med 2017;42(3):372–6.

56. Dimarakis I, Grant S, Corless R, et al. Impact of hepatic cirrhosis on outcome in adult cardiac surgery. Thorac Cardiovasc Surg 2015;63(1):58–66.

57. Shaheen AA, Kaplan GG, Hubbard JN, et al. Morbidity and mortality following coronary artery bypass graft surgery in patients with cirrhosis: a population-based study. Liver Int 2009;29(8):1141–51.

58. Bizouarn P, Ausseur A, Desseigne P, et al. Early and late outcome after elective cardiac surgery in patients with cirrhosis. Ann Thorac Surg 1999;67(5):1334–8.

59. Smith C, Nashef SAM, Roques F, et al. EuroSCORE II. Eur J Cardiothorac Surg 2012;41(4):734–45.

60. Aboud A, Opacic D, Gummert J, et al. Model for end-stage liver disease predicts mortality after pericardiectomy for constrictive pericarditis†. Interact Cardiovasc Thorac Surg 2018;27(6):813–8.

61. Jacob KA, Hjortnaes J, Kranenburg G, et al. Mortality after cardiac surgery in patients with liver cirrhosis classified by the Child-Pugh score. Interact Cardiovasc Thorac Surg 2015;20(4):520–30.

62. Morimoto N, Okada K, Okita Y. Results of cardiac surgery in advanced liver cirrhosis. Gen Thorac Cardiovasc Surg 2013;61(2):79–83.

63. Suman A, Barnes DS, Zein NN, et al. Predicting outcome after cardiac surgery in patients with cirrhosis: a comparison of Child-Pugh and MELD scores. Clin Gastroenterol Hepatol 2004;2(8):719–23.

64. Chou AH, Chen TH, Chen CY, et al. Long-term outcome of cardiac surgery in 1,040 liver cirrhosis patient- nationwide population-based cohort study. Circ J 2017;81(4):476–84.

65. Pollard RJ, Sidi A, Gibby GL, et al. Aortic stenosis with end-stage liver disease: prioritizing surgical and anesthetic therapies. J Clin Anesth 1998;10(3):253–61.
66. Dhoble A, Bhise V, Nevah MI, et al. Outcomes and readmissions after transcatheter and surgical aortic valve replacement in patients with cirrhosis: a propensity matched analysis. Catheter Cardiovasc Interv 2018;91(1):90–6.
67. Christmas AB, Wilson AK, Franklin GA, et al. Cirrhosis and trauma: a deadly duo. Am Surg 2005;71(12):996–1000.
68. Talving P, Lustenberger T, Okoye OT, et al. The impact of liver cirrhosis on outcomes in trauma patients: a prospective study. J Trauma Acute Care Surg 2013;75(4):699–703.
69. Langness S, Costantini TW, Smith A, et al. Isolated traumatic brain injury in patients with cirrhosis: do different treatment paradigms result in increased mortality? Am J Surg 2017;213(1):80–6.
70. Demetriades D, Constantinou C, Salim A, et al. Liver cirrhosis in patients undergoing laparotomy for trauma: effect on outcomes. J Am Coll Surg 2004;199(4):538–42.
71. de Goede B, Klitsie PJ, Lange JF, et al. Morbidity and mortality related to non-hepatic surgery in patients with liver cirrhosis; a systematic review. Best Pract Res Clin Gastroenterol 2012;26(1):47–59.
72. Georgiou C, Inaba K, Teixeira PG, et al. Cirrhosis and trauma are a lethal combination. World J Surg 2009;33(5):1087–92.
73. Bugaev N, Breeze JL, Daoud V, et al. Management and outcome of patients with blunt splenic injury and preexisting liver cirrhosis. J Trauma Acute Care Surg 2014;76(6):1354–61.
74. Cook MR, Fair KA, Burg J, et al. Cirrhosis increases mortality and splenectomy rates following splenic injury. Am J Surg 2015;209(5):841–7 [discussion: 847].
75. Sankar K, Moore CM. Transjugular intrahepatic portosystemic shuntstransjugular intrahepatic portosystemic ShuntsJAMA patient page. JAMA 2017;317(8):880.
76. Youn AM, Ko YK, Kim YH. Anesthesia and sedation outside of the operating room. Korean J Anesthesiol 2015;68(4):323–31.
77. Northup PG, Caldwell SH. Coagulation in liver disease: a guide for the clinician. Clin Gastroenterol Hepatol 2013;11(9):1064–74.
78. Shah NL, Intagliata NM, Northup PG, et al. Procoagulant therapeutics in liver disease: a critique and clinical rationale. Nat Rev Gastroenterol Hepatol 2014;11(11):675–82.
79. Rai R, Nagral S, Nagral A. Surgery in a patient with liver disease. J Clin Exp Hepatol 2012;2(3):238–46.
80. Stellingwerff M, Brandsma A, Lisman T, et al. Prohemostatic interventions in liver surgery. Semin Thromb Hemost 2012;38(3):244–9.
81. Kor DJ, Stubbs JR, Gajic O. Perioperative coagulation management–fresh frozen plasma. Best Pract Res Clin Anaesthesiol 2010;24(1):51–64.
82. Ng VL. Liver disease, coagulation testing, and hemostasis. Clin Lab Med 2009;29(2):265–82.
83. Csikesz NG, Nguyen LN, Tseng JF, et al. Nationwide volume and mortality after elective surgery in cirrhotic patients. J Am Coll Surg 2009;208(1):96–103.
84. Hamad MA, Thabet M, Badawy A, et al. Laparoscopic versus open cholecystectomy in patients with liver cirrhosis: a prospective, randomized study. J Laparoendosc Adv Surg Tech A 2010;20(5):405–9.
85. Carbonell AM, Wolfe LG, DeMaria EJ. Poor outcomes in cirrhosis-associated hernia repair: a nationwide cohort study of 32,033 patients. Hernia 2005;9(4):353–7.

86. McKay A, Dixon E, Bathe O, et al. Umbilical hernia repair in the presence of cirrhosis and ascites: results of a survey and review of the literature. Hernia 2009;13(5):461–8.
87. Marsman HA, Heisterkamp J, Halm JA, et al. Management in patients with liver cirrhosis and an umbilical hernia. Surgery 2007;142(3):372–5.
88. Mullin EJ, Metcalfe MS, Maddern GJ. How much liver resection is too much? Am J Surg 2005;190(1):87–97.
89. Teh SH, Christein J, Donohue J, et al. Hepatic resection of hepatocellular carcinoma in patients with cirrhosis: model of End-Stage Liver Disease (MELD) score predicts perioperative mortality. J Gastrointest Surg 2005;9(9):1207–15.

Anesthetic Considerations for Patients on Renal Replacement Therapy

Christine Acho, DO*, Anoop Chhina, MD, Dragos Galusca, MD

KEYWORDS

- Anesthesia • Renal replacement therapy • Renal failure • Perioperative

KEY POINTS

- As the population ages and improvements continue to be made in treating renal disease, the number of patients presenting for elective surgery on renal replacement therapy (RRT) will increase.
- An understanding of common laboratory derangements and comorbidities is essential for management of patients on RRT, as every aspect of the perioperative period is affected by renal disease.
- Patients with renal disease are at increased risk for adverse perioperative cardiac events. Perioperative management strategies should attempt to minimize this risk.
- Acute kidney injury is commonly encountered in intensive care unit patients and is associated with high morbidity and mortality. In cases of severe acute kidney injury, RRT remains the cornerstone of treatment.

BACKGROUND AND EPIDEMIOLOGY

As of 2014, over 100,000 Americans were diagnosed with end-stage renal disease (ESRD), in addition to the 662,000 Americans who were already living with ESRD.[1] Renal replacement therapy (RRT) to correct electrolyte abnormalities, optimize volume status, and remove toxins has improved mortality rates in ESRD since the early 2000s.[2] RRT can also be used in patients with acute kidney injury (AKI) who have severe disease.

As improvements continue to be made in the management of ESRD and AKI requiring RRT, the number of patients with these conditions presenting for surgery will increase. Every aspect of the perioperative period is affected by renal

Department of Anesthesiology, Pain Management & Perioperative Medicine, Henry Ford Hospital, 2799 West Grand Boulevard, Detroit, MI 48202, USA
* Corresponding author. Henry Ford Hospital E-435, 2799 West Grand Boulevard, Detroit, MI 48202.
E-mail address: cacho1@hfhs.org

Anesthesiology Clin 38 (2020) 51–66
https://doi.org/10.1016/j.anclin.2019.10.003   **anesthesiology.theclinics.com**
1932-2275/20/© 2019 Elsevier Inc. All rights reserved.

dysfunction, its associated comorbidities, and altered physiology secondary to RRT. Perioperative mortality and morbidity are known to be higher in patients with ESRD and AKI.[3–5] The goal of management should therefore be to minimize these risks.

In this review the authors primarily focus on the management of the patient with ESRD on RRT presenting for elective surgery. Special considerations for critically ill patients requiring acute RRT who present for surgery and patients with ESRD who present for emergency surgery is addressed briefly.

DEFINITIONS

In 2005, the Kidney Disease Improving Global Outcomes (KDIGO) summit developed a classification system for chronic kidney disease (CKD). Stage 5, also known as ESRD, is defined as a glomerular filtration rate (GFR) less than 15 mL/min/1.73 m^2 or any patient requiring dialysis regardless of their GFR (**Table 1**).[6]

Various definitions of AKI exist including the RIFLE (Risk, Injury, Failure, Loss of kidney function, and End-stage kidney disease), KDIGO, and Acute Kidney Injury Network criteria (**Tables 2** and **3**). In either classification system, there is a group of patients who will require dialysis regardless of laboratory findings.[7–9]

RENAL REPLACEMENT THERAPY OVERVIEW

RRT consists of a variety of modalities that (except for peritoneal dialysis) use an extracorporeal circuit to remove waste products and free water from the patient's bloodstream, thereby mimicking the natural function of the kidneys. RRT can be broadly broken down into 4 processes: hemodialysis (HD), hemofiltration, hemodiafiltration, and ultrafiltration. By understanding these processes, the clinician is able to better understand the various types of RRT (**Table 4**) and their unique implications.

HD is the main mechanism for the clearance of small solutes. A hemodialyzer generates a concentration gradient across a semipermeable membrane with the dialysate solution and the patient's blood. The removal of solutes depends on the diffusion of solutes across this membrane along their concentration gradient.[10–12]

Table 1 Classification of chronic kidney disease		
Stage	**GFR (mL/min/1.73 m^2)**	**Description**
1	>90	GFR normal to high
2	60–89	Kidney damage[a] and mild decrease in GFR
3	30–59	Moderate decrease in GFR
4	15–29	Sever decrease in GFR
5	<15 or requiring RRT	Kidney failure/ESRD

Abbreviations: ESRD, end-stage renal disease; GFR, glomerular filtration rate; RRT, renal replacement therapy.

  [a] Kidney damage ≥3 mo defined by structural or functional renal abnormalities, with or without decreased GFR or GFR less than 60 mL/min/1.73 m^2 for ≥3 mo.

Adapted from Kidney International Supplements. KDIGO Clinical Practice Guideline for Acute Kidney Injury. Vol 2, Issue 1, 2012. Available at: https://brundagegroup.com/wp-content/uploads/2018/09/KDIGO-AKI-Guideline.pdf. Accessed May 2 2019; and Mehta RL, Kellum JA, Shah SV, et al. Acute Kidney Injury Network: report of an initiative to improve outcomes in acute kidney injury. Crit Care 2007;11(2):R31.

Table 2
Kidney Disease Improving Global Outcomes and Acute Kidney Injury Network classification systems of acute kidney injury

Stage	Definition		Urine Output
	KDIGO	**AKIN**	
1	1.5–1.9 times increase in SCr *Or* $\geq$0.3 mg/dL increase in Scr	$\geq$1.5 times increase in Scr *Or* $\geq$0.3 mg/dL increase in Scr	<0.5 mL/kg/h for 6–12 h
2	2.0–2.9 times increase in Scr	$\geq$2.0 time increase in Scr	<0.5 mL/kg/h for $\geq$12 h
3	3.0 times increase in Scr *Or* $\geq$4.0 mg/dL with an increase >0.5 mg/dL *Or* Initiation of RRT	$\geq$3.0 increase in Scr *Or* $\geq$4.0 mg/dL with an increase >0.5 mg/dL *Or* Initiation of RRT	<0.3 mL/kg/h for $\geq$24 h *Or* Anuria for $\geq$12 h

Abbreviations: AKIN, Acute Kidney Injury Network; KIDGO, Kidney Disease Improving Global Outcomes; RRT, renal replacement therapy; SCr, serum creatinine.

Adapted from Kidney International Supplements. KDIGO Clinical Practice Guideline for Acute Kidney Injury. Vol 2, Issue 1, 2012. Available at: https://brundagegroup.com/wp-content/uploads/2018/09/KDIGO-AKI-Guideline.pdf. Accessed May 2 2019; and Mehta RL, Kellum JA, Shah SV, et al. Acute Kidney Injury Network: report of an initiative to improve outcomes in acute kidney injury. Crit Care 2007;11(2):R31; with permission.

PREOPERATIVE MANAGEMENT OF PATIENTS WITH END-STAGE RENAL DISEASE ON HEMODIALYSIS
Timing

There is limited information regarding ideal timing of HD and elective surgery. At our institution, the general recommendation is to schedule patients for surgery on their nondialysis days. HD before surgery is necessary to correct electrolyte abnormalities and improve volume status; however, too close a proximity to surgery may be associated with intraoperative hypotension.[13]

Vascular Access

Patients at risk for ESRD and those with ESRD require thoughtful consideration with regard to vascular access. The preferred HD access is the arterio-venous fistula (AVF), which requires the patient's native vein and artery for construction. The goal of strategic venous access is to help ensure the preservation of veins in patients with CKD or ESRD so that the creation of future AVFs may be more successful and of high quality.

Guidelines for obtaining venous access in patients with CKD and ESRD were developed with these considerations in mind. Peripheral venous catheters should be placed in the dorsal veins of the hands. In patients with an established AVF, the contralateral hand is the preferred site. If central venous access is needed, the internal jugular veins are preferred.[14] Special attention is required for patients who have established HD access. A tunneled central catheter (TCC) is placed in patients who require HD but have not yet established long-term access. At our institution we recommend limiting access of TCCs to minimize the risk of infection and indefinitely avoid accessing AVF and grafts. If a patient has an AVF or graft we recommended palpating for a thrill during surgery at frequent intervals to ensure adequate perfusion through the site.

Table 3
RIFLE (Risk, Injury, Failure, Loss of kidney function, and End-stage kidney disease) classification of acute kidney injury

Class	GFR (mL/min/1.73 m²)	Urine Output
Risk	1.5 times increase in SCr Or >25% decrease in GFR	<0.5 mL/kg/h for 6 h
Injury	2 times increase in serum Cr Or >50% decrease in GFR	<0.5 mL/kg/h for 12 h
Failure	3 times increase in serum Cr Or >75% decrease in GFR	<0.3 mL/kg/h for ≥24 h Or Anuria for ≥12 h
Loss	Complete loss of function >4 wk	
ESRD	Complete loss of function >3 mo	

Abbreviations: ESRD, end-stage renal disease; GFR, glomerular filtration rate; SCr, serum creatinine.

Adapted from Bellomo R, Ronco C, Kellum JA, et al. Acute renal failure— definition, outcome measures, animal models, fluid therapy and information technology needs: the Second International Consensus Conference of the Acute Dialysis Quality Initiative (ADQI) Group. Crit Care 2004;8(4):R206; with permission.

Common Electrolyte Abnormalities

Hyperkalemia

The ratio of intracellular to extracellular potassium is essential for the maintenance of the resting cell membrane potential. The smallest alterations in this relationship can cause changes in the function of excitable tissues. Therefore, potassium is tightly regulated. In brief, the renal system is responsible for the excretion of 90% of the body's potassium. The other 10% is regulated by gastrointestinal excretion and cellular uptake. Hyperkalemia in ESRD can be due to noncompliance with a renal diet, ineffective HD, and disorders of internal potassium balance.

In the perioperative period, hyperkalemia may also be due to fasting and medications. Fasting has been shown to be associated with hyperkalemia in ESRD, which is not seen in patients with preserved renal function. Medications most commonly implicated in hyperkalemia in ESRD include nonspecific and β_2-adrenergic antagonists and supratherapeutic levels of digoxin.[15]

The effect of hyperkalemia on the cardiovascular conduction system is the most worrisome clinical consequence. Classic electrocardiogram manifestations include peaked T-waves and prolongation of the PR and QRS intervals, which predispose the patient to fatal arrhythmias.[16] Treatment of hyperkalemia is reviewed later in this text.

Calcium and phosphate

Calcium and phosphate levels are regulated by the parathyroid glands, which secrete parathyroid hormone (PTH) in response to low serum calcium levels. PTH increases serum calcium by stimulating bone matrix turnover, promoting renal excretion of phosphorus and renal reabsorption of calcium, and stimulating the production of activated vitamin D.

In CKD, the failing nephrons are unable to activate vitamin D and excrete excess phosphorus; however, serum values remain normal secondary to increased PTH secretion. As CKD progresses to ESRD, nephrons are no longer functional and cannot

Table 4
Characteristics of renal replacement therapy modalities

	Intermittent Hemodialysis	Peritoneal Dialysis	SLED	CRRT
Mechanism of clearance	Diffusion across a semipermeable membrane	Diffusion across a semipermeable membrane (peritoneum)	Diffusion across a semipermeable membrane	CVVH: convection CVVHD: diffusion CVVHDF: both SCUF: ultrafiltration
Solute removal	Small solutes	Small solutes	Small solutes	CVVH: larger solutes CVVHD: small solutes CVVHDF: small & larger solutes SCUF: minimal
Fluid removal	Yes	Yes	Yes	CVVH: yes, replaced CVVHD: yes CVVHDF: yes, replaced SCUF: yes (up to 8 L/d)
Timing	Most commonly 3 d/wk Up to 4 h/session	Continuous	6–12 h/session No set frequency/wk	Continuous
Anticoagulation required	No	No	No/Yes[a]	Yes
Advantages	• Rapid solute correction and toxin removal • Decreased anticoagulation requirements • Cost-effective	• Improved hemodynamics • Vascular access not required • Technically simple	• Improved hemodynamics • Can be timed around procedures/studies • Decreased anticoagulation requirements	• Improved hemodynamics • Can target fluid removal specifically (SCUF)
Disadvantages	• Large and rapid fluid shifts can cause hemodynamic instability • *Dialysis Disequilibrium Syndrome*[b] • Vascular access required • Infection (bacteremia)	• Slower solute correction • No control over rate of fluid removal • Technical complications (membrane failure) • Infection (peritonitis)	• Slower solute correction • Technically more complex • Some level of anticoagulation may be required • Access site complications	• Slower solute correction • Anticoagulation required • Risk of hypothermia

Abbreviations: CCVHDF, continuous veno-venous hemodiafiltration; CRRT, continuous renal replacement therapy; CVVH, continuous veno-venous hemofiltration; CVVHD, continuous veno-venous hemodialysis; SCUF, slow continuous ultrafiltration; SLED, sustained low-efficiency dialysis.

[a] SLED may be done safely and effectively without anticoagulation; some institutions may use anticoagulation with SLED.

[b] Dialysis disequilibrium syndrome occurs due to rapid shifts in urea and other solutes leading to cerebral edema. Neurologic symptoms include headache, altered mental status, coma, and seizure.

Data from Refs.[10–12]

respond to PTH. Secondary hyperparathyroidism, hyperphosphatemia, and hypocalcemia become evident.[17,18]

Hyperphosphatemia is associated with increased cardiovascular morbidity and mortality. Treatment of hyperphosphatemia with high-dose calcium-containing phosphate binders may also contribute to cardiovascular complications by promoting vascular calcification via deposition of calcium-phosphate crystals.[19]

This process also occurs paradoxically in the setting of hypocalcemia, independently of hyperphosphatemia treatment. PTH acts to increase serum calcium levels by increasing bone matrix turnover, which promotes the formation of calcium-phosphate crystals and renal osteodystrophy. Special considerations when positioning and transferring patients during the perioperative period is needed secondary to this weakened bone matrix. Hypocalcemia is also associated with prolonged QT, arrhythmias, and muscle spasms.[17]

Metabolic Acidosis

The renal system plays a significant role in the maintenance and regulation of the extracellular pH by excreting nonvolatile acids and generating bicarbonate. These functions are reduced as the GFR declines to 40 to 50 mL/min leading to a metabolic acidosis. Eventually, as renal disease progresses to ESRD, an anion-gap metabolic acidosis develops secondary to the increased retention of phosphate and other anions.[20]

Calcium is released from the boney matrix in response to the acidosis to act as a buffer and prevent the development of a severe metabolic acidosis. This compensatory mechanism also contributes to renal osteodystrophy. Metabolic acidosis is associated with wasting of the skeletal muscles, hypoalbuminemia, and inflammation, all of which increase patient frailty. Increased mortality is associated with bicarbonate levels less than 22 mEq/L in patients with renal disease.[20–22]

Anemia of Chronic Kidney Disease

Erythropoietin (EPO) is produced by the kidneys and serves as a stimulus for bone marrow erythropoiesis. As renal function declines so does the production of EPO. In addition to decreased EPO, uremia has been shown to hinder bone marrow erythropoiesis.[23] In addition to fatigue and weakness, anemia further stresses the heart in an already susceptible population.

EPO, iron supplementation, and transfusions are used to treat and manage anemia in ESRD. Transfusions are still commonly used in the acute setting or in EPO refractory patients; however, since the introduction of EPO, the overall number of transfusions in ESRD has decreased.[24] Aggressive treatment of anemia with EPO has been associated with an increased risk of cerebrovascular accident (CVA). Aggressive correction of hemoglobin levels beyond 11 to 12 g/dL is not recommended.[25]

COMMON COMORBIDITIES
Neurologic

The prevalence of neurologic complications is disproportionally higher in patients with ESRD compared with the general population. Common comorbidities include cognitive impairment, CVA, autonomic dysfunction, and peripheral neuropathy. Factors unique to ESRD can directly cause, worsen, or accelerate these processes.[26]

Patients with ESRD have a relatively high risk of CVA and associated mortality rates compared with the general population. This increased risk has been attributed to vascular changes, accumulation of toxic metabolites, hypertension (HTN), and hemo-dynamic derangements which prime the cerebral tissue for ischemic events.[26,27] No specific guidelines regarding strategies to prevent CVA within the perioperative period have been made; therefore, prevention and management strategies recommended for other patients should be applied to patients with ESRD.

Autonomic dysregulation is a state of increased sympathetic and decreased para-sympathetic activity that is present in more than 50% of patients with ESRD. The exact mechanism of the phenomena is unknown but may be due to a decline in renal regu-lation of various hormonal mediators. Common clinical manifestations include delayed gastric emptying, impotence, higher resting heart rate, decreased heart rate variability, reduced exercise tolerance, and orthostatic hypotension.[26]

Cardiovascular

Cardiovascular disease in ESRD is often undiagnosed, undertreated, and associated with worse outcomes than patients with normal renal function. Over 50% of deaths in patients with CKD are due to major cardiac events.[28] An understanding of how renal disease negatively impacts the cardiovascular system is essential for the proper pre-vention, detection, and management of such events.

Type 4 cardiorenal syndrome, also known as chronic renocardiac syndrome, de-scribes a phenomenon whereby the physiologic derangements of renal disease lead to various cardiovascular complications. Features of ESRD including volume over-load, impaired vasodilation, vascular calcifications, and increased inflammatory markers have all been implicated in the development of left ventricular hypertrophy, congestive heart failure (CHF), arrhythmias, and coronary artery disease (CAD). As cardiac function continues to deteriorate, the sympathetic and renin-angiotensin-aldosterone systems become stimulated, further stressing the heart.[29,30]

CHF is the one of the most common cardiovascular complications seen in ESRD. An initial study done by Harnett and colleagues[31] found over 30% of their study popula-tion had CHF. Furthermore, these patients had a median survival of only 36 months. Both systolic and diastolic dysfunction are seen in ESRD for the reasons mentioned earlier.

CKD also is responsible for the development of accelerated CAD. In addition to tradi-tional CAD risk factors, patients with ESRD are at risk for the development of CAD sec-ondary to nontraditional risk factors such as chronic inflammation and vascular calcification. Over 50% of patients with ESRD have significant CAD, many of them without clinical symptoms secondary to high prevalence of DM and reduced functional capacity at baseline.[32] Perioperative cardiac risk assessment should still be based on the 2014 American College of Cardiology/American Heart Association guidelines.[33]

Respiratory

Pulmonary complications commonly seen in ESRD include pulmonary edema, effu-sion, and HTN. Pulmonary edema is not only related to increased hydrostatic pressure from fluid overload and the presence of CHF, but also due to decreased oncotic pres-sure from hypoalbuminemia.[34] Pulmonary HTN is unusually common in patients with ESRD and associated with an increased risk of all-cause mortality and adverse car-diac events.[35]

Endocrine

Glycemic management in patients with ESRD has proven to be challenging secondary to increased insulin resistance; however, patients with ESRD are susceptible to hypo-glycemic events. Derangements in metabolism, including the breakdown of insulin, which is normally done by the kidneys, and altered pharmacokinetics of various glycemic drugs contribute to this.[36] KDIGO currently recommends a target HbA1c of less than 7.0% for patients with CKD.[6]

INTRAOPERATIVE MANAGEMENT
Volume Assessment and Fluid Resuscitation

Hypervolemia and hypovolemia have both been associated with negative outcomes in patients with ESRD. Hypovolemia is associated with poor tissue perfusion, cardiovascular remodeling, and, as mentioned previously, intraoperative hypotension. Chronic hypervolemia, even when asymptomatic, is also associated with cardiac remodeling, CHF, and more frequent hospitalizations.[13,37–39]

Perioperative assessment of volume status of patients with ESRD is complex and poorly understood. First, it is important to understand that, although patients scheduled for elective surgery will have had HD the day before, they can present as hypo- or hypervolemic because the window for euvolemia is narrow. Secondly, HD does not ensure that euvolemia was achieved because the amount of ultrafiltrate to be removed is questionable.

Preoperative assessments including blood pressure, peripheral edema, pulmonary crackles, and cardiac natriuretic peptide may also not be sufficient. The use of bedside ultrasonography can be used for volume assessment as it is noninvasive, more accurate than auscultation and chest radiography, and can be completed in the preoperative bay. The presence of pulmonary B-lines, which are thickened interlobular septa secondary to fluid overload, and effusions are easily identified.[37–40] A very well written review on fluid assessment was done by Ekinci and colleagues.[39]

Research regarding intraoperative fluid assessment in ESRD is limited. Invasive monitoring has not been shown to improve outcomes in patients and is therefore not recommended as a standard guide for fluid resuscitation.[41] Information regarding which fluid to use for resuscitation of patients with ESRD is equally limited. A direct comparison of crystalloids versus colloids in patients with ESRD within the perioperative period has not been studied. The use of 5% albumin to normal saline (NS) in the treatment of dialysis-related hypotension showed no significant difference in outcomes or total volume of fluid given.[42]

NS and lactated Ringer's (LR) have been directly compared in several studies examining the optimal fluid choice for renal transplant patients. O'Malley and colleagues,[43] found 19% of renal transplant patients resuscitated with NS developed serum potassium levels >6 mEq/L compared with 0% in the LR group. This is explained by the development of a hyperchloremic metabolic acidosis associated with large-volume NS resuscitation, which is compensated for by exchanging extracellular hydrogen ions for intracellular potassium ions.[44]

Hemodynamic Goals and Monitoring

No specific hemodynamic goals for patients with ESRD have been published. Invasive monitoring has not been shown to improve clinical outcomes and is therefore not routinely recommended.[41] As with any patient, optimization of the patient's preload and afterload and considerations of additional comorbidities are essential.

As discussed earlier, the exact volume status of the patient remains largely unknown despite being on scheduled HD. Patients may actually be hypovolemic at the time of surgery. Hypovolemia is a common cause of hypotension during and after induction of anesthesia. HTN on the other hand is another common perioperative and intraoperative concern in patients with ESRD.

The pathophysiology of HTN in ESRD is associated with fluid overload, increased activity of the sympathetic nervous system, vascular calcification, and impaired vasodilation. Arterial stiffening is common in ESRD and is associated with isolated systolic HTN. These patients poorly tolerate reductions in diastolic blood pressure during surgery.[45,46] Fluid resuscitation when appropriate and the use of vasopressors should be used to augment intraoperative blood pressure.

Bleeding and Transfusion Management

Bleeding risk in CKD has been reported by several groups. In a meta-analysis done be Acedillo and colleagues,[47] patients with CKD was a risk factor for perioperative blood transfusion.[48] Changes in vascular structure, anemia, thrombocytopenia, platelet dysfunction, uremia, and alterations in the coagulation cascade have all been implicated as risk factors for bleeding.[48]

Some patients with ESRD are actual hypercoagulable and are prescribed antiplatelet and anticoagulants medications. There are no universal guidelines regarding the discontinuation of antiplatelet or anticoagulation therapy in ESRD within the perioperative period; however, a review published by Hughes and colleagues,[49] and the American College of Cardiology guidelines for periprocedural bridging therapy, are excellent resources.[50] No standard preoperative bleeding risk workup is recommended specifically for patients with ESRD. In patients in whom uremic bleeding may be of concern, bleeding time assay can be done to assess platelet function.

Methods used to manage bleeding in ESRD includes desmopressin (DDVAP), recombinant human factors, and transfusion of blood products. Desmopressin improves the hemostatic response and decreases fibrinolysis in uremic patients. Typical dosing is 0.3 µg/kg intravenously (IV) given at least 30 minutes to 1 hour before surgery.[51] Blood transfusions should be used when clinically appropriate, remembering a more conservative approach is favored.[52] Complications from blood product transfusions include infectious, noninfectious, immunogenic, and allogenic reactions. Limitation of transfusions is also important in patients with ESRD who are transplant candidates to minimize the incidence of alloimmunization.[48]

Intraoperative Medications with Renal Considerations

Inhalational agents

The most commonly used inhalation agents are isoflurane, sevoflurane, and desflurane. A previous study showed compound A, a product of the interaction between sevoflurane and carbon dioxide absorbents, was nephrotoxic in rats.[53] Since then, the use of sevoflurane in human subjects has failed to show a difference in renal function or clinical outcomes associated with the use of sevoflurane.[54] Today, all of the commonly used inhalational anesthetics are considered safe for use in renal patients.

Muscle relaxants and reversal

Succinylcholine is the only depolarizing muscle relaxant currently in use. It has both a quick onset and duration of action making it ideal for rapid sequence intubation and procedures that do not require prolonged relaxation. Serum potassium is known to transiently increase by 0.5 to 1.0 mmoL after the administration of succinylcholine. Despite this, the use of succinylcholine is safe for use in patients with CKD. Caution should also be used in patients with AKI, as their myocardium may not be able to tolerate this transient increase in potassium.[55] It is also important to keep in mind that renal failure is associated with decreased pseudocholinesterase activity, which can cause prolongation of the neuromuscular blockade.[56]

Of the nondepolarizing muscle relaxants, pancuronium is the most dependent on renal clearance. Prolongation of neuromuscular blockade with pancuronium in the presence of renal failure has been reported. Clearance and elimination of vecuronium and rocuronium are both altered in renal failure. The duration of neuromuscular blockade with either agent in the presence of renal disease results in prolonged neuromuscular blockade. Atracurium and cisatracurium do not depend on renal metabolism and are not associated with prolongated neuromuscular blockade in ESRD.[57,58]

Reversal of neuromuscular blockade is achieved by administration of an anticholinesterase, which requires the simultaneous administration of an antimuscarinic to prevent bradycardia. Neostigmine is the most common anticholinesterase used. Fifty percent of neostigmine undergoes renal excretion, prolonging its duration of action in renal patients. This is an important consideration because the duration of the antimuscarinic agent should match that of neostigmine to prevent delayed onset bradycardia. Glycopyrrolate has a similar duration of action in renal patients as neostigmine.[57,59]

Suggamadex is specifically designed for the reversal of rocuronium. The suggamadex-rocuronium complex depends on renal excretion. Staals and colleagues[60] showed that the concentration of the suggamadex-rocuronium complex was higher in renal patients up to 48 hours after surgery, but no patients experienced recurarization. Given the prolongation and unknown safety profile during this time period, suggamadex is currently not recommended for use in patients with severe renal impairment.[61]

Opioids

ESRD affects each opioid differently. Fentanyl, sufentanil, and hydromorphone can be safely used in patients with ESRD, but may require dose adjustments. Morphine, codeine, oxycodone, and meperidine are all medications that should be avoided in ESRD. These drugs undergo hepatic metabolism into various active metabolites that depend on renal excretion. The accumulation of these metabolites has been associated with adverse events. Morphine-6-glucoronide is an active metabolite of morphine and codeine, which accumulates causing respiratory depression. The use of oxycodone is also associated with respiratory depression in ESRD. Meperidine is unique, in that its active metabolite, normeperidine, is associated with seizures.[62]

Midazolam

The pharmacokinetics of midazolam are unaltered in patients with CKD; however, a recent study found that the half-life and clearance of midazolam and its metabolites were increased in intensive care unit (ICU) patients with AKI.[63,64]

Dexmedetomidine

The use of dexmedetomidine is considered to be safe in patients with renal disease. De Wolf and colleagues[65] showed that the pharmacokinetic profile was unchanged in renal disease. Patients with ESRD were not more prone to hypotension but were sedated slightly longer than patients with normal renal function.

ANESTHETIC IMPLICATIONS OF INTENSIVE CARE UNIT PATIENTS ON RENAL REPLACEMENT THERAPY

Continuous Renal Replacement Therapy or Intermittent Hemodialysis

AKI in ICU patients is associated with high morbidity and mortality. In cases of severe AKI, RRT remains the cornerstone of treatment. The timing of initiation of RRT remains controversial.[66] Traditionally, 2 modalities of RRT have been used in the ICU: continuous renal replacement therapy (CRRT) and intermittent hemodialysis (IHD). IHD is typically administered over 3 to 4 hours and mimics maintenance HD for ESRD. CRRT permits slow, but continuous removal of solutes and fluid, thereby conferring better hemodynamic tolerability. Sustained low-efficiency dialysis (SLED) represents the application of conventional HD technology, but is done over 8 hours with slower blood flows than IHD.

A recent meta-analysis by Nash and colleagues[67] showed no difference in mortality or dependence on dialysis when CRRT was compared with SLED or IHD.

Complications of continuous renal replacement therapy

Metabolic: increased solute clearance achieved by CRRT may cause unwanted loss of amino acids, vitamins, and catecholamines. Severe hypophosphatemia can also occur as a result of CRRT. Hypophosphatemia is associated with respiratory and cardiac depression, as well as immune dysfunction. It is important to monitor and proactively treat hypophosphatemia.

Anticoagulation: sufficient anticoagulation, without excessive risk of bleeding, is generally required to maintain filter and circuit patency. Unfractionated heparin is the most commonly used anticoagulant. The complications associated with systemic heparin administration stimulated interest in regional citrate anticoagulation (RCA). Compared with systemic heparin, RCA has been associated with less bleeding, increased filter lifespan, and reduced transfusion rates and need for antithrombin III/platelet supplementation.[66] It is important to know which anticoagulant is being used, especially if CRRT is to be continued intraoperatively.

Antibiotic dosing during CRRT: adequate antibiotic therapy is crucial in critically ill patients. CRRT can alter the pharmacokinetics of drugs. Dosing adjustments should to be based on plasma drug levels.

Anesthetic Implications of Continuous Renal Replacement Therapy

Preoperative assessment

Many patients on CRRT are critically ill. They may require ventilatory support and may be hemodynamically unstable, requiring vasopressor or inotropic support. The first question the anesthesiologist should answer when assessing the patient is "why is this patient on CRRT?" In many cases, the CRRT is being used to correct the metabolic sequelae of an underlying medical disorder. If CRRT is interrupted during transfer to the operating room (OR) or is not continued intraoperatively, the metabolic abnormalities will return and may complicate intraoperative management. A thorough evaluation of intravascular volume, total fluid balance, cardiac function, and electrolytes is essential for planning intraoperative anesthetic and hemodynamic management.[68] Finally, the anesthesiologist must determine when is the appropriate time to discontinue CRRT for surgery or if the surgery should be delayed.

Intraoperative management

Most often CRRT will be discontinued before transport to the OR; however, sometimes CRRT will be continued intraoperatively, most commonly during cardiac surgery or liver transplantation. For most CRRT systems, the optimal management requires discontinuation of the CRRT during transport and reinstitution when the patient arrives in the OR.

When CRRT is used during surgery, the anesthesiologist must pay close attention to total fluid administration, both in terms of quantity and specific replacement fluids. The therapeutic plan for CRRT that might have been appropriate for ICU management may no longer be appropriate in the OR.[68] Careful monitoring of arterial blood gases and electrolytes is essential to ensure normal acid-base balance. The provider should also be vigilant about monitoring the patient's vascular access and body temperature closely. Hypothermia is a frequently encountered problem and should be addressed to prevent deleterious effects on the coagulation system and hemodynamic stability.

Postoperative use
When CRRT is used in the postoperative period, flows and replacement fluid composition must be carefully titrated to account for intraoperative fluid shifts and blood loss. The patient must be closely monitored for evidence of postoperative coagulopathy or electrolyte abnormalities.

EMERGENCY SITUATIONS WITHOUT TIME FOR OPTIMIZATION
Management of Hyperkalemia

The urgency of treatment depends on the presence or absence of signs and symptoms associated with hyperkalemia, the severity of the potassium elevation, and the cause of hyperkalemia.

In cases of hyperkalemic emergency,[69] patients with clinical signs or symptoms of hyperkalemia (eg, muscle weakness or paralysis, cardiac conduction abnormalities, and cardiac arrhythmias), patients with severe hyperkalemia (serum potassium >6.5 mEq/L), and patients with moderate hyperkalemia (serum potassium >5.5 mEq/L), plus significant renal impairment and ongoing tissue breakdown or potassium absorption, treatment includes following:

- Stabilization of the cardiac cells: IV calcium
- Promote extracellular potassium to move intracellularly:
    Insulin and glucose
    Sodium bicarbonate (*if primarily metabolic acidosis*)
    β_2-Adrenergic agonists
- Removal of potassium from the body:
    Loop or thiazide diuretics
    Cation exchange resin
    Dialysis; preferably HD if severe

Hypertension and Cardiovascular Events

Cardiovascular disease remains the leading cause of morbidity and mortality among patients on dialysis. HTN is extremely prevalent in patients on dialysis. Patients with ESRD presenting for an emergency surgery may have uncontrolled HTN. The CRIC multicenter prospective research study conducted on maintenance HD patients found a U-shaped association between dialysis-unit-systolic blood pressure and risk of cardiovascular events, with the lowest risk of events at the range of 150 to 170 mm Hg.[70] It is pertinent to recognize and aggressively treat hypotension as well as hypertension.

DISCLOSURE

The authors have nothing to disclose.

REFERENCES

1. Centers for Disease Control and Prevention. National chronic kidney disease fact sheet, 2017. Atlanta (GA): US Department of Health and Human Services, Centers for Disease Control and Prevention; 2017.
2. Collins A, Foley R, Gilberston D, et al. The state of chronic kidney disease, ESRD, and morbidity and mortality in the first year of dialysis. Clin J Am Soc Nephrol 2009;4:S5–11.

3. Mathew A, Devereaux PJ, O'Hare A, et al. Chronic kidney disease and postoperative mortality: a systematic review and meta-analysis. Kidney Int 2008;73:1069–81.

4. Huber M, Ozrazgat-Baslanti T, Thottakkara P, et al. Cardiovascular-specific mortality and kidney disease in patients undergoing vascular surgery. JAMA Surg 2016;151:441–50.

5. Palant CE, Amdur RL, Chawla LS. Long-term consequences of acute kidney injury in the perioperative setting. Curr Opin Anaesthesiol 2017;30:100–4.

6. KDIGO 2012 Clinical Practice Guidelines for the Evaluation and Management of Chronic Kidney Disease. 2013;3(1). Available at: https://kdigo.org/wp-content/uploads/2017/02/KDIGO_2012_CKD_GL.pdf. Accessed May 2, 2019.

7. KDIGO Clinical Practice Guideline for Acute Kidney Injury. 2012;2 (Supplement 1). Available at: https://brundagegroup.com/wp-content/uploads/2018/09/KDIGO-AKI-Guideline.pdf. Accessed May 2, 2019.

8. Mehta RL, Kellum JA, Shah SV, et al. Acute Kidney Injury Network: report of an initiative to improve outcomes in acute kidney injury. Crit Care 2007;11:R31.

9. Bellomo R, Ronco C, Kellum JA, et al. Acute renal failure—definition, outcome measures, animal models, fluid therapy and information technology needs: the Second International Consensus Conference of the Acute Dialysis Quality Initiative (ADQI) Group. Crit Care 2004;8:R204.

10. Sinnakirouchenan R, Holley J. Peritoneal dialysis versus hemodialysis: risks, benefits, and access issues. Adv Chronic Kidney Dis 2011;18(6):428–32.

11. Neri M, Vila G, Garzotto F, et al. Nomenclature for renal replacement therapy in acute kidney injury: basic principles. Crit Care 2016;20(1):318.

12. Macedo E, Mehta R. Continuous dialysis therapies: core curriculum 2016. Am J Kidney Dis 2016;68:645–57.

13. Deng J, Lenart J, Applegate RL. General anesthesia soon after dialysis may increase postoperative hypotension—a pilot study. Heart Lung Vessel 2014;6:52–9.

14. Hoggard J, Saad T, Schon D, et al. Guidelines for venous access in patients with chronic kidney disease. Semin Dial 2008;21:186–91.

15. Ahmed J, Weisberg L. Hyperkalemia in dialysis patients. Semin Dial 2001;14:348–56.

16. Montford JR, Linas S. How dangerous is hyperkalemia? J Am Soc Nephrol 2017;28:3155–65.

17. Blaine J, Chonchol M, Levi M. Renal control of calcium, phosphate, and magnesium homeostasis. Clin J Am Soc Nephrol 2015;10:1257–72.

18. Felsenfeld A, Levine B, Rodriquez M. Pathophysiology of calcium, phosphorus, and magnesium dysregulation in CKD. Semin Dial 2015;28:564–77.

19. London GM, Marchais S, Guerin A, et al. Association of bone activity, calcium load, aortic stiffness and calcifications in ESRD. J Am Soc Nephrol 2008;19:1827–35.

20. Kraut J, Madias N. Metabolic acidosis of CKD: an update. Am J Kidney Dis 2016;67:307–17.

21. Kraut J, Madias N. Adverse effects of the metabolic acidosis of chronic kidney disease. Adv Chronic Kidney Dis 2017;24:289–97.

22. Raphael KL, Zhang Y, Wei G, et al. Serum bicarbonate and mortality in adults in NHANES III. Nephrol Dial Transplant 2013;28:1207–13.

23. Babitt J, Lin H. Mechanisms of anemia in CKD. J Am Soc Nephrol 2012;23:1631–4.

24. Goodnough LT, Strasburg D, Riddell JT, et al. Has recombinant human erythropoietin therapy minimized red-cell transfusions in hemodialysis patients? Clin Nephrol 1994;41:301–7.

25. KDIGO. KDIGO clinical practice guideline for anemia in chronic kidney disease. Kidney Int Suppl 2012;2(4):279–335. Available at: https://kdigo.org/wp-content/uploads/2016/10/KDIGO-2012-Anemia-Guideline-English.pdf. Accessed: May 13, 2019.

26. Arnold R, Issar T, Krishnan A, et al. Neurological complications in chronic kidney disease. JRSM Cardiovasc Dis 2016;5:1–13.

27. Dad T, Weiner DE. Stroke and chronic kidney disease: epidemiology, pathogenesis, and management across kidney disease stages. Semin Nephrol 2015;35(4):311–22.

28. Foley RN, Parfery PS, Sarnak MJ. Clinical epidemiology of cardiovascular disease in chronic renal disease. Am J Kidney Dis 1998;32:S112–9.

29. Ronco C, Haapio M, House A, et al. Cardiorenal syndrome. J Am Coll Cardiol 2008;52:1527–39.

30. Gansevoort R, Correa-Rotter R, Hemmelgarn B, et al. Chronic kidney disease and cardiovascular risk: epidemiology, mechanisms, and prevention. Lancet 2013;382:339–52.

31. Harnett J, Foley R, Kent G, et al. Congestive heart failure in dialysis patients: prevalence, incidence, prognosis and risk factors. Kidney Int 1995;47:884–90.

32. Cheung AK, Sarnak MJ, Yan G, et al. Atherosclerotic cardiovascular disease risks in chronic hemodialysis patients. Kidney Int 2000;58:353–62.

33. Fleisher LA, Fleischmann KE, Auerbach AD, et al. 2014 ACC/AHA guideline on perioperative cardiovascular evaluation and management of patients undergoing noncardiac surgery. J Am Coll Cardiol 2014;64:e77–137.

34. Peirson D. Respiratory complications in patients with renal failure. Respir Care 2006;51:413–22.

35. Sise ME, Courtwright AM, Channick RN. Pulmonary hypertension in patients with chronic and end-stage renal disease. Kidney Int 2013;84:682–92.

36. Perkovic V, Agarwal R, Fioretto P, et al. Management of patients with diabetes and CKD: conclusions from a "kidney disease: improving global outcomes" (KDIGO) controversies conference. Kidney Int 2016;90:1175–83.

37. Dekker M, Kooman J. Fluid status assessment in hemodialysis patients and the association with outcome: review of recent literature. Curr Opin Nephrol Hypertens 2018;27:188–93.

38. Dekker M, Marcelli D, Canaud B, et al. Impact of fluid status and inflammation and their interaction on survival: a study in an international hemodialysis patient cohort. Kidney Int 2017;91:1214–23.

39. Ekinci C, Karabork M, Siriopol D, et al. Effects of volume overload and current techniques for the assessment of fluid status in patients with renal disease. Blood Purif 2018;46:34–47.

40. Moore C, Copel J. Point-of-care-ultrasonography. N Engl J Med 2014;364:749–57.

41. Manoach S, Weingart S, Charchaflieh J. The evolution and current use of invasive hemodynamic monitoring for predicting volume responsiveness during resuscitation, perioperative and critical care. J Clin Anesth 2012;24:242–50.

42. Fortin PM, Bassett K, Musini VM. Human albumin for intradialytic hypotension in haemodialysis patients. Cochrane Database Syst Rev 2010;(11):CD006758.

43. O'Malley C, Frumento R, Hardy M. A randomized, double-blind comparison of lactated Ringer's solution and 0.9% NaCl during renal transplantation. Anesth Analg 2005;100:1518–24.
44. Khajavi MR, Etezadi F, Moharari R, et al. Effects of normal saline vs lactated Ringer's during renal transplantation. Ren Fail 2008;30:535–9.
45. Horl M, Horl W. Hemodialysis-associated hypertension: pathophysiology and therapy. Am J Kidney Dis 2002;39:227–44.
46. Lapage KG, Wouters PF. The patient with hypertension undergoing surgery. Curr Opin Anaesthesiol 2016;29:397–402.
47. Acedillo R, Shah M, Devereaux P, et al. The risk of perioperative bleeding in patients with chronic kidney disease: a systematic review and meta-analysis. Ann Surg 2013;258:901–13.
48. Tanhehco Y, Berns J. Red blood cell transfusion risks in patients with end-stage renal disease. Semin Dial 2012;25:539–44.
49. Hughes S, Szeki I, Nash MJ, et al. Anticoagulation in chronic kidney disease patients—the practical aspects. Clin Kidney J 2014;7(5):442–9.
50. Doherty JU, Gluckman TJ, Hucker W, et al. 2017 ACC expert consensus decision pathway for periprocedural management of anticoagulation in patients with non-valvular atrial fibrillation. J Am Coll Cardiol 2017;69:871–98.
51. Mannucci PM. Desmopressin (DDAVP) in the treatment of bleeding disorders: the first 20 years. Blood 1997;90:2515–21.
52. Herbet P, Wells G, Blajchman M, et al. A multicenter randomized controlled clinical trial of transfusion requirements in critical care. N Engl J Med 1999;340:409–17.
53. Gonsowski GT, Laster MJ, Eger EL, et al. Toxicity of compound A in rats: effect of 3-hour administrations. Anesthesiology 1994;80:556–65.
54. Conzen P, Kharasch E, Czerner S, et al. Low flow sevoflurane compared with low flow isoflurane anesthesia in patients with stable renal insufficiency. Anesthesiology 2002;97:578–84.
55. Thapa S, Brull SJ. Succinylcholine-induced hyperkalemia in patients with renal failure: an old question revisited. Anesth Analg 2000;91:237–41.
56. Norman S, del Greco F, Dietz A. Serum cholinesterase deficiency in renal failure. Trans Am Soc Artif Intern Organs 1969;15:328–31.
57. Craig RG, Hunter JM. Neuromuscular blocking drugs and their antagonists in patients with organ disease. Anaesthesia 2009;64:55–65.
58. Appiah-Ankman J, Hunter JM. Pharmacology of neuromuscular blocking drugs. Continuing Education in Anaesthesia Critical Care & Pain 2004;4:2–7.
59. Cronnelly R, Stanski D, Miller R, et al. Renal function and the pharmacokinetics o neostigmine in anesthetized man. Anesthesiology 1979;51:222–6.
60. Staals LM, Snoeck MJ, Driessen JJ, et al. Reduced clearance of rocuronium and suggamadex in patients with severe to end-stage renal failure: a pharmacokinetic study. Br J Anaesth 2010;104:31–9.
61. Merck & Co., Inc.. Bridion. 2015. Available at: https://www.accessdata.fda.gov/drugsatfda_docs/label/2015/022225lbl.pdf. Accessed May 17, 2019.
62. Dean M. Opioids in renal failure and dialysis patients. J Pain Symptom Manage 2004;28:497–504.
63. Vinik HR, Rever JG, Greenblatt DJ, et al. The pharmacokinetics of midazolam in chronic renal failure patients. Anesthesiology 1983;59:390–4.
64. Kirwan CJ, MacPhee IA, Lee T, et al. Acute kidney injury reduces the hepatic metabolism of midazolam in critically ill patients. Intensive Care Med 2012;38:76–84.

65. De Wolf AM, Fragen RJ, Avram MJ, et al. The pharmacokinetics of dexmedetomidine in volunteers with severe renal impairment. Anesth Analg 2001;93:1205–9.
66. Ronco C, Ricci Z, De Backer D, et al. Renal replacement therapy in acute kidney injury: controversy and consensus. Crit Care 2015;19:146.
67. Nash DM, Przech S, Wald R, et al. Systematic review and meta-analysis of renal replacement therapy modalities for acute kidney injury in the intensive care unit. J Crit Care 2017;41:138–44.
68. Petroni KC, Cohen NH. Continuous renal replacement therapy: anesthetic implications. Anesth Analg 2002;94:1288–97.
69. Ahee P, Crowe AV. The management of hyperkalaemia in the emergency department. Emerg Med J 2000;17:188–91.
70. Bansal N, McCulloch CE, Lin F, et al. Blood pressure and risk of cardiovascular events in patients on chronic hemodialysis: the CRIC Study (Chronic Renal Insufficiency Cohort). Hypertension 2017;70(2):435–43.

Anesthesia for Neurosurgical Emergencies

Shilpa Rao, MD[a],*, Rafi Avitsian, MD[b]

KEYWORDS

- Intracranial pressure • Cerebral perfusion pressure • Seizure management
- Trauma to spine

KEY POINTS

- Anesthesiologists have an important role in maintaining neuronal homeostasis during neurosurgical emergencies by ensuring adequate oxygenation, ventilation, and suitable hemodynamic conditions depending on the insult.
- Acute change in mental status is an important sign to recognizing central nervous system pathologic condition, and a systematic approach can aid in diagnosis and treatment.
- Measures for neuronal protection by ensuring adequate perfusion can improve outcome during neurosurgical emergencies.
- Many intracranial emergencies, including trauma and intracranial vascular emergencies, cause increased intracranial pressure and disrupt cerebral perfusion pressure.
- Avoiding secondary injury after spinal traumas and maintaining adequate perfusion to the spinal cord are the mainstay of anesthetic management of traumas to the spine.

INTRODUCTION

With the creation of subspecialty novel surgical modalities for various intracranial and spine pathologic conditions, neuroanesthesiologists have incorporated data from outcomes research to modify perioperative care and improve results. Timely intervention during life-threatening complications can impact outcomes. Neurons are very sensitive to ischemic and metabolic insults and may be irreversibly damaged if immediate action is not taken toward restoring their homeostasis. Herein, the authors describe anesthetic care of patients facing neurosurgical emergencies.

[a] Department of Anesthesiology, Yale School of Medicine and Yale New Haven Hospital, 333 Cedar Street, TMP 3, PO Box 208051, New Haven, CT 06520-8051, USA; [b] Department of General Anesthesiology, Cleveland Clinic Foundation, 9500 Euclid Avenue # E31, Cleveland, OH 44195, USA
* Corresponding author.
E-mail address: Shilpa.rao@yale.edu

Anesthesiology Clin 38 (2020) 67–83
https://doi.org/10.1016/j.anclin.2019.10.004
1932-2275/20/© 2019 Elsevier Inc. All rights reserved.

INTRACRANIAL EMERGENCIES
Approach to a Patient with Altered Mental Status

Neurosurgical procedures are unique in that the best monitoring modality is the neurologic examination and the most important sign includes an intact mental status. An altered mental status (AMS) can alert the neurosurgical team of the urgency with which a patient should be attended.

The Glasgow Coma Scale (GCS; **Table 1**) provides a practical method for assessment of impairment at different levels of the central nervous system (CNS) in accordance with response to respective stimuli. It is based on a 15-point scale for estimating and categorizing the extent and outcomes of brain injury. Intubation and airway protection are recommended when GCS is 8 or less, or in any significant decline in GCS. Generally, brain injury is classified as the following:

- Severe, GCS <8 to 9
- Moderate, GCS 8 to 12
- Minor, GCS ≥13

Tracheal intubation and severe facial/eye swelling make it difficult to test the verbal and eye responses. In these circumstances, the score is given as 1 with a modifier attached (either "t" for intubation or "c" for eyes closed).[1]

The GCS Pupils Score was recently described. It is calculated by subtracting the Pupil Reactivity Score (**Table 2**) from the calculated GCS to yield a total score. A combination of both of these scores is important to assess the nature of emergent intervention.

A change in mental status can be the presenting sign of CNS pathologic condition or can be seen during the course of treatment. A change in the mental status after treatment of a subarachnoid hemorrhage (SAH) can be a sign of a rebleeding or vasospasm, both of which need immediate intervention, such as angiography, for diagnosis and treatment, and/or neurosurgical intervention. Measures outlined in later discussion to reduce intracranial pressure (ICP) are commenced immediately. Acute exacerbation of certain medical conditions can also present with AMS change, and the causes can vary from endocrine problems (hypothyroidism, pituitary tumors) to substance abuse and medication errors.

Table 1
Calculating the Glasgow Coma Scale

	Parameter	Score
Eye opening to	Spontaneous	4
	Verbal command	3
	Pain	2
	None	1
Best verbal response	Oriented, conversing	5
	Disoriented	4
	Inappropriate words	3
	Incomprehensible words	2
	No verbal response	1
Best motor response	Follows verbal commands	6
	Localizes to pain	5
	Withdrawal to pain	4
	Abnormal flexion (decorticate)	3
	Abnormal extension (decerebrate)	2
	No motor response	1

Table 2 Calculating the pupil reactivity score	
Pupils Nonreactive to Light	**Score**
Both	2
One	1
Neither	0

A delayed emergence after craniotomy is considered a change in mental status because the patient does not reach an expected level of consciousness, thus suggesting a postoperative complication. Contributing factors include residual anesthetic and/or narcotics, inadequate reversal of neuromuscular blockade, ventilation and oxygenation problems, and electrolyte imbalances, such as hyponatremia, hypoglycemia, intracranial bleed, and subclinical seizures. Appropriate diagnosis may be aided by reviewing anesthetic elimination and muscle relaxation reversal, arterial blood gas (ABG) values, and computed tomography (CT) scan if needed.

An increased ICP from a space-occupying lesion (eg, tumor, bleeding) or hydrocephalus can also present primarily with AMS. Management is outlined in later discussion.

A review of the patient's medication is important to recognize medication-related AMS, including polypharmacy. Many anticonvulsants may cause sedation, which may be misinterpreted as altered consciousness. Metabolic causes of AMS are important and can worsen the prognosis of already existent intracranial pathologic condition. Hypoglycemia or hyperglycemia should be treated rapidly because both can severely worsen outcome. Electrolyte abnormalities may be iatrogenic, such as treatment of increased ICP, including mannitol, hypertonic saline, and diuretics. Infectious causes of AMS are categorized as systemic, specifically in elderly population, sepsis, or local infections of CNS. Rapid diagnosis and treatment of these infectious processes directly affect outcome.

Although investigating the cause of AMS is primarily with the neurosurgical team, it is important for the anesthesiologist to be aware of the possible iatrogenic causes because the treatment and management will directly need multiple and immediate interventions, which includes ensuring the airway is protected at all times. Intubation and mechanical ventilation may be required emergently, because the patient is at an increased risk of aspiration. After correction of hypoxia and hypercapnia, a more thorough review of history and examination can help in diagnosis and treatment as necessary.

Acute Increase in Intracranial Pressure

The cranium is a tight space with low compliance (or high elastic property), meaning a small change in volume can cause an increase in ICP. Increased ICP decreases blood supply, causing ischemia and edema with further increase in ICP. The 3 constituents of cranium include the brain, cerebrospinal fluid (CSF), and intracranial blood. An increase in any one of these components unless accompanied by a decrease in others will increase the ICP (the Monroe-Kelly doctrine).

Causes of acute increase in ICP include the following:

- Head trauma: various open or depressed skull fractures, intracranial hematomas, diffuse axonal injury, and so forth

- Diffuse cerebral edema: due to severe hypoxia, trauma, severe hypoglycemia, or any acute intracranial insult
  - A disruption and incompetency of the blood-brain barrier (BBB) will cause a flux of solutes and water from capillaries (vasogenic cerebral edema).
  - A disruption of neuronal hemostasis can cause cellular swelling (cytotoxic or cellular cerebral edema).
- Intracranial hemorrhage and intracranial vascular lesions: for example, cerebral aneurysms, arteriovenous malformations (AVM)
- Intracranial thrombosis: for example, thrombosis of the superior sagittal sinus
- Intracranial tumors, meningitis, or other intracranial infections
- Obstructive hydrocephalus
- Hypertensive emergencies, reperfusion injuries

Early signs of increasing ICP include AMS, restlessness, irritability, and confusion. With continued increase, voluntary movements, sensations, and extraocular movements will slow. In addition, with resulting sympathetic surge T-wave changes will develop on the electrocardiogram. As pressure increases near the medulla, the patient may experience projectile vomiting and cardiac arrhythmias ranging from supraventricular tachycardia to severe bradycardia, and this will progress to coma. When herniation of the brain is imminent, loss of extraocular movement will occur, with the pupils dilating, becoming unreactive and turning outward.[2] Along with clinical signs and symptoms, a CT scan (if time permits) is useful in diagnosing the extent of brain injury or bleed as well as midline shift and herniation.

Traumatic brain injury (TBI) can be associated with both epidural and subdural hematoma, along with other associated injuries. Epidural hematoma results from fracture of the temporal bone, resulting in laceration of underlying middle meningeal artery. There is an initial loss of consciousness, followed by a brief "lucid interval." Signs and symptoms of impending brain herniation and raised ICP will follow eventually, if untreated. CT scan findings include a convex lens-shaped hyperdensity due to blood accumulating between the skull bone and dura. In contrast, subdural bleeding occurs between the dura and arachnoid, without a definite "lucid interval" (Fig. 1).

An acute increase in ICP and impending brain herniation is a true neurosurgical emergency. In addition to a surgical decompression, concurrent medical treatment is necessary. The goal is maintenance of cerebral perfusion pressure, defined as the difference between mean arterial pressure (MAP) and ICP. Although increasing MAP can improve blood supply to the brain, it could be deleterious if the pathophysiology of increased ICP is intracranial bleeding or hypertensive crisis. Anesthesiologists play a vital role in the medical management of these patients, including measures to decrease the ICP, maintain cerebral perfusion, and implement brain-protective measures. The latter is through decreasing cerebral metabolic rate and oxygen need. Anesthetic induction and endotracheal intubation are important in protecting the airway from aspiration in an obtunded patient. Mechanical ventilation controls the end-tidal carbon dioxide and helps prevent additional increases in ICP owing to hypercarbia.

The anesthetic goals through induction are summarized as follows:

- Minimize hemodynamic responses to laryngoscopy and intubation
- Maintain cerebral perfusion pressure and oxygen supply to neurons
- Minimize C-spine movement during laryngoscopy and intubation
- Rapidly and safely secure the endotracheal tube

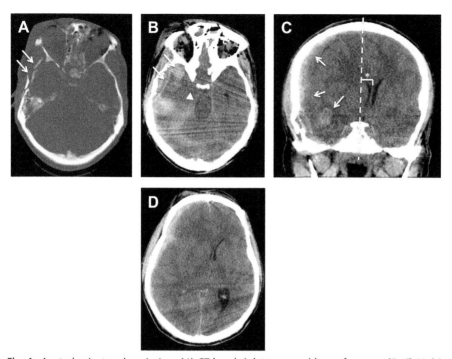

Fig. 1. Acute brainstem herniation. (*A*) CT head right temporal bone fracture. (*B*, *C*) Multi-compartmental hemorrhage right temporal contusion and acute subdural hematoma (SDH)/extradural hematoma (EDH) (*arrows*), (*C*) midline shift (*asterisk*), and (*D*) uncal herniation. (*Courtesy of* B. J. Cord, MD, PhD, New Haven, CT.)

It is recommended to have difficult airway equipment available because of the emergent nature of the surgery, with the possibility of inadequate airway assessment owing to AMS. Any induction agent can be used in appropriate doses, depending on the patient's hemodynamic status, although ketamine may further increase ICP. Hypotension is detrimental in TBI and must be avoided at all costs. A rapid sequence intubation and intubation protect the airway from possible aspiration of gastric contents and can be performed with manual in-line stabilization in an uncooperative patient. Nasotracheal intubation is avoided in patients with TBI, because of possible underlying basal skull fractures.

Apart from standard American Society of Anesthesiologists (ASA) monitors, invasive blood pressure (BP) monitoring is recommended and gives the ability to check serial ABG for hemoglobin, glucose, electrolytes, and such. A Foley catheter is required to monitor urine output; however, it should be placed after confirming there is no trauma to the ureter or bladder. Advanced monitoring techniques, such as transcranial Doppler, to assess cerebral blood flow (CBF) and velocities, and near-infrared spectroscopy (NIRS), to continuously monitor regional cerebral tissue oxygenation, can be used in select circumstances. Transthoracic echocardiography and/or Doppler can be used to assess underlying cardiac functional status and to rapidly diagnose venous air embolism.

As with any major emergency surgery, adequate intravenous access is required for rapid administration of fluids and medications, including vasoactive agents, as well as transfusion of blood products. Indications for placing a central venous catheter (CVC) include inadequate peripheral vascular access, need for infusion of vasoactive agents or hypertonic saline (3% or higher concentrations), a need for central venous blood pressure measurements (eg, large fluid shifts) or blood draws (eg, mixed venous oxygen saturation), a required access path for pulmonary vein or jugular bulb, chance for venous air embolism as well as for long-term venous access in the intensive care unit (ICU) (eg, total parenteral nutrition). It is safer to place the CVC under ultrasound guidance if there are signs of neck and chest trauma, which can shift anatomic landmarks. In addition to the time concerns, placement of a jugular line will almost certainly require movement of the cervical spine, which should be avoided in patients with TBI. Trendelenburg positioning for placement of CVC may be deleterious if ICP is high. Placement of a subclavian line has a higher risk of pneumothorax, which can rapidly increase $Paco_2$ and ICP. Hence, the risks and benefits must be carefully considered. Surgical decompression should not be delayed for the placement of these lines. Although a femoral CVC can increase chance of infection, at times, this may be the only possible option. A peripherally inserted CVC is also a suitable alternative.

If the patient already has an external ventricular drain (EVD) in situ, ICP can be monitored through the EVD transducer. The EVD is useful in determining cerebral perfusion pressure and facilitates drainage of CSF to reduce ICP. Placing a lumbar drain, lumbar CSF sampling, and subarachnoid access in patients with increased ICP can cause brain herniation and should be avoided (**Fig. 2**).

Patients with elevated ICP should be positioned head up, to maximize venous outflow from the head. It is important to avoid excessive flexion or rotation of the neck and restrictive neck taping and minimize stimuli that could induce Valsalva responses, such as endotracheal suctioning. Keeping patients appropriately sedated and relaxed while under anesthesia can decrease ICP by reducing metabolic demand, ventilator dyssynchrony, venous congestion, and the sympathetic responses.

Continued mechanical ventilation to lower $Paco_2$ to 26 to 30 mm Hg has been shown to rapidly reduce ICP through vasoconstriction and decrease the volume of intracranial blood; a 1-mm Hg change in $Paco_2$ is associated with a 3% change in CBF.[3] However, several recent studies recommend against hyperventilation in the first 24 hours after TBI.[4] During this period, even mild hyperventilation will cause vasoconstriction and ischemia in injured brain areas and worsen neurologic outcomes. The only time that hyperventilation can be considered in the first 24 hours is if ICP is critically high

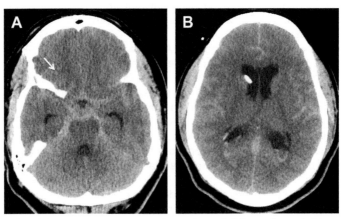

Fig. 2. (*A*) CT head demonstrates aneurysmal SAH (*arrow*). (*B*) EVD (*arrow*). (*Courtesy of* B. J. Cord, MD, PhD, New Haven, CT.)

and there is a concern for immediate herniation. Even in this scenario, the period of hyperventilation should be very brief.[4]

Patients with increased ICP should be kept euvolemic and normo-osmolar to hyper-osmolar by avoiding all free water (including D5W [5% dextrose in water], 0.45% saline, and enteral free water) and using only isotonic or slightly hypertonic fluids (such as normal saline). Serum osmolality should be kept greater than 280 mOsm/L, usually in the 295- to 305-mOsm/L range. Hyponatremia is common in the setting of elevated ICP, particularly in conjunction with SAH.

The value of colloid compared with crystalloid fluid resuscitation in patients with elevated ICP has been studied, but findings have been inconclusive. A subgroup analysis in 1 large study suggested that in patients with TBI, fluid resuscitation with albumin was associated with a higher mortality as compared with normal saline.[5]

Additional treatment strategies to reduce ICP include the following treatments.

Osmotic diuretics
    Mannitol at a dose of 1 g/kg (20% solution) reduces brain volume by drawing free water out of the brain tissue and into the circulation, to be excreted by the kidneys, thereby reducing ICP and improving CBF. Onset is within 15 to 20 minutes, and the duration of action is 4 to 8 hours. Some of the complications associated with mannitol therapy include volume depletion, initially hyponatremia and subsequently hypernatremia. If very high doses of mannitol are infused, or if the drug is given to patients with preexisting renal failure, mannitol is retained in the circulation. The ensuing increase in plasma osmolality results in the osmotic movement of water and potassium out of cells leading to extracellular fluid volume expansion (and possibly pulmonary edema), hyponatremia, metabolic acidosis (by dilution), and hyperkalemia[6,7]

Hypertonic saline
    Hypertonic saline has been used in a wide range of concentrations, from 3%, most commonly used as a continuous infusion, to 23.4%, which is typically used in intermittent boluses. When used as a continuous infusion, 3% NaCl may be titrated to a sodium goal of approximately 145 to 155 mEq/L. Hypertonic saline should be administered via a CVC for risk of extravasation. Short-term use via peripheral intravenous access is permissible in life-threatening ICP elevation while central access is obtained.

Cerebrospinal fluid drainage
    If the patient has a functioning EVD, CSF can be drained carefully to reduce ICP, and attention should be directed to avoid excessive drainage.

Glucose and electrolyte control
    Both hyperglycemia and hypoglycemia are associated with worsened outcome in a variety of neurologic conditions, including severe TBI, and hence, need to be avoided. Hyperglycemia is particularly common in these patients; hence, frequent glucose monitoring and control are imperative during the perioperative period. This has been presumed to be at least in part related to aggravation of secondary brain injury. Several mechanisms for this are proposed, including increased tissue acidosis from anaerobic metabolism, free radical generation, and increased BBB permeability.[8]
    Hyponatremia is commonly seen in a variety of CNS diseases and injury, usually due to syndrome of inappropriate secretion of antidiuretic hormone (SIADH) and cerebral salt wasting syndrome (CSW). CSW is diagnosed in a patient with polyuria, hypovolemia, hyponatremia (serum sodium <135 mEq/L), with a low-plasma

osmolality and elevated urine osmolality (>100 mosmol/kg). Treatment of CSW usually involves 3% hypertonic saline to increase serum sodium along with intravascular volume replacement. In contrast, in SIADH there is hypervolemia with hyponatremia, and the treatment is fluid restriction along with giving sodium.

Temperature control

Increased body temperature increases metabolic demand and blood flow and worsens outcomes in increased ICP. Early (within 2.5 hours) and short-term (48 hours after injury) prophylactic hypothermia is not recommended to improve outcomes in patients with diffuse injury.[9] Current approaches emphasize maintaining normothermia through the use of antipyretic medications, surface-cooling devices, or endovascular temperature management catheters, although induced normothermia using endovascular cooling and a continuous feedback-loop system has been shown to lower the fever burden and improve ICP control following TBI.[10]

Barbiturates

Pentobarbital and thiopental infusions may be used to manage elevated ICP refractory to other therapies. Although effective for the control of ICP, the use of barbiturate coma has not been shown to improve outcomes following TBI. These agents profoundly decrease cerebral metabolic demand, CBF, and cerebral blood volume.[11,12] Monitoring of EEG is necessary to ensure burst suppression when indicated.

Ultimately, surgical decompression is the mainstay of therapy for severe ICP elevation and can be lifesaving. There is a growing body of literature supporting the efficacy of decompressive craniectomy in certain clinical situations (see later discussion). It has been demonstrated that in patients with elevated ICP, craniectomy alone lowered ICP 15%, but opening the dura in addition to the bony skull resulted in an average decrease in ICP of 70%.[13]

Clinical trials of decompressive craniectomy in TBI suggest that the procedure is effective in controlling ICP and is lifesaving in patients who have failed medical therapy.

A randomized trial (DECRA) in 155 adults with severe diffuse TBI and ICP greater than 20 mm Hg for 15 minutes within a 1-hour period despite first-tier therapies compared bifrontal craniectomy with continued medical care. Patients in the craniectomy group, as compared with those in the standard-care group, had less time with ICP above the treatment threshold ($P<.001$), fewer interventions for increased ICP ($P<.02$ for all comparisons), and fewer ICU days ($P<.001$). However, patients undergoing craniectomy had worse scores on the Extended Glasgow Outcome Scale than those receiving standard care and a greater risk of an unfavorable outcome.[14]

The RESCUEicp trial used more broadly applicable eligibility criteria; 408 patients aged 10 to 65 years old with refractory ICP greater than 25 mm Hg for 1 to 12 hours despite medical therapy were randomized to continued medical therapy or craniectomy appropriate to the nature of injury. Outcomes at 1 year revealed that the surgical group had a higher rate of favorable outcomes (defined as better than lower severe disability or, ie, functionally independent within the home or better) of 45% versus 32%.[15]

Any acute CNS injury may trigger neurogenic pulmonary edema from massive sympathetic discharge. There is leakage of intravascular fluid into the alveoli and pulmonary interstitial space, leading to acute hypoxemia. Compared with cardiogenic pulmonary edema, these patients have lower preload. Often, these patients will continue to require postoperative mechanical ventilation with lung protection strategies (limitation of tidal volume to 6 mL/kg body weight). However, permissive hypercapnia and higher levels of positive end expiratory pressure need to be used cautiously in these patients with increased ICP.

Seizure and Status Epilepticus

Convulsive status epilepticus describes the more common form of emergency situation that can occur with prolonged or repeated tonic-clonic (grand mal) seizures. Most tonic-clonic seizures end within 1 to 2 minutes, but they may have postictal symptoms for much longer. Status epilepticus occurs when the patient does not recover consciousness between the seizure episodes or seizure persists despite therapy. Nonconvulsive status epilepticus is seen when long or repeated absence or when there is continuous focal impaired awareness (complex partial) seizures.

As with earlier emergency management priorities, airway protection is important in these scenarios, to prevent injuries, including tongue bite. The patient must be kept in a padded bed to prevent secondary injuries from falls and so forth. The first line of treatment is usually with benzodiazepines. Subsequent treatment with antiepileptics, such as phenytoin, valproic acid, and/or levetiracetam, will be required. A benzodiazepine infusion or barbiturate coma becomes necessary to stop seizures.

Neurosurgical intervention may be required if an underlying resectable cause is found. The anesthesiologist's role in treatment of status epilepticus is evaluation of need for intubation for airway protection and administration of antiepileptics in consultation with the neurologic team. Monitoring the hemodynamics and treatment accordingly are important.

In patients under general anesthesia, it may be clinically difficult to recognize a seizure. The hemodynamics may show tachycardia and hypertension as a result of sympathetic discharge, although in patients with associated cardiac dysfunction this may not be apparent, in addition to multiple other confounding situations with similar hemodynamic changes. ABG can confirm hypercarbia seen on end-tidal monitoring and elevated lactate levels, with no other underlying possible explanation.

Anticoagulation and Neurosurgical Emergencies

With an increasing number of patients being treated with oral anticoagulation for various other reasons, the number of patients requiring emergency neurosurgical intervention who are on anticoagulation or antiplatelet therapy has increased. Often, the clinical scenario involves a patient with acute AMS after a fall while on anticoagulation.

Some of the commonly used anticoagulants and their indications are noted in **Table 3**.

These patients require emergency reversal of anticoagulation as well as decompressive neurosurgery to evacuate the hematoma. Anesthesiologists are involved in the management of increased ICP as described above and reversal of anticoagulation.

Anticoagulant-associated intracranial hematoma carries a particularly poor prognosis, with a case fatality of up to 50% at 3 months.[16] It is important to review the patient's medications and their indications before reversal of anticoagulation. Given the high risk of hematoma expansion in the first few hours after onset in these patients on anticoagulation, it is imperative that prothrombin complex concentrate (PCC) is given without delay to maximize therapeutic effect. A large observational study of 853 vitamin K antagonist-intracerebral hemorrhage patients receiving PCC at 19 German centers has been recently published, demonstrating that treatment within 4 hours of

Table 3
Commonly used anticoagulants and their indications

Medication	Indication	Dose (Oral)	Interval
Warfarin	Prophylaxis and treatment of deep vein thrombosis (DVT) and pulmonary embolism (PE)	2.5 mg onwards	Once a day
Apixaban	Prevention of stroke in nonvalvular atrial fibrillation DVT prophylaxis after hip/knee surgery	5 mg	Twice daily
Rivaroxaban	Prevention of stroke in nonvalvular atrial fibrillation Prevention and treatment of DVT and PE DVT prophylaxis after hip/knee surgery	15 mg or 20 mg	Once a day
Dabigatran	Prevention of stroke in nonvalvular atrial fibrillation Prevention and treatment of DVT and PE DVT prophylaxis after hip/knee surgery	75 mg to 150 mg	Twice a day
Clopidogrel	Unstable angina/non-ST segment elevation myocardial infarction, dual antiplatelet therapy for coronary stent, concomitant with aspirin	300-mg loading dose, followed by 75 mg per day up to 12 mo	Once a day
Unfractionated heparin	Acute coronary syndromes, prevention or treatment of DVT, bridge therapy for atrial fibrillation	Titrate to maintain aPTT 2–2.5 times control	
Enoxaparin	Prevention or treatment of DVT, treatment of acute coronary syndromes, and bridge therapy for atrial fibrillation	1 mg/kg subcutaneously	Every 12 h

admission to hospital is associated with a significant reduction in hematoma enlargement, when compared with more delayed treatment (19.8% vs 41.5%)[17] (**Fig. 3**).

Intracranial Vascular Emergencies

Management of patients with ischemic stroke
Patients presenting with symptoms of acute ischemic stroke require immediate restoration of CBF to salvage residual ischemic brain tissue. Intravenous tissue plasminogen activator (alteplase) is the first line of therapy for reperfusion and improves functional outcome at 3 to 6 months when given within 4.5 hours of symptom onset.[18] Mechanical thrombectomy and removal of the inciting clot can be performed up to 24 hours from symptom onset.

Neuroanesthesiologists are involved in the management of these patients who are coming in for endovascular therapy, which is done for both diagnosis and treatment. Therapy can be performed under general anesthesia or monitored anesthesia care (MAC)/sedation. A quick and focused preanesthesia evaluation needs to be performed while the patient is being prepared for the procedure, to minimize delays in treatment.

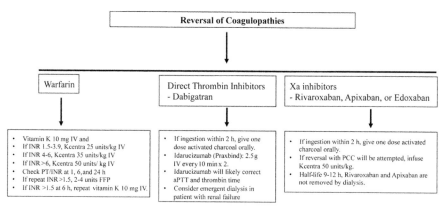

Fig. 3. The guidelines for reversing warfarin and non vitamin K antagonist oral anticoagulants coagulopathies in patients with symptomatic intracerebral hemorrhage (ICH). aPTT, activated partial thromboplastin time; FFP, fresh frozen plasma; INR, international normalized ratio; IV, intravenously; PT, prothrombin time. (*From* Dastur CK, Yu W. Current management of spontaneous intracerebral haemorrhage. Stroke and Vascular Neurology 2017;2:25; with permission.)

Recent studies have failed to show a better outcome with the use of sedation instead of general anesthesia for thrombectomy. The SIESTA trial[19] included 150 patients with acute ischemic stroke in the anterior circulation, and patients were randomly assigned to an intubated general anesthesia group and nonintubated conscious sedation group during stroke thrombectomy. The primary outcome was early neurologic improvement after 24 hours and was not significantly different in both the groups; hence, the findings do not support an advantage for the use of conscious sedation.

The General Or Local Anesthesia in Intra Arterial THerapy trial[20] compared general anesthesia and conscious sedation for anterior circulation ischemic stroke and found no worse clinical or tissue outcome after general anesthesia.

The authors recommend using MAC as the first line of anesthetic management in appropriate patients who are able to protect their airway and who are cooperative. Rapid need for conversion to general anesthesia should be kept in mind. The advantages of MAC include facilitation of immediate neurologic examination, able to proceed with rapid onset of treatment, and less hemodynamic variations than is seen in general anesthesia. At all times, standard ASA monitors and emergency drugs and equipment need to be immediately available. An invasive arterial BP monitoring is valuable because it can help in maintaining a tight BP control; however, the procedure should not be delayed if placing the arterial line takes valuable time. If the patient is exhibiting signs and symptoms of raised ICP, the management should proceed as outlined in earlier discussion (under the Management of increased ICP section).

Other important intraoperative considerations include the following:

- BP management: Sustained periods of hypotension worsen neurologic outcomes and must be avoided. Hypotension may require treatment with vasopressors, such as alpha agonists, for example, phenylephrine or norepinephrine infusions. Severe hypertension, especially after reperfusion, must be avoided because the reperfused tissue may be at risk for hemorrhagic transformation. Nicardipine and/or labetalol can be used for control of hypertension.

- Anticoagulation: intravenous heparin is administered during these procedures to minimize further thrombotic events, and heparin activity should be monitored by measuring activated clotting time (ACT), with the target ACT of 250 to 300 seconds.[21]
- These patients will require postoperative ICU admission and further monitoring.

Intracranial aneurysms and arteriovenous malformations

Most SAH cases are a result of intracranial aneurysm rupture. The symptoms can vary from headache (usually described as "the worst headache" in the patient's life) and neck rigidity or pain to focal neurologic deficiencies and/or AMS (see earlier discussion). Treatment can be either endovascular coiling or open microsurgical clipping.

Optimal timing of aneurysm surgery depends on the clinical status of the patient and associated factors. Early surgery (ie, <48–96 hours after SAH) is favored for candidates in good condition or those with unstable BP, seizures, mass effect from thrombus, large amounts of blood, or evidence of aneurysm growth or rebleeding. Early surgery carries an increased operative morbidity, although the risks of vasospasm and rebleeding are reduced considerably. Delayed surgery (ie, 10–14 days after SAH) may be considered for large aneurysms in difficult locations or for candidates in poor clinical condition. Surgery is indicated for ruptured or symptomatic aneurysms in patients without extenuating contraindications or considerably advanced age. Surgery generally is precluded if the clinical status is poor, corresponding to Hunt and Hess grade 4 or 5.[22]

However, a retrospective study reviewing 105 patients,[23] concluded that younger patients with good clinical grade were associated with a favorable neurologic outcome both at discharge and at 6 months after surgery, irrespective of timing, size of the aneurysm, and duration of surgery.

A hemodynamically stable induction and intubation avoids sympathetic discharge that can elevate BP and result in rebleeding. The management of associated increased ICP is outlined in earlier discussion. Endovascular treatment can be complicated with intraoperative aneurysm rupture, and the anesthesiologist should be ready to immediately decrease the ICP, reverse any anticoagulation, and prepare for an emergency craniotomy for decompression and clipping. It is recommended to have blood available for transfusion in cases of significant blood loss.

During open microsurgical clipping, constant communication with the surgeon is necessary for induced hypotension (during surgical dissection around the aneurysm), initiation of burst suppression and brain protection, and induced hypertension (when there is a need for a temporary clip) to allow collateral perfusion of areas of brain affected by the temporary clip.

One of the possible complications after SAH is cerebral vasospasm, which can necessitate emergent interventional angioplasty and/or injection of vasodilators. Anesthesiologists should concentrate on hemodynamic goals, including induced hypertension and maintaining adequate intravascular volume. Selective intraarterial injection of nicardipine during angiography can cause significant hemodynamic instability and requires supportive management by the anesthesiologist.[24]

Rupture of AVM can cause SAH with or without increased ICP and may need emergent surgical intervention. Anesthetic management is similar to treatment of intracranial aneurysms. Following excision of an AVM, there is a risk of cerebral edema as a result of eliminating the low-pressure venous flow of a high-pressure arterial abnormality with resultant of backflow of pressure. During AVM resection, the surgeon might need to place temporary clips on feeder arteries to visualize bleeding. Tight control of BP can help the operator identify and control arterial bleeding. To accomplish this, short-acting agents, such as nitroprusside or esmolol, should be considered. The theoretic risk of vasodilator-induced steal is outweighed by benefits of BP control on vasogenic edema and risk of bleeding. There may be a need to continue induced hypotension in the postoperative period to decrease the risk of brain edema from normal perfusion pressure breakthrough.[25]

Carotid artery stenosis

Carotid artery stenosis is manifested by neurologic signs and symptoms of inadequate intracranial hypoperfusion, such as transient ischemic attack or stroke, necessitating an urgent (if not emergent) need for treatment. The treatment can be an open endarterectomy or endovascular stenting. In both instances, there may not be adequate time for detailed evaluation and optimization of the patient.

The anesthesiologist should consider associated comorbidities that can affect vascular supply in other organs, including diabetes mellitus, hyperlipidemia, and smoking history. These comorbidities can put patients at risk of coronary artery disease, heart failure, renal insufficiency or failure, hypertension, and chronic obstructive pulmonary disease. Intravascular treatment of carotid stenosis can be performed under MAC, but there is always the possibility of complications that may need immediate conversion to general anesthesia and intubation. Deployment of the carotid stent may cause sudden bradycardia that although in most cases is self-limited but may need intervention if symptomatic. The open carotid endarterectomy can also be performed under regional anesthesia, providing an awake patient for continuous neurologic examination at the time of carotid artery cross-clamping. However, most neurosurgeons prefer operating under general anesthesia. The use of electroencephalography (EEG) is usually the method of choice for monitoring adequacy of collateral blood supply at the time of carotid cross-clamp because it can show slowing of EEG waveform if there is inadequate perfusion. The anesthesiologist can also use NIRS to confirm the adequacy of perfusion. Regardless of treatment method, invasive hemodynamic monitoring to diagnose hypotension as well as induced hypertension for better collateral flow at the time of cross-clamp is recommended. Furthermore, after endarterectomy or placement of carotid stent, a careful hemodynamic monitoring is necessary to avoid hypertension because this can cause hyperperfusion injury to the brain.

SPINAL CORD EMERGENCIES

The spinal cord, similar to brain, consists of neurons that are very sensitive to hypoperfusion and ischemia. Most spinal cord emergencies result from acute disruption of vascular supply to spinal cord. Emergencies include trauma, epidural or subdural hematomas (**Fig. 4**), abscesses, or degenerative disease or tumors causing unstable changes and pressure to spinal cord. Clinically, these can manifest as acute loss of sensory and/or motor functions at and below the level of injury.

The spinal cord receives the arterial supply from 2 posterior and 1 anterior spinal artery, and there are certain low-flow or watershed areas that have higher chance of injury with ischemia. Regardless of pathologic condition, the goal is to maintain the spinal cord perfusion pressure (SCPP) to minimize worsening of neurologic symptoms and to avoid secondary injury from moving, which can transect the spinal cord or further reduce its blood supply.

One of the common intraoperative complications is bleeding, which can be difficult to control. Intravenous tranexamic acid is established as an efficacious hemostatic agent in spine surgeries.[26] Emergent thoracic spine procedures may necessitate lung isolation; in addition, most complex spine procedures need invasive monitoring, including arterial line and central venous access for vasoactive medication infusions.

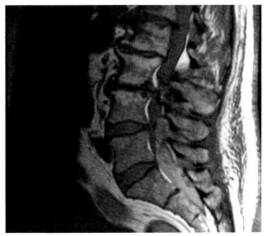

Fig. 4. Epidural hematoma extending from the mid L4 level dorsally through the tip of the thecal sac at about S2-S3.

The authors discuss later the approach to unstable cervical spine and anesthetic considerations during intraoperative neuromonitoring.

Unstable Cervical Spine

Excluding a cervical spine injury would necessitate meeting the following criteria. Under the NEXUS guidelines, when an acute blunt force injury is present, the following criteria need to be assessed:

- There is no midline posterior cervical tenderness.
- There is no evidence of intoxication, and the patient is alert and oriented.
- There are no focal neurologic deficits.
- There are no other painful distracting injuries (eg, long bone fracture).

If the patient does not meet all of the above criteria, a cervical spine radiograph series needs to be performed; however, plain films are inadequate in completely ruling out C-spine injury. A CT or MRI scan may be required to definitely rule out fracture or ligamentous injury.

During the initial assessment phase, the cervical spine is immobilized in a hard collar, until medically cleared.

Goals of anesthetic and airway management in these patients include the following:

- Assessment of respiratory function, as respiration may be compromised in high cervical spinal cord injuries, necessitating intubation for airway protection. Extreme care and caution must be taken in order to minimize movement of the cervical spine during intubation. If the patient is able to tolerate it, an awake fiber-optic intubation with appropriate topicalization remains the preferred method of safely securing the airway. In some acute situations needing immediate intubation, manual inline stabilization protects the cervical spine during intubation.
- Large-bore intravenous access, which is required for fluid resuscitation, especially during the initial spinal shock. If central venous access is planned, the subclavian vein may be preferred over the internal jugular vein.
- Arterial catheter/invasive hemodynamic monitoring.

- Avoidance of hypotension; hypotension can be detrimental in spinal cord injuries. It is recommended to maintain MAP greater than 85 to 90 mm Hg, to maintain SCPP.
- Care must be taken at all times to maintain C-spine immobility during patient transport, transfer to the operating room table, and during positioning of the patient.

Administration of high-dose methylprednisolone for the treatment of acute spinal cord injury is no longer recommended.

INTRAOPERATIVE LOSS OF NEUROMONITORING SIGNALS

Neuromonitoring techniques are extensively used in various surgeries involving the spinal cord as well as for resection of intracranial lesions, to ensure safety and viability of signal transduction pathways during the intraoperative period. Specific techniques include intraoperative EEG, evoked-potential monitoring, electromyography, and so forth. Anesthetic agents have significant impact on the amplitude and latency of these signals. It is important to maintain a stable and compatible anesthetic technique in order to facilitate successful monitoring, thereby ensuring a successful surgery and outcome. Intraoperative loss of these signals or an acute change in the amplitude and/or latency warrants immediate attention from all the involved personnel. Some of the causes of acute change in signals include hypotension, acute hypoxia, hypothermia, change in anesthetic medications, severe anemia, or position injury of the nerve under monitoring. Surgical factors include excessive traction on or around the susceptible area, nerve injury, and so forth. It is important to recognize these potential causes and treat them immediately in order to prevent long-term morbidity. The surgeon should be notified immediately to correct any surgical cause of these changes.

NEUROSURGICAL EMERGENCIES IN PEDIATRIC PATIENTS

Pediatric patients pose a unique set of challenges to the anesthesiologist, when presented with an acute neurosurgical emergency. The challenges are due to differences in the disease pathophysiology between children and adults as well as smaller body habitus, reduced blood volume, and decreased ability to cope with stress, especially in neonates. In addition, signs and symptoms of increased ICP may often be nonspecific or difficult to assess in a very young child. The following is an overview of the common causes of neurosurgical emergencies and their management:

- Severe head trauma: increased intracranial pressure and possible herniation can occur because of skull fractures with or without associated intracranial hematoma. Immediate surgical intervention is necessary, along with medical management of increased ICP.
- Rupture of cerebral arteriovenous malformation, which necessitatrd immediate surgical intervention. Perioperative BP control is important in this setting.
- Intraoperative hemodynamic instability, especially with surgeries around the brainstem, usually resolves with cessation of stimulation. At times, treatment with intravenous glycopyrrolate and/or atropine may be required. Very rarely, injected epinephrine and/or transcutaneous pacing is necessary.
- Seizures and status epilepticus management should be performed as noted above.
- Meningocele and meningomyelocele are usually diagnosed in utero, before birth, with ultrasound. Meningoceles can occur anywhere along the craniocaudal tract. Delivery of the baby is planned in a tertiary medical center with dedicated

neonatal ICU as well as pediatric neurosurgical and care team facilities. Treatment involves surgical closure of the defect within a day or 2 after birth, to prevent infection and protect the exposed spinal cord and meninges.

DISCLOSURE

The authors have nothing to disclose.

REFERENCES

1. Available at: http://www.traumaticbraininjury.com/symptoms-of-tbi/glasgow-comascale/. Accessed May 10, 2019.
2. Molnar C, Nemes C, Szabo S, et al. Harvey Cushing, a pioneer of neuroanesthesia. J Anesth 2008;22(4):483–6.
3. McLone D. Pediatric neurosurgery: surgery of the developing nervous system. 4th edition. Philadelphia: W.B. Saunders; 2001. p. 626.
4. Godoy DA, Seifi A, Garza D, et al. Hyperventilation therapy for control of posttraumatic intracranial hypertension. Front Neurol 2017;8:250.
5. SAFE Study Investigators, Australian and New Zealand Intensive Care Society Clinical Trials Group, Australian Red Cross Blood Service. Saline or albumin for fluid resuscitation in patients with traumatic brain injury. N Engl J Med 2007; 357:874.
6. Manninen PH, Lam AM, Gelb AW, et al. The effect of high-dose mannitol on serum and urine electrolytes and osmolality in neurosurgical patients. Can J Anaesth 1987;34:442.
7. Fanous AA, Tick RC, Gu EY, et al. Life-threatening mannitol-induced hyperkalemia in neurosurgical patients. World Neurosurg 2016;91:672.e5.
8. Rovlias A, Kotsou S. The influence of hyperglycemia on neurological outcome in patients with severe head injury. Neurosurgery 2000;46:335.
9. Available at: https://braintrauma.org/uploads/03/12/Guidelines_for_Management_of_Severe_TBI_4th_Edition.pdf. Accessed May 10, 2019.
10. Puccio AM, Fisher MR, Jankowitz BT, et al. Induced normothermia attenuates intracranial hypertension and reduces fever burden after severe traumatic brain injury. Neurocrit Care 2009;11:82.
11. Roberts I, Sydenham E. Barbiturates for acute traumatic brain injury. Cochrane Database Syst Rev 2012;(12):CD000033.
12. Brain Trauma Foundation, American Association of Neurological Surgeons, Congress of Neurological Surgeons, Joint Section on Neurotrauma and Critical Care, AANS/CNS, Bratton SL, Chestnut RM, Ghajar J, et al. Guidelines for the management of severe traumatic brain injury. XI. Anesthetics, analgesics, and sedatives. J Neurotrauma 2007;24(Suppl 1):S71.
13. Jourdan C, Convert J, Mottolese C, et al. Evaluation of the clinical benefit of decompression hemicraniectomy in intracranial hypertension not controlled by medical treatment. Neurochirurgie 1993;39:304 [in French].
14. Cooper DJ, Rosenfeld JV, Murray L, et al. Decompressive craniectomy in diffuse traumatic brain injury. N Engl J Med 2011;364:1493.
15. Hutchinson PJ, Kolias AG, Timofeev IS, et al. Trial of decompressive craniectomy for traumatic intracranial hypertension. N Engl J Med 2016;375:1119.
16. Meretoja A, Strbian D, Putaala J, et al. SMASH-U: a proposal for etiologic classification of intracerebral hemorrhage. Stroke 2012;43:2592–7.

17. Kuramatsu JB, Gerner ST, Schellinger PD, et al. Anticoagulant reversal, blood pressure levels, and anticoagulant resumption in patients with anticoagulation-related intracerebral hemorrhage. JAMA 2015;313:824–36.

18. Lees KR, Bluhmki E, von Kummer R, et al. Time to treatment with intravenous alteplase and outcome in stroke: an updated pooled analysis of ECASS, ATLANTIS, NINDS, and EPITHET trials. Lancet 2010;375(9727):1695.

19. Schönenberger S, Uhlmann L, Hacke W, et al. Effect of conscious sedation vs general anesthesia on early neurological improvement among patients with ischemic stroke undergoing endovascular thrombectomy: a randomized clinical trial. JAMA 2016;316(19):1986–96.

20. Simonsen CZ, Yoo AJ, Sørensen LH, et al. Effect of general anesthesia and conscious sedation during endovascular therapy on infarct growth and clinical outcomes in acute ischemic stroke: a randomized clinical trial. JAMA Neurol 2018;75(4):470–7.

21. Lazzaro MA, Novakovic RL, Alexandrov AV, et al. Developing practice recommendations for endovascular revascularization for acute ischemic stroke. Neurology 2012;79(13 Suppl 1):S243.

22. Liebeskind DS. Cerebral aneurysms. Treatment and management. Available at: https://emedicine.medscape.com/article/1161518-treatment#d8. Accessed May 10, 2019.

23. Chee LC, Siregar JA, Ghani ARI, et al. The factors associated with outcomes in surgically managed ruptured cerebral aneurysm. Malays J Med Sci 2018;25(1): 32–41.

24. Avitsian R, Fiorella D, Soliman MM, et al. Anesthetic considerations of selective intra-arterial nicardipine injection for intracranial vasospasm: a case series. J Neurosurg Anesthesiol 2007;19(2):125–9.

25. Avitsian R, Schubert A. Anesthetic considerations for intraoperative management of cerebrovascular disease in neurovascular surgical procedures. Anesthesiol Clin 2007;25(3):441–63.

26. Winter SF, Santaguida C, Wong J, et al. Systemic and topical use of tranexamic acid in spinal surgery: a systematic review. Global Spine J 2016;6(3):284–95.

Anesthesia for Obstetric Disasters

Kristen L. Fardelmann, MD*, Aymen Awad Alian, MBBCh

KEYWORDS

- Maternal mortality • Maternal cardiac arrest • Postpartum hemorrhage
- HELLP syndrome • Amniotic fluid embolism • High neuraxial blockade
- Local anesthetic systemic toxicity

KEY POINTS

- In the United States, increases in cardiovascular disease, cardiomyopathy, and cerebrovascular accidents are significantly contributing to the increase in maternal mortality.
- Over the past 30 years, maternal mortality secondary to obstetric hemorrhage, hypertensive disorders of pregnancy, and anesthetic complications has improved.
- Obstetric hemorrhage remains the leading contributor to maternal cardiac arrest in the United States.
- Knowledge of best practices in obstetric anesthesia is critical to effectively manage obstetric hemorrhage, hypertensive emergency, HELLP syndrome, amniotic fluid embolism, high neuraxial blockade, local anesthetic systemic toxicity, and the difficult obstetric airway.

MATERNAL MORTALITY

In 1986, the Centers for Disease Control and Prevention initiated surveillance of maternal deaths.[1] Pregnancy-related death is defined as the "death of a woman while pregnant or within 1 year of the end of a pregnancy that was caused by pregnancy or its physiologic effects, a complication of the pregnancy or its management."[1] Between 1987 and 2013, maternal mortality in the United States increased from 7.2 to 18.0 deaths per 100,000 live births.[1]

Traditional causes of maternal mortality, such as hemorrhage, hypertensive disorders of pregnancy, and anesthesia complications, are declining. Changes in data acquisition and maternal comorbid disease, including increasing maternal age, obesity, hypertension, diabetes, and chronic heart disease, have been suggested as contributors to increased mortality.[2–5] **Fig. 1** depicts the changes in cause of maternal mortality between 1987 to 1990 and 2011 to 2013.[2]

Department of Anesthesiology, Yale School of Medicine, 333 Cedar Street, PO Box 208051, New Haven, CT 06520-8051, USA
* Corresponding author.
E-mail address: kristen.fardelmann@yale.edu

Anesthesiology Clin 38 (2020) 85–105
https://doi.org/10.1016/j.anclin.2019.10.005   anesthesiology.theclinics.com
1932-2275/20/© 2019 Elsevier Inc. All rights reserved.

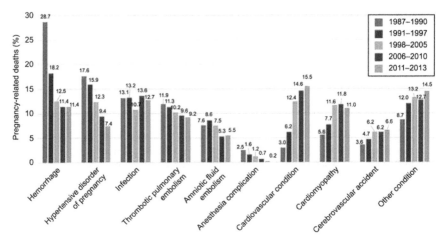

Fig. 1. Population-level, cause-specific proportionate pregnancy-related mortality (%) for 1987 to 1990 and 2011 to 2013. (*Adapted from* Creanga AA, Syverson C, Seed K, et al. Pregnancy-Related Mortality in the United States, 2011-2013. Obstet Gyneco 2017;130(2):366-373; with permission.)

Racial and ethnic disparities are prevalent, with 43.5 deaths per 100,000 live births of non-Hispanic black women followed by other races, non-Hispanic white women, and Hispanic women at 14.4, 12.7, and 11.0, respectively.[2] Differences in socioeconomic status and payer classification play a role in maternal morbidity with foreign-born parturients contributing to 50% of maternal mortality in Hispanic and women of other race.[2,6]

Despite the unclear and multifactorial contributors, it is important to assess the cause of maternal mortality to direct education and best practices and to improve maternal and fetal outcomes.

CARDIAC ARREST IN PREGNANCY

Although rare, maternal cardiac arrest may lead to significant maternal and fetal morbidity and mortality. Population-based data in the United States, the United Kingdom, and Canada reveal an estimated incidence between 1:12,000 and 36,000 hospitalizations for delivery with survival rates to hospital discharge between 40.7% and 71.3%.[7–10]

Maternal risk factors for cardiac arrest in pregnancy include parturients who are greater than 35 years of age, gestational age less than 37 weeks, multiparity (≥4 births), non-Hispanic black parturients, and Medicaid patients. Maternal and obstetric comorbid conditions associated with cardiac arrest are outlined in **Table 1**.[8–10] Hemorrhage remains the leading contributor of maternal cardiac arrest in the United States with other precipitating causes outlined in **Table 2**.[8–10] Survival is dependent on cause with the highest survival seen with aspiration pneumonitis, anaphylaxis, local anesthetic systemic toxicity (LAST), magnesium toxicity, and anesthesia complications.[8] Survival was less likely if cardiac arrest occurred outside the hospital, if the patient was moved before perimortem cesarean delivery (PMCD), or if PMCD was delayed.[10]

Guidelines and recommendations (**Table 3**) for the treatment of cardiac arrest in pregnancy are provided by the American Heart Association and the Society for

Table 1	
Comorbidities associated with cardiac arrest in pregnancy	
Maternal conditions	• Pulmonary hypertension • Malignancy • Cardiovascular disease ○ Hypertensive disorders of pregnancy • Liver disease • Diseases of the nervous system • Lower-respiratory tract diseases • Systemic lupus erythematous • Chronic renal disease • Sickle cell disease • Drug abuse/dependence • Gestational diabetes
Obstetric conditions	• Stillbirth • Cesarean delivery • Severe preeclampsia/eclampsia • Morbidly adherent placenta • Placental abruption • Polyhydramnios • Placenta previa

Data from Refs.[8–10]

Obstetric Anesthesia and Perinatology.[11–13] Suboptimal knowledge and management of cardiac arrest in pregnancy have been identified in several studies with multidisciplinary simulation and more frequent teaching/certification critical to improving delivery of evidence-based care.[7,14–16]

OBSTETRIC COMPLICATIONS
Obstetric Hemorrhage

Maternal hemorrhage is the leading cause of cardiac arrest during hospitalization for delivery in the United States.[8,17] Survival of maternal hemorrhage continues to improve but is associated with blood transfusion and hysterectomy.[2,18,19] The American College of Obstetricians and Gynecologists' reVITALize program has recently redefined postpartum hemorrhage (PPH) as "total blood loss greater than or equal to 1000 mL or blood loss accompanied by signs or symptoms of hypovolemia within 24 hours after delivery regardless of mode of delivery."[17]

Independent of the risk factors for PPH by diagnosis, maternal age less than 20 and greater than 35 years, delivery at hospitals with less than 271 annual deliveries, Hispanic ethnicity, and Asian/Pacific Islander ancestry are additional risk factors.[2,17,19,20]

The etiology of PPH is multifactorial[17–19]:
- Uterine atony (70-80% of cases)
- Retained placenta (10%)
- Coagulopathy (5%)
- Trauma

Labor that is prolonged or induced, especially with prolonged use of oxytocin for augmentation or induction, increases risk of uterine atony.[17–19] Pregnancies complicated by maternal multiparity, chorioamnionitis, multiple gestation, polyhydramnios, macrosomia, uterine fibroids, stillbirth, and preeclampsia also increase

Table 2
Precipitating causes of maternal cardiac arrest

Cause	Mhyre et al,[8] 2017 (%)	Beckett et al,[9] 2014 (%)	Balki et al,[10] 2017 (%)
Hypovolemia/hemorrhage	—	16.7	—
Postpartum	27.9	—	39.2
Antepartum	16.8	—	15.4
Intrapartum	—	—	4.9
Cardiac	—	7.7	—
Heart failure	13.3	2.6	31.5
Acute myocardial infarction	3.1	—	1.0
Aortic dissection/rupture	0.3	2.6	1.4
Cardiac tamponade	—	1.3	—
Embolism	—	—	5.9
AFE	13.3	17.9	12.6
Venous thromboembolism	7.1	14.1	—
Sepsis	11.2	1.3	8.7
Anesthesia complications	7.8	21.8	12.6
Eclampsia	6.1	—	6.9
Cerebrovascular disorder	4.4	3.8	4.6
Trauma	2.6	—	3.1
Obstetric trauma	—	—	12.2
Hypoxia	—	5.1	—
Aspiration pneumonitis	7.1	—	—
Pulmonary edema	2.4	—	4.6
Status asthmaticus	1.1	1.3	—
Toxic drug	—	1.3	—
Magnesium toxicity	1.4	—	—
Anaphylaxis	0.3	1.3	—
Pulmonary artery rupture	—	1.7	—

Data from Refs.[8–10]

risk for uterine atony.[17–19] Cesarean delivery with or without labor, especially if performed under general anesthesia in comparison to neuraxial anesthesia, is associated with uterine atony.[17–19] Significant trauma leading to PPH is seen with lacerations, hematomas, uterine rupture, episiotomy, precipitous delivery, and operative vaginal delivery.[17–19] Morbidly adherent placentation, previous uterine surgery, placenta previa, and succenturiate placenta have been identified as risk factors for retained placenta.[17–19] Coagulopathy may be due to an underlying inherited clotting disorder or use of anticoagulation but may also be a result of maternal and pregnancy related complications including amniotic fluid embolism, hemorrhage, placental abruption, fetal demise, infection, preeclampsia/eclampsia/HELLP syndrome, or dilutional.[17–19]

Anesthetic management of PPH is reviewed (**Table 4**) and emphasizes early activation of obstetric hemorrhage protocols, use of goal-directed blood product replacement, and appropriate use of agents that increase uterine muscle tone (uterotonic agents).[17,21–26]

Table 3 Management of maternal cardiac arrest	
Intervention:	**Specific Recommendations:**
CALL FOR HELP and Initiate Basic Life Support/Advanced Cardiovascular Life Support Obstetric Anesthesiologist, Obstetrician, and Neonatal Intensive Care Unit Team	
High-quality chest compressions	• Supine positioning with backboard • Hand placement: Place heel of 1 hand on the lower half of sternum and the heel of the other on top of the first hand in parallel • Rate: 100 per minute • Depth: At least 2 inches (allow for recoil) • Compression:ventilation of 30:2 • Minimize interruptions (<10 s) • Change providers every 2 min or as needed

Early defibrillation	• Place automated external defibrillator: Anterolateral pad placement
	  ○ Lateral pad under left breast tissue
	• Energy requirements are the same as in nonobstetric patients
	  ○ Biphasic shock: 120–200 J
	• Resume high-quality cardiopulmonary resuscitation (CPR) after defibrillation
	• Do not delay defibrillation for removal of fetal monitors

Left uterine displacement	• Continuous manual displacement
	  ○ Lift uterus up and off maternal vessels
	  ○ Perform if uterus is at or above the umbilicus

Airway management	• Anticipate difficult airway • Minimize trauma • Ventilate with 8–10 breaths/min • Monitor for continuous capnography • Use endotracheal tube of small inner diameter
Medications	• Use usual ACLS drug doses • Discontinue intravenous (IV) magnesium ○ Give IV/intraosseous (IO) calcium chloride 10 mL in 10% solution or calcium gluconate 30 mL in 10% solution
Volume assessment	• Assess for hypovolemia/hemorrhage • IV access above the diaphragm
PMCD	• If return of spontaneous circulation does not occur by 4 min, initiate PMCD with goal of delivery by 5 min ○ Uterus should extend at or above the umbilicus and remain in LUD • Do not delay PMCD for transportation to operating room • Do not delay for appropriate antiseptic technique • Do not delay for equipment; only a scalpel is needed
Fetal assessment	• Fetal assessment should not be performed during resuscitation • Remove or detach fetal monitors as soon as possible to facilitate PMCD
Immediate postarrest care	• Refer to articles referenced for further reading

Data from Refs.[11–13]

Table 4 Anesthetic management of postpartum hemorrhage	
CALL FOR HELP!	
Early assessment	• Quantify estimated blood loss
Hemodynamics	• Consider invasive blood pressure monitoring (should not delay other interventions) • Vasopressor administration to maintain systolic blood pressure >90 mm Hg
Obtain adequate IV/IO access	• Above the diaphragm

Fluid and blood product resuscitation	• Activate massive transfusion protocol
	• Inconsistent recommendations exist for fixed ratio transfusions:
	  ○ Suggested total transfusion red blood cell (RBC):plasma ratio of 2:1 (NPMS)
	  ○ Administer apheresis platelets every 6–8 units of RBCs (NPMS)
	• Consider early fibrinogen Administration
	  ○ Cryoprecipitate
	  ○ Fibrinogen concentrate

Point-of-care coagulation testing	Early coagulation assessment with goal-directed product replacement • ROTEM/thromboelastography (TEG) • Laboratory coagulation evaluation
Tranexamic acid	• Dose: 1 g administered IV over 10–15 min. A second dose may be administered 30 min later if hemorrhage persists or within 24 h if hemorrhage returns • Most effective if administered within 3 h of hemorrhage event
Uterotonic agents	• Oxytocin • Methylergonovine • 15-methyl prostaglandin F_{2alpha} • Misoprostol

Cell salvage	• Safe and effective in obstetrics
	  ○ Current techniques have limited concerns for:
	    ■ AFE
	      • Leukocyte depletion filters
	    ■ Maternal alloimmunization
	      • Rho (D) immune globulin administration

Other considerations	• Maintain normothermia • Manage electrolyte abnormalities ○ Calcium replacement

Data from Refs.[17,21–26]

The pillar of medical management in PPH secondary to uterine atony includes the use of four uterotonic agents:

- Oxytocin
- Methylergonovine
- 15-methyl prostaglandin F_{2alpha}
- Misoprostol

Primarily administered via intravenous infusion, oxytocin is dosed between 10-40 units per 1000 mL over 30-60 minutes and titrated to adequate uterine tone.[17,21] If administered via intramuscular route, a one-time dose of 10 units is given.[17,21] Side effects include nausea, vomiting, hyponatremia, decreased blood pressure, and increased heart rate.[17,21] Caution should be taken in patients with hypersensitivity to oxytocin and with intravenous bolus administration as this may lead to hemodynamic instability.[17,21] Methylergonovine is administered via an intramuscular dose of 200 mcg every 2-4 hours.[17,21] The side effect profile includes nausea, vomiting, and hypertension.[17,21] Caution should be taken in patients with a hypertensive disorder of pregnancy, chronic hypertension, or heart disease due to the possibility of severe hypertensive response and the end organ risks of hypertensive crisis including cerebral hemorrhage in these clinical scenarios.[17,21] 15-methyl prostaglandin F_{2alpha} is dosed intramuscular or intramyometrial at 250 mcg as frequently as every 15 minutes with a maximum of 8 doses in 24 hours.[17,21] Common effects of 15-methyl prostaglandin F_{2alpha} include nausea, vomiting, diarrhea, fever, headache, and shivering. Caution should be taken in patients with asthma, cardiac disease, pulmonary disease, pulmonary hypertension, and hepatic disease.[17,21] Severe bronchospasm may be seen with the use of 15-methyl prostaglandin F_{2alpha}.[17,21] Finally, misoprostol, formulated in 100-200 mcg tablets, is a one-time dosed medication administered via buccal/sublingual or per rectum route in 400-1000 mcg doses.[17,21] Nausea, vomiting, diarrhea, fever, and headache are common side effects of misoprostol administration with cautioned use in patients with hypersensitivity to this medication.[17,21]

In 2015, the National Partnership for Maternal Safety (NPMS) created an evidence based maternal hemorrhage safety bundle (https://safehealthcarefor everywoman.org) with the goal to improve maternal outcomes through implementation in all birthing facilities within the United States.[22]

Amniotic Fluid Embolism/Anaphylactoid Syndrome of Pregnancy

Amniotic fluid embolism (AFE) is a rare, but potentially devastating event with an estimated incidence between 1.7 and 6.6 per 100,000 maternities and mortality of 0.3 to 1.7 per 100,000 maternities.[27–32] Parturients greater than 35 years of age, multiple gestation pregnancy, placenta previa, induction of labor, cesarean delivery, and instrumental vaginal delivery have been associated with AFE.[27,28]

The suspected cause is characterized by entrance of fetal tissue into the maternal circulation leading to activation of the immune system and an anaphylactoid response.[31,32]

AFE is a clinical diagnosis of exclusion with potential signs and symptoms (**Table 5**) and no absolute diagnostic criteria.[30–32] Rotational thromboelastometry (ROTEM) has been suggested as a point-of-care test to aid diagnosis and management (**Fig. 2**).[33,34] Tryptase, C3 and C4 levels, Sialyl-Tn, C1 esterase inhibitor, and insulin-like growth factor binding protein-1 are a few examples of potential diagnostic biomarkers.[30,32,35] However, the application of these acute phase reactants for diagnostic purposes is controversial because levels are likely abnormal in many critically ill parturients.[30,31] In 2016, the Society for Maternal-Fetal Medicine created recommendations for diagnosis and treatment of AFE (**Table 6**).[31]

Anesthetic management (**Table 7**) consists of supportive care and includes treatment of cardiac and respiratory collapse and hematologic abnormalities.[30–32] Two case reports suggest a role of atropine, ondansetron, and ketorolac administration in treatment of AFE; however, further evaluation is warranted.[36,37]

Table 5
Clinical signs and symptoms of amniotic fluid embolism

Neurologic	*Cardiovascular*

• Altered mental status
  • Disorientation, restlessness, agitation, numbness/tingling
• Seizure
• Unresponsiveness
	• Chest pain
	• Lightheadedness
	• Hypotension
	• Arrhythmia
	• Heart failure
	  ○ Initial phase: Right ventricular failure
	  ○ Secondary phase: Left ventricular failure
	• Pulmonary hypertension
	• Cardiac arrest

Respiratory	*Hematologic*
• Shortness of breath • Hypoxia • Pulmonary edema • Respiratory insufficiency/failure • Acute respiratory distress syndrome	• Maternal hemorrhage • Coagulopathy • Disseminated intravascular coagulation

Data from Refs.[30–32]

Hypertensive Emergency in Pregnancy

Severe hypertension is a significant contributor to maternal mortality with cerebrovascular hemorrhage, myocardial ischemia, and congestive heart failure unfortunate consequences. Diagnostic criteria for hypertensive emergency in pregnancy include a systolic blood pressure greater than 160 mm Hg and/or diastolic blood pressure greater than 110 mm Hg at least 15 minutes apart.[38,39]

Goals of therapy include decreasing blood pressure to less than 155 to 160/100 to 110 mm Hg to prevent severe maternal morbidity and mortality while maintaining adequate uteroplacental perfusion and fetal oxygenation.[39–41] **Table 8** outlines appropriate medication management options for the pregnant patient.[38–40] Timing is critical with early recognition and intervention within 30 to 60 minutes having the potential to decrease preventable complications.[38]

Intracranial hemorrhage remains the leading cause of death during hypertensive emergency in pregnancy.[42] Over a 60-year period, early antenatal detection and improved, protocoled clinical management have all contributed to the decrease in maternal death from 9.74 to 0.09 per 100,000 maternities secondary to hypertensive disorders of pregnancy in the United Kingdom.[38,42] In 2017, the NPMS created a consensus bundle for hypertensive emergency during pregnancy and the postpartum period (https://safehealthcareforeverywoman.org/) to assist all labor and delivery units in the United States with protocol development and implementation.[38]

HELLP Syndrome

HELLP is an acronym for the clinical features of this obstetric condition often accompanying preeclampsia and hallmarked by microangiopathic hemolytic anemia, elevated liver enzymes, and low platelets (**Table 9**).[43] Because of the rarity and inconsistent diagnostic criteria, the incidence is difficult to assess, but there is obvious significant maternal and fetal morbidity and mortality with mortality estimated around 1% for the parturient (**Table 10**).[43–45] Parturients greater than 35 years of age, who are nullipara, with a hypertensive disorder in a previous

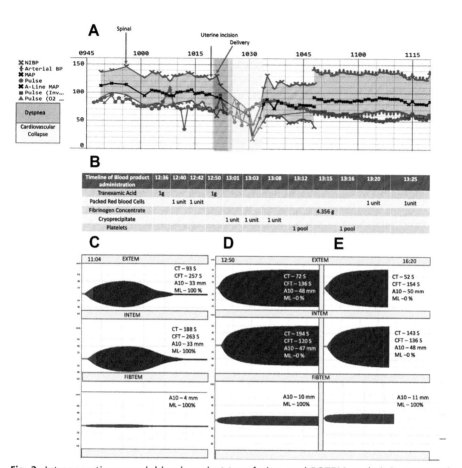

Fig. 2. Intraoperative record, blood product transfusion, and ROTEM analysis in suspected AFE. Severe bradycardia with profound hypotension (*A*). Coagulation profile and blood sample for ROTEM analysis were sent given increased intraoperative bleeding. Blood products administered (*B*). ROTEM results confirmed disseminated intravascular coagulation with hyperfibrinolysis and a consumption of coagulation factors (*C*). Fibrinogen concentrate was used as a bridge to treat hypofibrinogenemia while awaiting cryoprecipitate. Follow-up ROTEM analysis revealed improvement of coagulation (*D*, *E*). A10, amplitude 10 minutes after clotting time; BP, blood pressure; CFT, clot formation time; CT, clotting time, MAP, mean arterial pressure; ML, maximum lysis; NIBP, non-invasive blood pressure.

pregnancy, and with a multiple gestation pregnancy are at increased risk of HELLP syndrome.[45]

Key components of anesthetic management are detailed in **Table 11**.[43,45] Because of risks associated with both general anesthesia and neuraxial anesthesia in the setting of HELLP syndrome, early neuraxial placement should be considered in all patients. High-dose dexamethasone or betamethasone has been used to improve clinical and laboratory findings, including platelet count, to allow for neuraxial anesthesia placement, prolongation of pregnancy for fetal lung maturity, and increased possibility of cervical ripening and successful vaginal delivery.[43,46,47] Some studies have shown clinically significant improvement in maternal and fetal morbidity; however, a reduction in maternal and neonatal mortality has not been found.[43,46,47] In a Cochrane Review

Table 6
Society for Maternal-Fetal Medicine recommendations for diagnosis and treatment of amniotic fluid embolism

	Evidence Grade
We recommend consideration of AFE in the differential diagnosis of sudden cardiorespiratory collapse in the laboring or recently delivered woman.	1C
We do not recommend the use of any specific diagnostic laboratory test to either confirm or refute the diagnosis of AFE; at the present time, AFE remains a clinical diagnosis.	1C
We recommend the provision of immediate high-quality cardiopulmonary resuscitation with standard BCLS and ACLS protocols in patients who develop cardiac arrest associated with AFE.	1C
We recommend that a multidisciplinary team, including anesthesia, respiratory therapy, critical care, and maternal-fetal medicine, should be involved in ongoing care of women with AFE.	Best Practice
Following cardiac arrest with AFE, we recommend immediate delivery in the presence of a fetus ≥23 wks gestation.	2C
We recommend the provision of adequate oxygenation and ventilation and, when indicated by hemodynamic status, the use of vasopressors and inotropic agents in the initial management of AFE. Excessive fluid administration should be avoided.	1C
Because coagulopathy may follow cardiovascular collapse with AFE, we recommend early assessment of clotting status and early aggressive management of clinical bleeding with standard massive transfusion protocols.	1C

Adapted from Society for Maternal-Fetal Medicine (SMFM), Pacheco LD, Saade G, et al. Amniotic fluid embolism: diagnosis and management. Am J Obstet Gynecol 2016;215(2):B23; with permission.

published in 2010, the most significant improvement in platelet count was seen with dexamethasone use when compared with betamethasone and with the antenatal initiation of corticosteroid therapy.[46]

Martin[48] discusses the "3 tenets" of HELLP syndrome management as potent glucocorticoids, intravenous magnesium sulfate, and systolic blood pressure control.[48] Of utmost importance is systolic blood pressure control because hypertensive emergency and maternal intracranial hemorrhage have been the leading contributors to maternal mortality in the setting of HELLP syndrome.

ANESTHESIA COMPLICATIONS
High Neuraxial Anesthesia Blockade

High neuraxial anesthesia blockade (HNAB) may occur in the setting of epidural anesthesia via unintentional injection of local anesthetic into the subarachnoid or subdural space, migration of an epidural catheter into the subdural or subarachnoid space, or overdose of local anesthetic in the spinal or epidural space. The Serious Complications Repository Project identifies the incidence of high neuraxial block as 1:4336 obstetric anesthetics with unrecognized spinal catheters identified in 1:15,435 obstetric anesthetics.[49] Twenty percent (11/55) of regional anesthetic liability claims in obstetrics between 2000 and 2011 were a result of HNAB.[50] Obesity, use of spinal technique after failed epidural

Table 7
Management of amniotic fluid embolism

CALL FOR HELP!	
Cardiovascular	*Respiratory*
• BLS/ACLS	• 100% Oxygen
○ High-quality CPR/early defibrillation	○ Goal oxygen saturation >90%
○ Left uterine displacement	• Consider advanced airway
○ Obtain adequate IV/IO access	○ Avoid hypoxia, hypercarbia, acidemia
○ Consider vasopressor/inotropic support	○ Low tidal volume
■ Norepinephrine, dobutamine,	○ High respiratory rate
milrinone, vasopressin	○ High positive end-expiratory pressure
• Consider limiting fluid administration	• Consider inhaled nitric oxide
• Consider echocardiogram evaluation	• Consider aerosolized prostacyclin
• Consider extracorporeal membrane oxygenation	
Hematologic	*Fetal Considerations*
• Early evaluation for coagulopathy	• Call neonatology service
○ Thromboelastography	• Delivery
■ ROTEM/TEG	○ Assisted second-stage vaginal delivery
○ Laboratory evaluation	○ Cesarean delivery
■ Complete blood count, prothrombin	○ PMCD
time/international normalized ratio,	■ Delivery goal within 5 min of cardiac
partial thromboplastin time,	arrest
fibrinogen	
• Goal directed treatment of hemorrhage/ coagulopathy	
○ Activate massive transfusion protocol	
■ Red blood cell transfusion	
■ Cryoprecipitate transfusion	
■ Fresh frozen plasma transfusion	
■ Platelet transfusion	
○ Fibrinogen concentrate	
○ Tranexamic acid	
○ Aggressive treatment of uterine atony	
○ Surgical intervention	
Future/Novel Treatments	
• Plasma exchange	
• High-dose corticosteroids	
• C1 esterase inhibitors	
• Ketorolac	
• Atropine	
• Ondansetron	

Data from Refs.[30–32]

anesthesia, height less than 60 inches, epidural anesthesia after wet tap, and spinal deformities are risk factors for high neuraxial blockade in the obstetric patient.[49,50]

Signs and symptoms of HNAB are outlined in **Table 12** and consist of neurologic, cardiovascular, respiratory, and fetal components. Anesthetic management of HNAB is outlined in **Table 13**.[51] It is important to recognize that all patients with signs and symptoms of HNAB may still have awareness. Providing continuous communication and reassurance to the patient is essential in addition to early consideration of sedative-hypnotic agents such as midazolam.

Table 8
Medication management of hypertensive emergency in pregnancy

Medication	Dose/Route/Frequency	Onset of Action	Considerations	Therapy Level
Initiate treatment within 30–60 min				
Labetalol	20 → 40 → 80 mg IV every 10 min × 3 subsequent doses (maximum [max] dose: 220 mg IV)	5–10 min	• Neonatal bradycardia • Neonatal hypoglycemia • Precaution for patients with asthma, heart disease, and heart failure	First line
Hydralazine	5–10 → 10 mg IV every 20 min × 2 subsequent doses (max dose: 20 mg IV)	10–20 min	• Risk of maternal hypotension, tachycardia • Neonatal thrombocytopenia	First line
Nifedipine	10 → 20 → 20 mg orally every 20 min × 3 subsequent doses	10–20 min	• Increases maternal heart rate • Precaution in women with coronary artery disease, diabetes mellitus, or aortic stenosis • Increased risk of sudden cardiac arrest in women >45 y of age	First line (No IV access needed)
Consult an Anesthesiologist				
Nicardipine	Infusion of 5 mg/h with increase of 2.5 mg/h every 5 min to maximum of 15 mg/h	10–15 min		Second line
Esmolol	Infusion		• Transient fetal bradycardia	Second line

Data from Refs.[38–40]

Table 9	
Diagnostic features of HELLP syndrome	
Hemolysis	• Abnormal peripheral blood smear • Bilirubin level >1.2 mg/dL • Lactic dehydrogenase >600 IU/L
Elevated liver enzymes	• Aspartate aminotransferase ≥70 IU/L • Lactic dehydrogenase >600 IU/L
Low platelets	• Platelet count <100,000/mm^3

Data from Sibai BM. Diagnosis, Controversies, and Management of the Syndrome of Hemolysis, Elevated Liver Enzymes, and Low Platelet Count. Obstet Gynecol 2004;103(5 Pt 1):981-991.

Table 10			
Maternal morbidity associated with HELLP syndrome			
Disseminated intravascular coagulation	Pulmonary edema	Subcapsular liver hematoma/liver hemorrhage	Acute respiratory distress syndrome
Placental abruption	Acute renal failure	Liver failure	Sepsis
Stroke	Death	Preterm delivery	Retinal detachment
Cerebral edema	Laryngeal edema		

Data from Refs.[43–45]

Table 11	
Anesthetic management of HELLP syndrome	
Hypertension	• See section earlier in the text entitled 'Hypertensive Emergency in Pregnancy' • Goal blood pressure <155–160/100–110 mm Hg
Seizure prophylaxis	• IV magnesium sulfate

Hematologic abnormalities	• Risk for hemorrhage
	  ○ Obtain adequate IV access
	  ○ Prepare RBC for transfusion
	• Platelet count
	  ○ Consider dexamethasone administration to increase platelet count
	  ○ Platelet transfusion:
	    ■ Hemorrhage
	    ■ Platelet count <20,000/mm^3
	• Assess coagulation
	  ○ ROTEM

Anesthetic risk assessment	• General anesthesia
	  ○ Risk of hypertensive emergency and difficult airway
	• Neuraxial anesthesia
	  ○ Risk of spinal-epidural hematoma

Data from Sibai BM. Diagnosis, Controversies, and Management of the Syndrome of Hemoly-sis, Elevated Liver Enzymes, and Low Platelet Count. Obstet Gynecol 2004;103(5 Pt 1):981-991; and Fitz-patrick KE, Hinshaw K, Kurinczuk JJ, et al. Risk Factors, Management, and Outcomes of Hemolysis, Elevated Liver Enzymes, and Low Platelets Syndrome and Elevated Liver Enzymes, Low Platelets Syndrome. Obstet Gynecol 2014;123(3):618-627.

Table 12	
Signs and symptoms of high neuraxial anesthesia blockade	
Neurologic	• Motor and sensory blockade • Agitation • Inability to communicate • Loss of consciousness
Cardiovascular	• Hypotension • Bradycardia • Cardiac arrest
Respiratory	• Dyspnea • Apnea
Fetus	• Nonreassuring fetal tracing

Data from Wong CA. Epidural and Spinal Analgesia: Anesthesia for Labor and Vaginal Delivery. In: Chestnut DH, Wong CA, Tsen LC, et al., editors. Chestnut's Obstetric Anesthesia, 6th edition. Philadelphia: Elsevier; 2020.

Local Anesthetic Systemic Toxicity

The incidence of LAST is reported between 0.34 and 1.9/1000 peripheral nerve blocks.[52] The Serious Complication Repository Project reports 1 obstetric cardiac arrest attributed to LAST from a nonneuraxial intravascular injection.[48] Recent case reports in parturients have involved the use of TAP (transversus abdominis plane) blocks for postcesarean analgesia.[53–56]

Pregnancy is a risk factor for LAST with potential mechanisms, including increased availability of free drug in the setting of decreased protein binding, increased risk of arrhythmia from the effects of estradiol and progesterone on cardiomyocyte physiology, increased neuronal sensitivity to local anesthetics lowering the seizure threshold, and increased epidural vein distention with possible increased intravascular uptake and/or catheter migration.[52,55]

The presentation of LAST is variable with no obvious progression of signs or symptoms (**Table 14**).[52] Onset may occur immediately as a consequence of intravascular injection or more commonly be delayed 30 to 60 minutes from slow systemic uptake.[52]

Table 13	
Management of high neuraxial anesthetic blockade	
CALL FOR HELP! Alert Obstetricians!	
Neurologic	• Continue communication with patient • Consider sedative-hypnotic
Cardiovascular	• Continuous electrocardiogram and vital signs monitoring • Left uterine displacement • Administer IV fluid resuscitation • Vasopressor support ○ Epinephrine
Respiratory	• Provide 100% oxygenation and ventilation • Consider intubation
Fetal	• Continuous fetal heart rate monitoring

Adapted from Wong CA. Epidural and Spinal Analgesia: Anesthesia for Labor and Vaginal Delivery. In: Chestnut DH, Wong CA, Tsen LC, et al., editors. Chestnut's Obstetric Anesthesia, 6th edition. Philadelphia: Elsevier; 2020.

Table 14	
Signs and symptoms of local anesthetic systemic toxicity	
Central nervous system	Nonspecific: Metallic taste, paresthesias, perioral numbness, diplopia, auditory changes, tinnitus, dizziness
	Excitation: Altered mental status, psychiatric symptoms, agitation, confusion, muscle twitching, seizures
	Depression: Drowsiness, lethargy, coma, respiratory arrest
Cardiovascular system	Tachycardia, hypertension, tachyarrhythmias, hypotension, conduction blockade, bradycardia, asystole, ventricular tachycardia, ventricular fibrillation, or torsades de pointes

Data from Neal JM, Barrington MJ, Fettiplace MR, et al. The Third American Society of Regional Anesthesia and Pain Medicine Practice Advisory on Local Anesthetic Systemic Toxicity: Executive Summary 2017. Reg Anesth Pain Med 2018;43(2):113-123.

Techniques applied to prevent LAST include use of the lowest effective dose, incremental aspiration and injection, intravascular markers, ultrasound guidance, and identification of at-risk patients.[52,57] In 2017, the American Society of Regional Anesthesia and Pain Medicine published an updated version of the LAST checklist, which highlights significant components of resuscitation (**Box 1**).[52,58]

Difficult Airway

Failed tracheal intubation remains a significant concern for anesthesiologists with an estimated incidence of 2.6 to 4.5 per 1000 general anesthetics in the obstetric patient

---

Box 1
Key components of local anesthetic systemic toxicity treatment

- Discontinue local anesthetic injection

- Call for HELP!

- Administer lipid emulsion 20% therapy:
  - Bolus administered over 2 to 3 minutes:
    - Weight greater than 70 kg: 100 mL
    - Weight less than 70 kg: 1.5 mL/kg
  - Infusion administered over 15 to 20 minutes:
    - Weight greater than 70 kg: 200 to 250 mL
    - Weight less than 70 kg: 0.25 mL/kg/min
  - If patient remains unstable:
    - Rebolus once or twice and double infusion rate
  - Maximum dose: 12 mL/kg

- If indicated:
  - Start BLS/ACLS
    - Reduce epinephrine boluses: ≤1 μg/kg
    - Avoid vasopressin, calcium channel blockers, β-blockers, and local anesthetics
  - Airway management: Provide 100% oxygen and ventilation as needed
  - Seizure management: Benzodiazepines

Data from Neal JM, Barrington MJ, Fettiplace MR, et al. The Third American Society of Regional Anesthesia and Pain Medicine Practice Advisory on Local Anesthetic Systemic Toxicity: Executive Summary 2017. Reg Anesth Pain Med 2018;43(2):113-123; and Neal JM, Woodward CM, Harrison TK. The American Society of Regional Anesthesia and Pain Medicine Checklist for Managing Local Anesthetic Systemic Toxicity: 2017 Version. Reg Anesth Pain Med 2018;43(2):150-153.

Table 15
Physiologic respiratory changes in pregnancy

Physiologic Change	Consequence
Vascular engorgement and mucosal edema	Increased airway bleeding and edema Increased Mallampati score Worsening airway examination with progression of pregnancy and labor
Decreased functional residual capacity	Early desaturation
Increased oxygen demand	Early desaturation
Reduced lower esophageal sphincter tone	Increased risk of aspiration
Delayed gastric emptying • Pain in labor • Opioid administration	Increased risk of aspiration
Enlarged breast tissue	Difficult laryngoscope insertion

Data from Mushambi MC, Kinsella SM, Popat M, et al. Obstetric Anaesthetists' Association and Difficult Airway Society guidelines for the management of difficult and failed tracheal intubation in obstetrics. Anaesthesia 2015;70(11):1286-1306.

(GA) and 2.3 per 1000 GA for cesarean section.[59,60] Maternal mortality secondary to failed intubation is estimated at 2.3 per 100,000 GA for cesarean section with hypoxemia and aspiration leading causes.[59] Admission to the neonatal intensive care unit is independently associated with failed intubation and poor maternal oxygenation.[59] Data from the UK Obstetric Surveillance System suggest increasing age, higher body mass index (BMI), and a recorded Mallampati score greater than 1 as independent predictors of failed tracheal intubation with every 1-kg/m^2 increase in BMI correlating with a 7% increased risk of failed tracheal intubation for obese women.[60] A recent prospective study suggests neck circumference greater than 39.5 cm, chest circumference/sternomental distance greater than 7.1, and pregnancy weight gain of greater than 11.7 kg as new predictors of difficult intubation during obstetric GA.[61]

Physiologic changes in pregnancy contribute to difficult airway management (**Table 15**).[62] Because the pressure of emergent GA induction is paramount in the setting of maternal and/or fetal distress, early evaluation, optimization of positioning, and availability of necessary equipment are essential (**Table 16**).[63] Although the

Table 16
Management of obstetric patients at risk for general anesthesia

Early airway assessment	• Early communication with obstetricians for patients at risk of difficult airway
Aspiration prevention	• Consider restriction of oral intake beyond clear liquids in patients at high risk for emergency cesarean delivery • Consider administration of antacids, H2-receptor antagonists, and metoclopramide
Neuraxial anesthesia	• Consider early neuraxial placement in patients with anticipated difficult airway

Data from Practice guidelines for obstetric anesthesia: an updated report by the American Society of Anesthesiologists Task Force on Obstetric Anesthesia and the Society for Obstetric Anesthesia and Perinatology. Anesthesiology 2016;124:270-300.

Table 17
Key components of airway management in the parturient

Preinduction	• Ensure presence of advanced airway devices and suction • Optimize patient positioning • Early preoxygenation • Rapid sequence induction
Laryngoscopy	• Minimize attempts (<3) • Reassess positioning • Consider alternative laryngoscope device • Subsequent attempts by experienced providers

Failed tracheal intubation	• Call for help
	• Maintain oxygenation
	  ○ Facemask ventilation
	  ○ Supraglottic airway device

Cannot intubate, cannot ventilate	• Call for help • Surgical airway • Prepare for cardiac arrest and PMCD
Cesarean delivery	• Consider awakening patient if surgery is not emergent

Data from Mushambi MC, Kinsella SM, Popat M, et al. Obstetric Anaesthetists' Association and Difficult Airway Society guidelines for the management of difficult and failed tracheal intubation in obstetrics. Anaesthesia 2015;70(11):1286-1306.

optimal scenario is to provide surgical anesthesia without manipulation of the airway via neuraxial techniques, when required, it is essential to know the key components of difficult airway management in the parturient (**Table 17**).[62]

DISCLOSURE

The authors have nothing to disclose.

REFERENCES

1. Centers for Disease Control and Prevention. Pregnancy related mortality surveillance. Available at: https://www.cdc.gov/reproductivehealth/maternalinfanthealth/pregnancy-mortality-surveillance-system.htm. Accessed January 3, 2019.
2. Creanga AA, Syverson C, Seed K, et al. Pregnancy-related mortality in the United States, 2011-2013. Obstet Gynecol 2017;130(2):366–73.
3. Creanga AA, Berg CJ, Ko JY, et al. Maternal mortality and morbidity in the United States: where are we now? J Womens Health (Larchmt) 2014;23(1):3–9.
4. Joseph KS, Lisonkova S, Muraca GM, et al. Factors underlying the temporal increase in maternal mortality in the United States. Obstet Gynecol 2017;129: 91–100.
5. Callaghan WM, Creanga AA, Kuklina EV. Severe maternal morbidity among delivery and postpartum hospitalizations in the United States. Obstet Gynecol 2012; 120:1029–36.
6. Creanga AA, Bateman BT, Kuklina EV, et al. Racial and ethnic disparities in severe maternal morbidity: a multistate analysis, 2008-2010. Am J Obstet Gynecol 2014;210(5):435.e1-8.
7. Zelop CM, Einav S, Mhyre JM, et al. Characteristics and outcomes of maternal cardiac arrest: a descriptive analysis of Get with the guidelines data. Resuscitation 2018;132:17–20.

8. Mhyre JM, Tsen LC, Einav S, et al. Cardiac arrest during hospitalization for delivery in the United States, 1998-2011. Anesthesiology 2014;120:810–8.
9. Beckett VA, Knight M, Sharpe P. The CAPS Study: incidence, management and outcomes of cardiac arrest in pregnancy in the UK: a prospective, descriptive study. BJOG 2017;124:1374–81.
10. Balki M, Liu S, Leon JA, et al. Epidemiology of cardiac arrest during hospitalization for delivery in Canada: a nationwide study. Anesth Analg 2017;124:890–7.
11. Jeejeebhoy FM, Zelop CM, Lipman S, et al. Cardiac arrest in pregnancy: a scientific statement from the American Heart Association. Circulation 2015;132: 1747–73.
12. Lipman S, Cohen S, Einav S, et al. The Society for Obstetric Anesthesia and Perinatology consensus statement on the management of cardiac arrest in pregnancy. Anesth Analg 2014;118:1003–16.
13. Hui D, Morrison LJ, Windrim R, et al. The American Heart Association 2010 guidelines for the management of cardiac arrest in pregnancy: consensus recommendations on implementation strategies. J Obstet Gynaecol Can 2011;33(8): 858–63.
14. Lipman SS, Daniels KI, Carvalho B, et al. Deficits in the provision of cardiopulmonary resuscitation during simulated obstetric crises. Am J Obstet Gynecol 2010; 203:179.e1-5.
15. Hards A, Davies S, Salman A, et al. Management of simulated maternal cardiac arrest by residents: didactic teaching versus electronic learning. Can J Anaesth 2012;59:852–60.
16. Adams J, Cepeda Brito JR, Baker L, et al. Management of maternal cardiac arrest in the third trimester of pregnancy: a simulation-based pilot study. Crit Care Res Pract 2016;2016:5283765.
17. Committee on Practice Bulletins-Obstetrics, Shields LE, Goffman D, Caught AB. ACOG practice bulletin number 183: postpartum hemorrhage. Obstet Gynecol 2017;130(4):e168–86.
18. Kramer MS, Berg C, Abenhaim H, et al. Incidence, risk factors, and temporal trends in severe postpartum hemorrhage. Am J Obstet Gynecol 2013;209: 449.e1-7.
19. Bateman BT, Berman MF, Riley LE, et al. The epidemiology of postpartum hemorrhage in a large, nationwide sample of deliveries. Anesth Analg 2010;110: 1368–73.
20. Bryant A, Mhyre JM, Leffert LR, et al. The association of maternal race and ethnicity and the risk of postpartum hemorrhage. Anesth Analg 2012;115: 1127–36.
21. Lyndon A, Lagrew D, Shields L, et al. Improving health care response to obstetric hemorrhage version 2.0. A California quality improvement toolkit. Stamford (CA): California Maternal Quality Care Collaborative; Sacramento (CA): California Department of Public Health; 2015.
22. Main EK, Goffman D, Scavone BM, et al. National partnership for maternal safety: consensus bundle on obstetric hemorrhage. Anesth Analg 2015;121:142–8.
23. Shaylor R, Weiniger CF, Austin N, et al. National and international guidelines for patient blood management in obstetrics: a qualitative review. Anesth Analg 2017;124:216–32.
24. WOMAN Trial Collaborators. Effect of early tranexamic acid administration on mortality, hysterectomy, and other morbidities in women with postpartum hemorrhage (WOMAN): an international, randomized, double-blind, placebo-controlled trial. Lancet 2017;389:2105–16.

25. Pacheco LD, Hanking GDV, Saad AF, et al. Tranexamic acid for the management of obstetric hemorrhage. Obstet Gynecol 2017;130:765–9.

26. Goucher H, Wong CA, Patel SK, et al. Cell salvage in obstetrics. Anesth Analg 2015;121:465–8.

27. Fitzpatrick KE, Tuffnell D, Kurinczuk JJ, et al. Incidence, risk factors, management and outcomes of amniotic-fluid embolism: a population-based cohort and nested case-control study. BJOG 2016;123:100–9.

28. Knight M, Berg C, Brocklehurst P, et al. Amniotic fluid embolism incidence, risk factors and outcomes: a review and recommendations. BMC Pregnancy Childbirth 2012;12:7.

29. Bonnet MP, Zlotnik D, Saucedo M, et al, for the French National Experts Committee on Maternal Mortality. Maternal death due to amniotic fluid embolism: a national study in France. Anesth Analg 2018;126:175–82.

30. Clark SL. Amniotic fluid embolism. Obstet Gynecol 2014;123:337–48.

31. Society for Maternal-Fetal Medicine (SMFM), Pacheco LD, Saade G, Hankins GDV, et al. SMFM Clinical Guidelines No. 9: amniotic fluid embolism: diagnosis and management. Am J Obstet Gynecol 2016;215:B16–24.

32. Sultan P, Seligman K, Carvalho B. Amniotic fluid embolism: update and review. Curr Opin Anesthesiol 2016;29:288–96.

33. Loughran JA, Kitchen TL, Sindhakar S, et al. Rotational thromboelastometry (ROTEM)-guided diagnosis and management of amniotic fluid embolism. Int J Obstet Anesth 2019;38:127–30.

34. Pujolle E, Mercier FJ, Le Gouez A. Rotational thromboelastometry as a tool in the diagnosis and management of amniotic fluid embolism. Int J Obstet Anesth 2019; 38:146–7.

35. Legrand M, Rossignol M, Dreux S, et al. Diagnostic accuracy of insulin-like growth factor binding protein-1 for amniotic fluid embolism. Crit Care Med 2012;40(7):2059–63.

36. Rezai S, Hughes AC, Larsen TB, et al. Atypical amniotic fluid embolism managed with a novel therapeutic regimen. Case Rep Obstet Gynecol 2017;2017:8458375.

37. Copper PL, Otto MP, Leighton BL. Successful management of cardiac arrest from amniotic fluid embolism with ondansetron, metoclopramide, atropine, and ketorolac: a case report. 2013. SOAP Abstract S47.

38. Bernstein PS, Martin JN Jr, Barton JR, et al. National Partnership for Maternal Safety: consensus bundle on severe hypertension during pregnancy and the postpartum period. Obstet Gynecol 2017;130:347–57.

39. American College of Obstetrics and Gynecology Committee Opinion No. 767: emergent therapy for acute-onset, severe hypertension during pregnancy and the postpartum period. Obstet Gynecol 2019;133:e174–80.

40. Dyer RA, Swanevelder JL, Bateman BT. Hypertensive disorders. In: Chestnut DH, Wong CA, Tsen LC, et al, editors. Chestnut's obstetric anesthesia. Philadelphia: Elsevier; 2019. p. 840–78.

41. Martin JN Jr, Thigpen BD, Moore RC, et al. Stroke and severe preeclampsia and eclampsia: a paradigm shift focusing on systolic blood pressure. Obstet Gynecol 2005;105(2):246–54.

42. Conti-Ramsden F, Knight M, Green M, et al. Reducing maternal deaths from hypertensive disorders: learning from confidential inquiries. BMJ 2019;364:1230.

43. Sibai BM. Diagnosis, controversies, and management of the syndrome of hemolysis, elevated liver enzymes, and low platelet count. Obstet Gynecol 2004;103: 981–91.

44. Sibai BM, Ramadan MK, Usta I, et al. Maternal morbidity and mortality in 442 pregnancies with hemolysis, elevated liver enzymes, and low platelets (HELLP syndrome). Am J Obstet Gynecol 1993;169:1000–6.
45. Fitzpatrick KE, Hinshaw K, Kurinczuk JJ, et al. Risk factors, management, and outcomes of hemolysis, elevated liver enzymes, and low platelets syndrome and elevated liver enzymes, low platelets syndrome. Obstet Gynecol 2014;123:618–27.
46. Woudstra DM, Chandra S, Hofmeyr GJ, et al. Corticosteroids for HELLP (hemolysis, elevated liver enzymes, low platelets) syndrome in pregnancy. Cochrane Database Syst Rev 2010;(9):CD008148.
47. Martin JN, Rose CH, Briery CM. Understanding and managing HELLP syndrome: the integral role of aggressive glucocorticoids for mother and child. Am J Obstet Gynecol 2006;195:914–34.
48. Martin JN. Milestones in the quest for best management of patients with HELLP syndrome (microangiopathic hemolytic anemia, hepatic dysfunction, thrombocytopenia). Int J Gynaecol Obstet 2013;121:202–7.
49. D'Angelo R, Smiley RM, Riley ET, et al. Serious complications related to obstetric anesthesia: the serious complication repository project of the Society for Obstetric Anesthesia and Perinatology. Anesthesiology 2014;120:1505–12.
50. Davies JM, Stephens LS. Obstetric anesthesia liability concerns. Clin Obstet Gynecol 2017;60(2):431–46.
51. Wong CA. Epidural and spinal analgesia: anesthesia for labor and vaginal delivery. In: Chestnut DH, Wong CA, Tsen LC, et al, editors. Chestnut's obstetric anesthesia. Philadelphia: Elsevier; 2019. p. 474–539.
52. Neal JM, Barrington MJ, Fettiplace MR, et al. The Third American Society of Regional Anesthesia and Pain Medicine practice advisory on local anesthetic systemic toxicity. Reg Anesth Pain Med 2018;43:113–23.
53. Weiss E, Jolly C, Dumoulin JL, et al. Convulsions in 2 patients after bilateral ultrasound-guided transversus abdominis plane blocks for cesarean analgesia. Reg Anesth Pain Med 2014;39:248–51.
54. Naidu RK, Richebe P. Probable local anesthetic systemic toxicity in a postpartum patient with acute fatty liver of pregnancy after a transversus abdominis plane block. A A Case Rep 2013;1:72–4.
55. Griffiths JD, Le NV, Grant S, et al. Symptomatic local anaesthetic toxicity and plasma ropivacaine concentrations after transversus abdominis plane block for caesarean section. Br J Anaesth 2013;110(6):996–1000.
56. Bern S, Weinberg G. Local anesthetic toxicity and lipid resuscitation in pregnancy. Curr Opin Anesthesiol 2011;24:262–7.
57. Barrington MJ, Kluger R. Ultrasound guidance reduces the risk of local anesthetic systemic toxicity following peripheral nerve blockade. Reg Anesth Pain Med 2013;38:289–99.
58. Neal JM, Woodward CM, Harrison TK. The American Society of Regional Anesthesia and Pain Medicine checklist for managing local anesthetic systemic toxicity: 2017 version. Reg Anesth Pain Med 2018;43:150–3.
59. Kinsella SM, Winton AL, Mushambi MC, et al. Failed tracheal intubation during obstetric general anesthesia: a literature review. Int J Obstet Anaesth 2015;24:356–74.
60. Quinn AC, Milne D, Columb M, et al. Failed tracheal intubation in obstetric anaesthesia: 2 yr national case-control study in the UK. Br J Anaesth 2013;110(1):74–80.

61. Jarraya A, Choura D, Mejdoub Y, et al. New predictors of difficult intubation in obstetric patients: a prospective observational study. Trends in Anaesthesia and Critical Care 2019;24:22–5.
62. Mushambi MC, Kinsella SM, Popat M, et al. Obstetric Anaesthetists' Association and Difficult Airway Society guidelines for the management of difficult and failed tracheal intubation in obstetrics. Anaesthesia 2015;70:1286–306.
63. Practice guidelines for obstetric anesthesia: an updated report by the American Society of Anesthesiologists Task Force on Obstetric Anesthesia and the Society for Obstetric Anesthesia and Perinatology. Anesthesiology 2016;124:270–300.

Perioperative Management of Patients with Sepsis and Septic Shock, Part I

Systematic Approach

Nibras Bughrara, MD[a,b,*], Stephanie Cha, MD[c,d],
Radwan Safa, MD[a,b], Aliaksei Pustavoitau, MD, MHS[e]

KEYWORDS

- Sepsis • Septic shock • Anesthesia management • Resuscitation
- Goal directed therapy

KEY POINTS

- Sepsis and septic shock are common medical emergencies, with high associated mortality and health care expenses.
- Sepsis is the presence of life-threatening organ dysfunction caused by dysregulated host response to infection.
- Septic shock is identified by persistent hypotension requiring vasopressor to maintain a mean arterial pressure of 65 mm Hg and serum lactate level of greater than 2 mmol/L despite adequate fluid resuscitation.
- The pillars for managing patients with septic shock are early recognition and administration of appropriate antimicrobial therapy, hemodynamic resuscitation, and timely source control.
- Anesthesiologists frequently encounter sepsis in their practice when source control is required; thus, they are uniquely equipped to positively impact survival because they possess the skills set for hemodynamic resuscitation, invasive monitoring, and organ systems support.

[a] Department of Anesthesiology, Albany Medical College, 47 New Scotland Avenue, MC 131, Albany, NY 12208, USA; [b] Department of Surgery, Albany Medical College, 47 New Scotland Avenue, MC 131, Albany, NY 12208, USA; [c] Division of Cardiothoracic Anesthesiology, Johns Hopkins University School of Medicine, 1800 Orleans Street, Suite 6216, Baltimore, MD 21287, USA; [d] Division of Critical Care, Johns Hopkins University School of Medicine, 1800 Orleans Street, Suite 6216, Baltimore, MD 21287, USA; [e] Division of Adult Critical Care Medicine, Johns Hopkins University School of Medicine, 600 North Wolfe Street, Meyer 297, Baltimore, MD 21287, USA
* Corresponding author. 47 New Scotland Avenue, MC 131, Albany, NY 12208.
E-mail address: bughran@amc.edu
Twitter: @BughraraNibras (N.B.)

Anesthesiology Clin 38 (2020) 107–122
https://doi.org/10.1016/j.anclin.2019.10.013
anesthesiology.theclinics.com
1932-2275/20/© 2019 Elsevier Inc. All rights reserved.

INTRODUCTION

Sepsis and septic shock have an estimated incidence of 1 million cases in the United States alone, making it increasingly likely for anesthesiologists to encounter such a patient.[1] In addition to a mortality rate exceeding 40% in septic shock,[2] sepsis is the most expensive condition treated and billed to Medicare.[3,4] Restoration of adequate organ perfusion along with timely antimicrobial agents and source control are the pillars of sepsis and septic shock management. Perioperative physicians play a key role in facilitating timely source control and managing patient hemodynamics to maintain adequate tissue perfusion, thereby having a direct impact on the outcomes of this vulnerable patient population.

DEFINITIONS

In 2002, the Society of Critical Care Medicine and European Society of Intensive Care Medicine created a collaborative global initiative, the Surviving Sepsis Campaign (SSC), with the goal to reduce morbidity and mortality from sepsis and septic shock worldwide. Over the years, the SSC developed and revised twice sepsis definitions. Currently, sepsis is defined as "infection complicated by life threatening organ dysfunction due to dysregulated host response." We describe the evolution of sepsis definitions.

Sepsis 1.0 definitions were based on systemic inflammatory response syndrome (SIRS) criteria combined with suspected infection. The presence of organ dysfunction defined severe sepsis. The main problem with SIRS criteria was their lack of specificity; for example, many patients preoperatively who experience anxiety with associated tachycardia and tachypnea do not have sepsis.[5]

Sepsis 2.0 definitions mandated the presence of organ dysfunction to call infection sepsis, but kept SIRS criteria in the definition, thus, eliminating severe sepsis concept. The definition of septic shock stayed similar to sepsis 1.0 definitions, with the addition of elevated serum lactate.[6]

Sepsis 3.0 definitions removed SIRS criteria. Instead, the Sequential Organ Failure Assessment (SOFA) score was used to define organ dysfunction, with sepsis being defined by increase in the score by 2 or equal to 2 if baseline SOFA score is not known. For screening purposed, quick SOFA score, based on 3 criteria describing neurologic (Glasgow Coma Scale of <15), cardiovascular (systolic blood pressure of <100 mm Hg), and respiratory (respiratory rate of >22/min) dysfunction can be used clinically to identify patients at high risk for sepsis. Septic shock was defined as the initiation and sustained need for vasopressor treatment to maintain a mean arterial pressure of greater than 65 mm Hg or a serum lactate level of greater than 2 $mmol/L^{-1}$.[7]

PATHOPHYSIOLOGY OF SEPTIC SHOCK

The associated excessive production of nitric oxide and other vasodilating substances depresses metabolic autoregulation of vascular tone,[8] in addition to frequently decreased levels of endogenous vasopressin,[9] all leading to a decrease in systemic vascular resistance and systemic blood pressure consistent with distributive shock. When adequately fluid resuscitated patients present with warm skin, bounding pulse and wide pulse pressure, and when their baseline cardiac function is normal increased cardiac output (CO) results. Vasodilation affects both arterial and venous systems. Venous system becomes a large reservoir of blood and, in the absence of fluid resuscitation, cardiac preload decreases. Central hypovolemia is further exacerbated by the damage to the endothelial glycocalyx with loss of intravascular fluid into the extravascular compartment, presenting clinically with tissue edema. Not infrequently, myocardial contractility suffers. All these changes in preload, myocardial contractility, and afterload combined lead to significant reduction in oxygen delivery to tissues.

Septic shock alters tissue metabolism through its effects on mitochondrial function. Failure of energy metabolism presents with lactic acidosis.[10] The cumulative effects of hypoxia and cellular injury produce significant organ dysfunction including cardiovascular dysfunction (for details refer to Nibras Bughrara and colleagues' article, "Perioperative Management of Patient with Sepsis and Septic Shock, Part II: Ultrasound Support for Resuscitation," in this issue), central nervous dysfunction (delirium), lung injury (acute respiratory distress syndrome [ARDS]), acute kidney injury, coagulopathy, ileus and hepatic dysfunction, followed by prolonged recovery, which can last for weeks. The longer the patient stays in shock the more damage tissues sustain.

SURVIVING SEPSIS CAMPAIGN CARE BUNDLES

To standardize care, SSC published and serially updated management guidelines[11–14] and developed sepsis care bundles. Greater compliance (31.3% compared with 10.9% 2 years prior across 165 sites internationally) was associated with decrease in in-hospital mortality from 37.0% to 30.8%.[15] At present, the hour-1 bundle replaced 3- and 6-hour bundles to emphasizes the emergent nature of management of sepsis and septic shock and includes quality of care markers vital to improving patient outcomes. The components of hour-1 bundle are:

1. Measure, and if elevated level, remeasure lactate;
2. Obtain blood cultures;
3. Administer appropriate antimicrobials;
4. Resuscitate with volume; and
5. Vasopressors.

The fundamental rationale of the hour-1 bundle is the emphasis on the early delivery of all necessary components of care, with SSC realizing that not all of them may be achieved in the first hour of recognition (**Table 1**). Our recommendations in management of sepsis and septic shock follow framework outlined by the SSC guidelines.

Table 1		
SSC previously recommended 3- and 6-hour bundles and current hour-1 care bundle[a]		
3-Hour Bundle	**6-Hour Bundle**	**Hour-1 Bundle[b]**
Measure lactate	Start vasopressor for refractory	Measure lactate, remeasure if
Culture before	hypotension (MAP of <65)	initial lactate is >2 mmol/L
giving antibiotics	If hypotension persists evaluate:	Cultures before giving antibiotics
Administer broad	CVP	Administer broad spectrum
spectrum antibiotics	ScvO₂	antibiotics
Administer 30 mL/kg	Bedside cardiovascular	Begin rapid administration of
crystalloid for	ultrasound examination	30 mL/kg crystalloids for
hypotension or	Dynamic assessment of fluid	hypotension or lactate
increased lactate	responsiveness	≥4 mmol/L
	Remeasure lactate if elevated	Start vasopressors if patient is
		hypotensive during or after
		fluid resuscitation to maintain
		MAP ≥65 mm Hg

Abbreviations: CVP, central venous pressure; MAP, mean arterial pressure; ScvO₂, central venous oxygen saturation.
[a] Replaced the 3- and 6-hour bundles in 2018.
[b] Time zero is defined as the time of recognition of sepsis (meeting all elements of sepsis).

SOURCE CONTROL AND ANTIMICROBIAL THERAPY

Early initiation of appropriate antimicrobial agents and interventions to control the infectious source like drainage or debridement are the fundamental principles in managing patients with sepsis and septic shock. These complementary components of care decrease the microbial load and its toxic burden, subsequently decreasing inflammatory response, cellular dysfunction, and tissue injury.[8]

In the first 6 hours, delay in initiating effective antimicrobial therapy increases the mortality rate by 7% per hour.[16] Failure to deliver appropriate antimicrobial therapy results in 5-fold increase in in-hospital mortality in patients with septic shock when compared with patients who received inappropriate antibiotic therapy.[17] Although appropriate cultures (including 2 sets of blood cultures from 2 separate sites) should be obtained before administering antimicrobial therapy, the initiation of antimicrobial medications should not be delayed if there is a delay in obtaining cultures. The clinical approach to the initiation of antimicrobial therapy involves targeting the most likely and most resistant pathogen at the presumed infectious source, further supported by institutional antibiograms, and on occasion requiring coverage with antibiotics from different classes. For example, soft tissue infections tend to be predominantly caused by gram-positive bacteria and including empirical methicillin-resistant *Staphylococcus aureus* coverage is an important consideration. In the operating room (OR), it is important to administer antibiotics according to the schedule so that no doses are missed.

The second principle of antimicrobial therapy is to reduce antimicrobial resistance, this could be achieved by de-escalation, that is, narrowing down the antibiotics spectrum based on the culture results and limiting treatment duration to what can be supported by the literature.

To achieve control of the infection source, patients with sepsis and septic shock should undergo timely intervention, commonly accomplished through minimally invasive means either at the bedside, interventional radiology suite or OR. Damage control with the focus on source control is the guiding principle, with subsequent hemodynamic stabilization in the intensive care unit (ICU). Definitive surgery should only be performed after the patient recovered from septic shock.

The 2 most common clinical settings for surgical source control are peritonitis and soft tissue infections. Timely control of the infection source is associated with decreases in mortality in patients with generalized postoperative peritonitis (mortality was 18% in the immediate control, 43% in the delayed control, and 100% in the no control groups),[18] early debridement in patients with necrotizing fasciitis was associated with improved survival, whereas delaying surgery for more than 24 hours was associated with increased mortality.[19]

HEMODYNAMIC RESUSCITATION

Resuscitation of patients with septic shock are based on optimizing CO by early intravenous fluids administration, vasopressor and sometimes, inotrope infusions.

Early goal-directed therapy (EGDT) is the underlying principle with set resuscitation targets involving central venous pressure (CVP) of 8 to 12 for volume administration, mean arterial pressure of greater than 65 for vasopressor infusion, and central venous oxygen saturation of greater than 70%. Adhering to these targets has shown for a 16% decrease in mortality.[11] A decade later, when EGDT was compared with usual care (when management is left to physicians' discretion and central line insertion for central venous pressure and mixed venous oxygen saturation measurements were not mandated), there were no differences in mortality between the groups.[13–15] This could be because providers since the initial study broadly adhered to the fundamental concept of EGDT, delivering fluids early, even before randomization.

Intravenous Fluids

Giving appropriate volumes of fluid early is important to avoid tissue hypoperfusion and resulting organ dysfunction.[12–15] The SSC guidelines recommend initial administrations of at least 30 mL/kg of intravenous crystalloids within the first 3 hours. Patients who achieve the 3-hour bundle care goals have less hypotension and a 5% decrease in mortality.[20]

Although intravenous fluids improve organ perfusion, excessive fluid is associated with myocyte overstretch and worsening pulmonary and interstitial edema, all leading to increase in mortality.[21]

After the initial fluid resuscitation, additional fluids must be guided by frequent reassessment of hemodynamic status, with no single measurement being a definitive evidence of adequate fluid resuscitation. Markers of tissue perfusion and balance between oxygen supply and demand, such as mixed or central venous oxygen saturation or serum lactate concentrations, can be helpful. Static parameters like central venous pressure are poor predictors of fluid responsiveness.[22] Dynamic parameters have much better performance. Change in CO to passive leg raising test can be evaluated preoperatively. Stroke volume variation and pulse pressure variation of more than 12% are consistent with fluid responsiveness during positive-pressure ventilation in the anesthetized patients, where the conditions for proper assessment are easily met (controlled mechanical ventilation with no spontaneous efforts, large tidal volume of more than 8 mL/kg, respiratory rate of <30 bpm, and sinus rhythm assuming absence of right heart failure).[23]

When choosing intravenous fluid balanced crystalloids are preferred over 0.9% saline owing to a lower incidence in major adverse kidney events,[24] and over albumin owing to its expense and lack of clear advantage over crystalloids.[25] Resuscitation with starch is associated with increase need for renal replacement therapy (RRT) and should be avoided.[26]

Vasoactive Agents

Patients with persistent hypotension (mean arterial pressure of <65) despite adequate volume resuscitation require vasoactive agent(s) initiated early for greater shock control and to reduce incidence of pulmonary edema and arrhythmias.[27] The available options are catecholamines (norepinephrine [NE], dopamine, epinephrine), alpha-1 agonist phenylephrine, vasopressin and angiotensin II (ATII).

NE stimulates alpha- and beta1-adrenergic receptors and causes mostly vasoconstriction with some inotropic effect. Dopamine stimulates both adrenergic and dopaminergic receptors, with its predominant effects being dose dependent: in lower doses (3–10 μg/kg/min) it increases heart rate and CO, whereas in higher doses (>10 μg/kg/min) it causes vasoconstriction. Dopamine's side effects include arrhythmias and immunosuppression via prolactin. Notably, even in doses of 1 to 3 μg/kg/min it increases renal blood flow and urine output dopamine does not improve renal function.[28] When outcomes of patients with shock who receive NE and dopamine are compared, both groups have similar mortality for patients with septic shock,[29] however, patients in the dopamine group have more arrhythmias, particularly supraventricular. Thus, NE is the first-line therapy according to the SSC guidelines and must be initiated early, because mortality in patients with septic shock increases by 5.3% for every hour of delay in initiating NE to reach a goal mean arterial pressure of greater than 65.[30]

Vasopressin is an endopeptide that works at peripheral vasopressin receptors. Vasopressin causes vasoconstriction in renal efferent arterioles, which in turn increases the glomerular filtration rate. Some patients with septic shock experience vasopressin deficiency secondary to decrease in secretion. Despite these benefits, vasopressin infusion up to 0.06 units/min used early in patients with septic shock[31] did not decrease mortality or kidney failure-free days by 28 days, even though patients in vasopressin group required RRT less frequently. When vasopressin infusion (0.01–0.03 units/min) is added to NE when it reaches at least 5 μg/min, its effect is comparable with increasing the dose of NE infusion alone in patients with septic shock, even though it does not decrease mortality,[32] except in patients with less severe shock.

ATII is a part of the renin–angiotensin–aldosterone system, an additional hormonal system that is responsible for restoration of systemic blood pressure during hypotension. ATII is an effective vasopressor and reduces requirements for other vasopressors in patients with vasodilatory shock and normal or high CO who received more than 0.2 μg/kg/min of NE.[33] In a subgroup of patients with acute renal failure (ARF) the time to discontinuation of RRT through day 7 was shorter in the ATII group,[34] suggesting a benefit of ATII in these patients. However, patients who received ATII also had increased incidence of thromboembolic events (12.5% vs 5.0%). Overall, although ATII seems to be effective, uncertainty about its use in patients with low CO (as it was studied only in patients with normal to high CO) and safety concerns prevents its recommendation for routine use in patients with septic shock.

Inotropic medications can be selectively used in patients with septic shock who develop low CO. According to SSC, dobutamine is the first-line drug of choice; however, epinephrine can be considered. When epinephrine was compared with combination of NE and dobutamine for the management of septic shock, there was no difference in mortality as well as in safety outcomes.[35]

Monitors

Owing to their tenuous hemodynamic status, patients with septic shock require invasive blood pressure monitoring and frequently central venous access for the administration of vasoactive medications. In addition to blood pressure monitoring, arterial catheter allows serial evaluation of blood gases. Invasive arterial pressure monitoring also allows assessment of pulse pressure variation as a measure of fluid responsiveness.

INTRAOPERATIVE MANAGEMENT

Patients with septic shock are hemodynamically unstable; therefore, the risks of proceeding to the OR are only justified in urgent or emergent situations. Although time for perioperative optimization is limited, assessment of and adjustment of volume status and appropriate early administration of antibiotics should be routinely attended to (**Table 2**).

Induction of anesthesia must be controlled with the primary goal of minimizing hypotension and myocardial depression. The often-quoted tenet of titrate to effect is especially relevant in the patient with septic shock. Usually, lower doses of commonly used drugs are appropriate. Ketamine and etomidate are the only induction medications that might maintain hemodynamics at typical induction doses.

Ketamine is an NMDA-receptor agonist with sedative-hypnotic and analgesic properties. It is a sympathomimetic with direct negative inotropic activity, providing with hemodynamic stability in the physiologically unstressed patient; the sympathomimetic effect offsets any direct negative inotropic effect.[36] The negative inotropic effects of

Table 2
Perioperative management of patients with sepsis or septic shock

Management Domain	Management Plan
Preoperative care Hour-1 bundle	Measure lactate level Obtain appropriate cultures including 2 blood cultures from 2 different sites Administer appropriate broad-spectrum antimicrobial therapy Hemodynamic resuscitation with volume and vasopressors
Monitors	Use FOCUS to identify the hemodynamic phenotype if able Invasive arterial blood pressure monitoring, PPV, and continuous CO Central venous catheter Blood gases and serum lactate and ScvO$_2$ Urinary catheter for urine output monitoring
Volume resuscitation	Balanced crystalloids are preferred over 0.9% saline and albumin 30 mL/kg initial bolus Avoid starch solutions
Vasoactive and inotropic agents	Target MAP of >70–75 mm Hg before induction NE is the first line; titrate up to 35–90 μg/min Vasopressin up to 0.06 U/min Epinephrine up to 20–50 μg/min Dopamine and dobutamine also could be used Consider ATII (patients with normal or high CO)
Metabolic resuscitation	Hydrocortisone 100 mg IV bolus then 50 mg IV every 6 h Vitamin C Thiamine
Blood products	Transfuse PRBC to a goal hemoglobin of >7 Transfuse and keep platelets >50
Ventilator management	Lung protective strategies with TV 6 mL/kg of predicted body weight, minimal PEEP of 5, recruitment maneuvers Severe ARDS patient with high ventilator requirements should be transported and continued supported using ICU ventilators intraoperatively
Anesthetic plan	Choose the safest induction agent, titrate to effect and use as little as possible

Abbreviations: IV, intravenous; MAP, mean arterial pressure; PEEP, positive end-expiratory pressure; PPV, pulse pressure variation; ScvO$_2$, central venous oxygen saturation.

ketamine must be weighed more heavily in patients with septic shock because these patients may be catecholamine depleted. Ketamine is also a bronchodilator and immunomodulator, which can suppress cytokine production in a rat model of septic shock[37] as well as suppress neutrophil function.[38]

Etomidate, an imidazole derivative, is a GABA$_A$ receptor agonist. Etomidate does not cause vasodilation or myocardial suppression and provides hemodynamic stability during induction of anesthesia. A relevant side effect of etomidate is transient acute adrenal suppression through inhibition of 11β-hydroxylase,[39] although the clinical significance of this effect is not well-established. Although etomidate does not increase mortality in critically ill patients with any type of shock[40] use of etomidate for induction was associated with increased 28-day mortality specifically in patients with septic shock.[41] Thus, when using etomidate, a presumed etomidate-related increase in mortality months in the future must be weighed against the immediate threat to perfusion posed by an unstable induction. Additionally, transient adrenal suppression can be managed with steroid supplementation once the diagnosis is suspected.

Propofol, when titrated carefully in conjunction with vasopressors, remains a viable option for induction in the hemodynamically unstable septic patient. Propofol also has immunomodulatory effects, including the inhibition of a tumor necrosis factor-alpha–induced oxidative burst in neutrophils.[42]

Analgesia is a central component of any balanced anesthetic. Historically, opioids are the analgesic agents of choice. With the exception of remifentanil, all opioids undergo hepatic metabolism and renal excretion, making their effects and duration of action variable in the setting of hepatic or renal insufficiency, both of which are common in patients with septic shock. Remifentanil, which is metabolized by nonspecific tissue and plasma esterases, is therefore a reasonable choice for anesthetic adjunct. Remifentanil has minimal effects on myocardial contractility and decreases the minimal alveolar concentration of volatile anesthetics, all of which have vasodilating effects. One needs to be careful with the hypotension associated with remifentanil. In contrast, morphine should be avoided in patients with sepsis. Data from animal studies suggests that morphine may exacerbate sepsis by promoting sustained hyperinflammation.[43] Morphine's pharmacodynamics also make it a poor choice in patients with sepsis and organ dysfunction because morphine is hepatically metabolized to an active intermediate that is cleared renally.

NEUROMUSCULAR BLOCKING AGENTS

Sepsis-associated end-organ injury, particularly hepatic and renal dysfunction, impacts the pharmacokinetics of neuromuscular blocking agents (NMBA). The aminosteroid NMBAs (rocuronium, vecuronium, and pancuronium) are metabolized by the liver and excreted by the kidneys. Altered clearance and volume of distribution in the setting of renal and hepatic dysfunction lead to accumulation of the NMBA and its active metabolites.[44] In the patient with sepsis, the aminosteroid NMBAs have a much more variable duration of action compared with benzylisoquinolone NMBAs (atracurium and cisatracurium). Owing to their spontaneous clearance by Hoffman elimination, these NMBAs are preferred in patients with hepatic or renal dysfunction.

Succinylcholine, a depolarizing NMBA, is metabolized by plasma cholinesterases, making its metabolism and clearance independent of hepatic or renal function. However, the use of succinylcholine can result in acute hyperkalemia leading to cardiac arrhythmias. The risk of a significant hyperkalemia is greatest in conditions leading to upregulation of the acetylcholine receptor, including prolonged immobilization and burns, and in setting of acidosis.

In many cases, patients with sepsis are considered to have full stomach and rapid sequence induction and endotracheal intubation may be warranted with the associated risk of hemodynamic instability. Succinylcholine and rocuronium could be used to facilitate intubation during the rapid sequence. Concurrent titration of vasopressor agent bolus could alleviate hemodynamic effects of anesthetic agents; application of concentrated lidocaine to the airway and administration of remifentanil are other alternatives.

SEPTIC ENCEPHALOPATHY

Septic encephalopathy, a transient and reversible brain dysfunction, affects 30% to 70% of patients with sepsis.[45] Brain dysfunction is driven by inflammatory, ischemic, and neurotoxic processes, and ranges from delirium to coma. The development of delirium in critically ill patients is associated with increased mortality, ICU and hospital length of stay, increased health care costs, and increased rates of short- and long-term cognitive dysfunction.[46] When present, delirium may signal ongoing systemic hypoperfusion. The Society of Critical Care Medicine recommends routine monitoring of delirium through validated tools such as the Confusion Assessment Method of the Intensive Care Unit and implementation of the Awakening and Breathing Coordination, Choice of drugs, Delirium monitoring and management, Early mobility, and Family engagement bundle of care, which has demonstrated improved survival and delirium-free days.[47] Pharmacologic therapy may be used for symptom control, however, clinical trials consistently fail to demonstrate preventative or therapeutic benefit of antipsychotic medications in patients with delirium.[48]

LUNG INJURY AND VENTILATOR MANAGEMENT

Intraoperative ventilator management should aim to minimize lung injury. Data driving lung protective ventilation derives mainly from patients with ARDS. The largest trial demonstrated a 9% absolute mortality reduction (31% vs 39.8%) in patients with ARDS ventilated with 6 mL/kg predicted body weight versus 12 mL/kg predicted body weight, targeting a plateau pressure of less than 30 cm H_2O.[49] Low tidal volume techniques risk hypercapnia and exceptions may be necessary in special patient populations, for example, profound metabolic acidosis, short stature, right ventricular failure, high intracranial pressure, sickle cell crisis, or patients with very stiff chest/abdominal walls. Additional consideration involves targeting a driving pressure (plateau positive end-expiratory pressure [PEEP]) of less than 12 to 15 cm H_2O.[50] In patients with moderate or severe ARDS, a higher PEEP strategy is associated with lower mortality compared with a lower PEEP strategy.[51] Finally, for those with poor oxygenation and severe ARDS, recruitment maneuvers (re-recruitment of alveoli through transient increase in transpulmonary pressure) may be considered, although they should be performed with caution given the risk for profound hypotension.[52] During the perioperative period, the combination of low tidal volume ventilation, use of PEEP, and intermittent recruitment maneuvers in patients with no underlying lung disease also improve pulmonary outcomes (atelectasis, infection, and ARDS) and decrease hospital length of stay.

BLOOD TRANSFUSION

Blood component transfusion may become necessary owing to intraoperative surgical complications resulting in bleeding. Transfusions themselves can lead to immune suppression and transfusion-associated lung injury, which may exacerbate the pathophysiology of sepsis.

Current SSC recommendations advise red blood cell transfusion for a hemoglobin of less than 7.0 mg/dL in the absence of myocardial ischemia, hypoxemia, or acute hemorrhage.[53] This recommendation is based on similar 90-day mortality, rate of ischemic events, and use of life support in patients transfused for a hemoglobin trigger of 7.0 mg/dL versus 9.0 mg/dL.[54]

Sepsis may result in significant coagulopathy and ultimately, disseminated intravascular coagulation. Correction of coagulopathy is best guided by laboratory data or point-of-care testing, particularly viscoelastic testing such as thromboelastography and thromboelastometry.[55] Fresh frozen plasma should not be transfused in the absence of bleeding or planned invasive procedures.[56] Platelet transfusion may be considered if the absolute platelet count is less than 10,000/mL in the absence of bleeding, less than 20,000/mL if a significant risk for bleeding is present, and less than 50,000/mL when clinically active bleeding is present or invasive procedures are planned.[56]

LIVER FAILURE

The incidence of sepsis-associated liver dysfunction and failure ranges from 34% to 46% and 1.3% to 22%, respectively, and is greater in patients with preexisting liver dysfunction. Liver dysfunction is a predictor of sepsis-associated mortality.[57] Laboratory data may reflect abnormalities of liver synthesis (abnormal coagulation panel, platelet count), impaired clearance (lactemia), impaired gluconeogenesis and glycogenolysis (hypoglycemia), or acute cellular injury (elevated transaminases). In addition, elevation of serum bilirubin may signal hepatic dysfunction and is an important component of ICU prognostic scores, such as the SOFA score.

Intraoperative considerations include careful drug selection to avoid agents primarily dependent on hepatic metabolism and alertness to developing coagulopathy.[58] Point-of-care testing may help to guide the management of coagulopathy, and invasive continuous monitoring may assist in maintaining normotension and euvolemia. Currently, there are no specific therapies routinely recommended for hepatic protection.

RENAL FAILURE

ARF occurs in 23% of patients with severe sepsis and 51% patients in septic shock, and the combination of ARF and sepsis is associated with a 70% mortality.[59] ARF is now defined by the KDIGO classification system as an increase in serum creatinine of more than 3 times baseline or 4.0 mg/dL or greater, or the initiation of RRT.[60] The pathophysiology of ARF in sepsis is driven by cytokine-mediated induction of nitric oxide synthesis and decreased systemic vascular resistance, with an associated resistance to exogenous vasopressors and increase in plasma concentrations of endogenous vasoconstrictor hormones (catecholamines, ATII, and endothelin), leading to renal vascular vasoconstriction.

There are several preventative measures that have been studied. EGDT has demonstrated a decrease in multiorgan dysfunction scores. The treatment of hyperglycemia and the use of corticosteroids may lessen the severity of acute renal injury. Routine use of sodium bicarbonate therapy is not recommended in patients with pH of 7.15 or greater.[61] Intraoperative dosing of anesthetic agents should account for impaired renal function.

In patients with sepsis requiring RRT, there are no data to suggest a mortality benefit of its administration (continuous vs intermittent),[62] intensity (low dose vs high dose [>30 mL/kg/h]),[63] or timing (early vs late initiation).[64] In regard to timing of RRT before surgery, current data suggest RRT the day before surgery, with a greater incidence of hypotension if performed within 7 hours of surgery.[65]

GLYCEMIC CONTROL

Hyperglycemia is associated with a number of adverse cellular and clinical effects, including myocardial oxygen imbalance, endothelial dysfunction, and impaired immune function, all exacerbated in sepsis. Although initially intensive insulin therapy demonstrated mortality benefit,[66] all current data suggest no difference in mortality[67] or increase in mortality[68] in patients receiving intensive insulin therapy compared with standard insulin therapy, and an appropriate glycemic target is less than 180 mg/dL to avoid hyperglycemia.

ADRENAL INSUFFICIENCY

Corticosteroids may be beneficial in the treatment of septic shock if adequate fluid resuscitation and vasopressor therapy are unable to restore hemodynamic stability with contradictory results regarding a decrease in 28-day mortality.[69] When administering corticosteroids, the recommended dose is 200 mg hydrocortisone per day, with tapering of dose after discontinuation of vasopressors. Corticosteroids are not recommended prophylactically because there is no evidence for decreasing the incidence of sepsis and septic shock, and their use can be associated with significant increases in hyperglycemia and hypernatremia.[69]

VITAMIN C AND THIAMINE

Vitamin C and thiamine may improve the pathophysiology of sepsis. Vitamin C plays a role in the maintenance of endothelial integrity, and its depletion contributes to increased capillary permeability.[70] In burn patients, vitamin C decreases 24-hour total fluid gain and duration of mechanical ventilation.[71] Thiamine (vitamin B_1) is often depleted in septic patients, and is thought to play a role in maintaining mitochondrial homeostasis and lactate clearance.[72] When combined with hydrocortisone, vitamin C and thiamine were associated with shortening the duration of vasopressor therapy and decreased mortality.[73] Vitamin C, however, should be administered with caution, because it may exacerbate acute kidney injury through dose-dependent oxalate excretion.[74]

NONPHARMACOLOGIC SUPPORT

Hemodynamically unstable septic patients with cardiac dysfunction can be considered for mechanical cardiac support. Although an intra-aortic balloon pump may be beneficial in patients on high doses of pharmacologic support, its use may worsen already low systemic vascular resistance. Extracorporeal membrane oxygenation has limited application, because the survival of patients receiving extracorporeal membrane oxygenation support for refractory septic shock is low (22%), with 0% survival for those initiated with extracorporeal membrane oxygenation of greater than 30.5 hours after the onset of shock.[32] Extracorporeal endotoxin removal remains largely experimental.[75,76]

TRANSITION OF CARE TO THE INTENSIVE CARE UNIT

Definitive source control is the cornerstone of sepsis management, may require surgery, and should occur within 6 to 12 hours after diagnoses (see section above on Source control and antimicrobial therapy). In addition, sepsis can develop intraoperatively owing to complications (leak, contamination, translocation). Providers should maintain high awareness of sepsis, because its recognition is confounded by concomitant inflammatory response to surgery-induced tissue injury. Patients with sepsis and septic shock tend to get worse for hours or even days before they get better, informing the decision to extubate.

Postoperatively, the patient is commonly transported to the ICU, and providers must be prepared to recognize and manage dangerous changes in physiology. This requires transporting with adequate monitoring, airway management devices, and medications. Similarly, OR–ICU handoffs are critically important to ensure team recognition of sepsis, and achieving hour-1 bundle elements of care. **Table 3** lists important elements of OR–ICU handoffs.

Table 3
Information elements discussed during transition of care from the OR to ICU

Category	Information Elements
Monitoring and support	Introduction of team members Monitors used Airway, lines and tubes Intraoperative ventilator settings Current continuous infusions or fluid therapies Surgical drains and instructions for management (eg, suction)
Patient history	Patient-specific information: age, weight, allergies, past medical/surgical history, relevant recent laboratory tests/vital signs. Specifically discuss risk factors that may challenge resuscitation (eg, cardiopulmonary disease, renal disease) History of present illness, including current suspected infectious source Surgery performed Important OR events and findings: airway management, complications (ie, bleeding source, contamination events, perforation)
Resuscitation/trends	Fluid totals: estimated blood loss, urine output, fluid intake, blood component transfusions Trend of vasopressor administration Targets of resuscitation, that is, MAP, CVP, lactate, urine output, FOCUS Relevant trends in laboratory data
Follow-up items	Time-sensitive elements: antibiotic dosing, microbiology cultures Anticipated causes for hemodynamic instability

Abbreviations: CVP, central venous pressure; FOCUS, focused cardiac ultrasound; MAP, mean arterial pressure.

DISCLOSURE

N. Bughrara, R. Safa, and S. Cha have nothing to disclose. A. Pustavoitau is an advisor and part owner of Coaptech, LLC, a company specializing in coaptive ultrasound.

REFERENCES

1. Gaieski DF, Edwards JM, Kallan MJ, et al. Benchmarking the incidence and mortality of severe sepsis in the United States. Crit Care Med 2013;41(5):1167–74.
2. Angus DC, Poll TVD. Severe sepsis and septic shock. N Engl J Med 2013;369(9): 840–51.
3. Centers for Medicare & Medicaid Services. Table 01 national health expenditures; aggregate and per capita amounts, annual percent change and percent distribution: selected calendar years 1960-2014. Available at: https://www.cms. gov/Research-Statistics-Data-and-Systems/Statistics-Trends-and-Reports/Natio nalHealthExpendData/Downloads/Tables.zip. Accessed May 9, 2019.
4. Martin GS, Mannino DM, Eaton S, et al. The epidemiology of sepsis in the United States from 1979 through 2000. N Engl J Med 2003;348(16):1546–54.
5. Bone RC, Balk RA, Cerra FB, et al. Definitions for sepsis and organ failure and guidelines for the use of innovative therapies in sepsis. The ACCP/SCCM Consensus Conference Committee. American College of Chest Physicians/Society of Critical Care Medicine. Chest 1992;101(6):1644–55.

6. Levy MM, Fink MP, Marshall JC, et al. 2001 SCCM/ESICM/ACCP/ATS/SIS International Sepsis Definitions Conference. Crit Care Med 2003;31(4):1250–6.
7. Singer M, Deutschman CS, Seymour CW, et al. The third international consensus definitions for sepsis and septic shock (sepsis-3). JAMA 2016;315(8):801–10.
8. Kumar A. An alternate pathophysiologic paradigm of sepsis and septic shock: implications for optimizing antimicrobial therapy. Virulence 2013;5(1):80–97.
9. Landry DW, Levin HR, Gallant EM, et al. Vasopressin deficiency contributes to the vasodilation of septic shock. Circulation 1997;95(5):1122–5.
10. Brealey D, Karyampudi S, Jacques TS, et al. Mitochondrial dysfunction in a long-term rodent model of sepsis and organ failure. Am J Physiol Regul Integr Comp Physiol 2004;286(3):R491–7.
11. Rivers E, Nguyen B, Havstad S, et al. Early goal-directed therapy in the treatment of severe sepsis and septic shock. N Engl J Med 2001;345(19):1368–77.
12. Goal-directed resuscitation for patients with early septic shock. N Engl J Med 2014;371(16):1496–506.
13. A randomized trial of protocol-based care for early septic shock. N Engl J Med 2014;370(18):1683–93.
14. Mouncey PR, Osborn TM, Power GS, et al. Trial of early, goal-directed resuscitation for septic shock. N Engl J Med 2015;372(14):1301–11.
15. Levy MM, Dellinger RP, Townsend SR, et al. The Surviving Sepsis Campaign: results of an international guideline-based performance improvement program targeting severe sepsis. Crit Care Med 2010;38(2):367–74.
16. Kumar A, Roberts D, Wood K, et al. Duration of hypotension before initiation of effective antimicrobial therapy is the critical determinant of survival in human septic shock. Crit Care Med 2006;34(6):1589–96.
17. Kumar A, Ellis P, Arabi Y, et al. Initiation of inappropriate antimicrobial therapy results in a fivefold reduction of survival in human septic shock. Chest 2009;136(5):1237–48.
18. Mulier S, Penninckx F, Verwaest C, et al. Factors affecting mortality in generalized postoperative peritonitis: multivariate analysis in 96 patients. World J Surg 2003;27(4):379–84.
19. Wong CH, Chang HC, Pasupathy S, et al. Necrotizing fasciitis: clinical presentation, microbiology, and determinants of mortality. J Bone Joint Surg Am 2003;85(8):1454–60.
20. Levy MM, Gesten FC, Phillips GS, et al. Mortality changes associated with mandated public reporting for sepsis. The Results of the New York State Initiative. Am J Respir Crit Care Med 2018;198(11):1406–12.
21. Boyd JH, Forbes J, Nakada T-A, et al. Fluid resuscitation in septic shock: a positive fluid balance and elevated central venous pressure are associated with increased mortality. Crit Care Med 2011;39(2):259–65.
22. Marik PE, Cavallazzi R. Does the central venous pressure predict fluid responsiveness? an updated meta-analysis and a plea for some common sense. Crit Care Med 2013;41(7):1774–81.
23. Monnet X, Marik PE, Teboul JL. Prediction of fluid responsiveness: an update. Ann Intensive Care 2016;6(111):1–11.
24. Semler M, Self W, Wanderer J, et al. Balanced crystalloids versus saline in critically ill adults. N Engl J Med 2018;378:829–39.
25. A comparison of Albumin and Saline for fluid resuscitation in the intensive care unit. N Engl J Med 2004;350(22):2247–56.

26. Haase N, Perner A, Hennings LI, et al. Hydroxyethyl starch 130/0.38–0.45 versus crystalloid or albumin in patients with sepsis: systematic review with meta-analysis and trial sequential analysis. BMJ 2013;346:f839.
27. Bai X, Yu W, Ji W, et al. Early versus delayed administration of norepinephrine in patients with septic shock. Crit Care 2014;18(532):1–8.
28. Low-dose dopamine in patients with early renal dysfunction: a placebo-controlled randomized trial. Lancet 2000;356(9248):2139–43.
29. De Backer D, Biston P, Devriendt J, et al. SOAP II Investigators. Comparison of dopamine and norepinephrine in the treatment of shock. N Engl J Med 2010; 362(9):779–89.
30. Varpula M, Tallgren M, Saukkonen K, et al. Hemodynamic variables related to outcome in septic shock. Intensive Care Med 2005;31:1066–71.
31. Gordon AC, Mason AJ, Thirunavukkarasu N, et al. The VANISH Investigators. Effect of early vasopressin vs norepinephrine on kidney failure in patients with septic shock: the VANISH randomized clinical trial. JAMA 2016;316(5):509–18.
32. Russel JA, Walley KR, Singer J, et al. The VASST Investigators. Vasopressin versus norepinephrine infusion in patients with septic shock. N Engl J Med 2008;358:877–87.
33. Khanna A, English S, Wang X, et al. Angiotensin II for the treatment of vasodilatory shock. N Engl J Med 2017;377:419–30.
34. Tumlin JA, Murugan R, Deane AM, et al. Outcomes in patients with vasodilatory shock and renal replacement therapy treated with intravenous angiotensin II. Crit Care Med 2018;46(6):949–57.
35. Annane D, Vignon P, Renault A, et al. Norepinephrine plus dobutamine versus epinephrine alone for management of septic shock: a randomized trial. Lancet 2007;370(9588):676–84.
36. Sprung J, Schuetz SM, Stewart RW, et al. Effects of ketamine on the contractility of failing and nonfailing human heart muscles in vitro. Anesthesiology 1998;88(5): 1202–10.
37. Taniguchi T, Shibata K, Yamamoto K, et al. Ketamine inhibits endotoxin-induced shock in rats. Anesthesiology 2001;95(4):928–32.
38. Melamed R, Bar-Yosef S, Shakhar G, et al. Suppression of natural killer cell activity and promotion of tumor metastasis by ketamine, thiopental, and halothane, but not by propofol: mediating mechanisms and prophylactic measures. Anesth Analg 2003;97(5):1331–9.
39. Pledger D, Kong A. Adrenocortical function in critically ill patients 24 h after a single dose of etomidate. Anaesthesia 1999;54(9):861.
40. Bruder EA, Ball IM, Ridi S, et al. Single induction dose of etomidate versus other induction agents for endotracheal intubation in critically ill patients. Cochrane Database Syst Rev 2015;(1):CD010225.
41. Chan CM, Mitchell AL, Shorr AF, et al. Etomidate is associated with mortality and adrenal insufficiency in sepsis: a meta-analysis. Crit Care Med 2012;40(11):2945.
42. Weiss M, Buhl R, Medve M, et al. Tumor necrosis factor-alpha modulates the selective interference of hypnotics and sedatives to suppress N-formyl-methionyl-leucyl-phenylalanine-induced oxidative burst formation in neutrophils. Crit Care Med 1997;25(1):128–34.
43. Banerjee S, Meng J, Das S, et al. Morphine induced exacerbation of sepsis is mediated by tempering endotoxin tolerance through modulation of miR-146a. Sci Rep 2013;3(1):1977.
44. Craig RG, Hunter JM. Neuromuscular blocking drugs and their antagonists in patients with organ disease. Anaesthesia 2009;64(Suppl 1):55.

45. Eidelman LA. The spectrum of septic encephalopathy. JAMA 1996;275(6):470.
46. Ely EW, Speroff T, Gordon SM, et al. Delirium as a predictor of mortality in mechanically ventilated patients in the intensive care unit. JAMA 2004;291(14): 1753–62.
47. Barnes-Daly MA, Phillips G, Ely EW. Improving hospital survival and reducing brain dysfunction at seven California community hospitals: implementing PAD guidelines via the ABCDEF bundle in 6,064 patients. Crit Care Med 2017;45(2): 171–8.
48. Girard TD, Exline MC, Carson SS, et al. Haloperidol and ziprasidone for treatment of delirium in critical illness. N Engl J Med 2018;379(26):2506–16.
49. Brower RG, Matthay MA, Morris A, et al. Ventilation with lower tidal volumes as compared with traditional tidal volumes for acute lung injury and the acute respiratory distress syndrome. N Engl J Med 2000;342(18):1301–8.
50. Amato MBP, Meade MO, Slutsky AS, et al. Driving pressure and survival in the acute respiratory distress syndrome. N Engl J Med 2015;372(8):747–55.
51. Meade M, Mercat A, Brower RG, et al. Higher vs lower positive end-expiratory pressure in patients with acute lung injury. Lung 2010;303(9):865–73.
52. Fan E, Wilcox ME, Brower RG, et al. Recruitment maneuvers for acute lung injury: a systematic review. Am J Respir Crit Care Med 2008;178(11):1156–63.
53. Rygård SL, Holst LB, Wetterslev J, et al. Long-term outcomes in patients with septic shock transfused at a lower versus a higher haemoglobin threshold: the TRISS randomised, multicentre clinical trial. Intensive Care Med 2016;42(11): 1685–94.
54. Quinlan M. A randomized trial of protocol-based care for early septic shock. J Emerg Med 2014;47(2):256–7.
55. Shore-Lesserson L, Manspeizer HE, DePerio M, et al. Thromboelastography-guided transfusion algorithm reduces transfusions in complex cardiac surgery. Anesth Analg 1999;88(2):312–9.
56. Liumbruno G, Bennardello F, Lattanzio A, et al. Recommendations for the transfusion of plasma and platelets. Blood Transfus 2009;7(2):132–50.
57. Yan J, Li S, Li S. The role of the liver in sepsis. Int Rev Immunol 2014;33(6): 498–510.
58. Starczewska MH, Mon W, Shirley P. Anaesthesia in patients with liver disease. Curr Opin Anaesthesiol 2017;30(3):392–8.
59. Schrier RW, Wang W. Acute renal failure and sepsis. N Engl J Med 2004;351(2): 159–69.
60. Zarbock A, Kellum JA. Acute kidney injury in cardiac surgery. Crit Care Nephrol Third Ed 2017;28(1):250–4.e2.
61. Kellum MJ, Kennedy KW, Barney R, et al. Cardiocerebral resuscitation improves neurologically intact survival of patients with out-of-hospital cardiac arrest. Ann Emerg Med 2008;52(3):244–52.
62. Bellomo R, Cass A, Cole, et al. Intensity of continuous renal-replacement therapy in critically ill patients. N Engl J Med 2009;361(17):1627–38.
63. Pavlesky PM, Zhang JH, O'Connor TZ, et al. Intensity of renal support in critically ill patients with acute kidney injury. N Engl J Med 2008;359(1):7–20.
64. Zarbock A, Kellum JA, Schmidt C, et al. Effect of early vs delayed initiation of renal replacement therapy on mortality in critically ill patients with acute kidney injury: the ELAIN randomized clinical trial. JAMA 2016;315(20):2190–9.
65. Deng J, Lenart J, Applegate RL. General anesthesia soon after dialysis may increase postoperative hypotension - A pilot study. Hear Lung Vessel 2014; 6(1):52–9.

66. Van den Berghe G, Wouters P, Weekers F, et al. Intensive insulin therapy in critically ill patients. N Engl J Med 2001;345:1359–67.
67. Song F, Zhong L-J, Han L, et al. Intensive insulin therapy for septic patients: a meta-analysis of randomized controlled trials. Biomed Res Int 2014;2014:1–10.
68. Griesdale DEG, De Souza RJ, Van Dam RM, et al. Intensive insulin therapy and mortality among critically ill patients: a meta-analysis including NICE-SUGAR study data. CMAJ 2009;180(8):821–7.
69. Venkatesh B, Finfer S, Cohen J, et al. Adjunctive glucocorticoid therapy in patients with septic shock. N Engl J Med 2018;378(9):797–808.
70. Zhou G, Kamenos G, Pendem S, et al. Ascorbate protects against vascular leakage in cecal ligation and puncture-induced septic peritonitis. Am J Physiol Regul Integr Comp Physiol 2011;302(4):R409–16.
71. Tanaka H, Matsuda T, Miyagantani Y, et al. Reduction of resuscitation fluid volumes in severely burned patients using ascorbic acid administration. Arch Surg 2000;135:326–31.
72. Woolum JA, Abner EL, Kelly A, et al. Effect of thiamine administration on lactate clearance and mortality in patients with septic shock. Crit Care Med 2018;46(11): 1747–52.
73. Marik PE, Khangoora V, Rivera R, et al. Hydrocortisone, vitamin C, and thiamine for the treatment of severe sepsis and septic shock: a retrospective before-after study. Chest 2017;151(6):1229–38.
74. de Grooth HJ, Manubulu-Choo WP, Zandvliet AS, el al. Vitamin C pharmacokinetics in critically ill patients: a randomized trial of four IV regimens. Chest 2018;153(6):1368–77.
75. Park TK, Yang JH, Jeon K, et al. Extracorporeal membrane oxygenation for refractory septic shock in adults. Eur J Cardiothorac Surg 2014;47(2):e68–74.
76. Bruenger F, Kizner L, Weile J, et al. First successful combination of ECMO with cytokine removal therapy in cardiogenic septic shock: a case report. Int J Artif Organs 2015;38(2):113–6.

Perioperative Management of Patients with Sepsis and Septic Shock, Part II

Ultrasound Support for Resuscitation

Nibras Bughrara, MD[a,b,*], Jose L. Diaz-Gomez, MD[c,d],
Aliaksei Pustavoitau, MD, MHS[e]

KEYWORDS

- Sepsis • Septic shock • Anesthesia management • Resuscitation
- Echocardiography • Point-of-care ultrasound • Hemodynamic phenotypes

KEY POINTS

- Patients with sepsis and septic shock develop complex derangements of their cardiovascular system, described by unique phenotypes.
- Hemodynamic phenotypes are clustered into three groups: small or normal ventricular cavity/normal or hyperactive ventricular systolic function, enlarged left ventricular cavity with or without right ventricular enlargement/decreased global contractility, and isolated right atrial and right ventricular dilation with normal or hyperactive left ventricular function.
- Point-of-care ultrasound efficiently identifies distinct hemodynamic phenotypes in septic shock through qualitative assessment of information from the subcostal four-chamber view, subcostal inferior vena cava view, and upper lung views.
- Recognition of hemodynamic phenotype with point-of-care ultrasound and analysis of pulse pressure variability provides anesthesiologist with information on myocardial performance, fluid responsiveness and tolerance, vasoactive and inotropic therapies, and specific additional interventions for optimal patient outcomes.

 Video content accompanies this article at www.anesthesiology.theclinics.com.

---

[a] Department of Anesthesiology, Albany Medical College, 47 New Scotland Avenue, MC 131, Albany, NY 12208, USA; [b] Department of Surgery, Albany Medical College, 47 New Scotland Avenue, MC 131, Albany, NY 12208, USA; [c] Cardiovascular Critical Care, Professional Development, Education, and Clinical Research, Critical Care Medicine, Division of Cardiovascular Anesthesia, Texas Heart Institute – Baylor St. Luke's Medical Center, 6720 Bertner Avenue, Suite 0-520, Houston, TX 77030, USA; [d] Critical Care Echocardiography and Point of Care Ultrasound, Baylor College of Medicine, Houston, TX, USA; [e] Division of Adult Critical Care Medicine, Johns Hopkins University School of Medicine, 600 North Wolfe Street, Meyer 297, Baltimore, MD 21287, USA
* Corresponding author. Department of Anesthesiology, Albany Medical College, 47 New Scotland Avenue, MC 131, Albany, NY 12208.
E-mail address: bughran@amc.edu
Twitter: @BughraraNibras (N.B.)

Anesthesiology Clin 38 (2020) 123–134
https://doi.org/10.1016/j.anclin.2019.11.001
anesthesiology.theclinics.com

SEPSIS-INDUCED MYOCARDIAL DYSFUNCTION

Pathophysiology of septic shock involves alterations of volume dynamics, central hemodynamics, and microcirculation. Patients with septic shock commonly experience myocardial dysfunction, by some estimates reaching 100% when LV systolic and diastolic, right ventricular (RV), and combined dysfunction are accounted for in this intriguing entity.[1]

Sepsis-induced cardiomyopathy traditionally describes an LV systolic dysfunction and occurs in 40% to 50% of patients with septic shock.[2] It is characterized by reduced global LV ejection fraction (LVEF) to less than 50% or a 10% decrease compared with baseline.[3] Despite its widespread use, LVEF is preload-dependent and is not a predictor of mortality.[4] Sepsis-induced cardiomyopathy does not have a specific treatment; it is entirely reversible in survivors with full recovery usually occurring in 7 to 10 days.[4] Alternatively, the longitudinal strain is independent of preload conditions and is more sensitive in diagnosing LV dysfunction in sepsis.[5,6] Strain correlates significantly with mortality.[7]

Patients with sepsis-induced cardiomyopathy commonly have elevated troponin levels, which is associated with increased mortality.[8] A promising treatment is the use of β-blockers in patients with septic shock, which were demonstrated to reduce mortality.[9]

Catecholamine-mediated cardiomyopathy (ie, takotsubo syndrome) is another cause of LV dysfunction in patients with sepsis and septic shock. It is reversible and characterized by apical ballooning and hypercontractile base. Commencement of exogenous catecholamines might worsen ongoing cardiomyopathy. Indeed, levosimendan, a calcium channel sensitizer, is used for hemodynamic support in these patients.[10]

Sepsis-induced myocardial dysfunction can also present as LV diastolic dysfunction, with grade I diastolic dysfunction (abnormal LV relaxation and stiffness without an elevation in filling pressure, which in sepsis could be an indicator of underresuscitation) associated with increased mortality in septic shock, whereas grades II and III diastolic dysfunction are without such association.[11]

RV dysfunction usually accompanies LV dysfunction, but it can also develop in isolation because of increased pulmonary vascular resistance (PVR) in the setting of acute respiratory distress syndrome (ARDS).[12] A decrease in RV systolic function is associated with a worse prognosis.[13,14]

Finally, new-onset atrial fibrillation is a common complication in sepsis and associated with prolonged length of stay and increased mortality.[15] Amiodarone is the treatment of choice.[16]

ROLE OF FOCUSED CARDIAC ULTRASONOGRAPHY

Unlike the complete echocardiography, POCUS and focused cardiac ultrasound (FOCUS; cardiac application of POCUS) is performed and interpreted at the bedside by the same provider in a quick and goal-oriented fashion and is learned after short training. In a recent pilot study by our group, anesthesiology residents received a 4-day instruction under direct supervision to obtain FOCUS examination. The goal of the FOCUS examination was to evaluate cardiac chamber size and contractility and IVC view to assess diameter and variability with respiration. Similar to previous reports on intensivists receiving limited training, our residents were able to obtain at least one useful image in 97% of the patients.[17,18] When comparing only the subcostal view with FOCUS, we found that the subcostal view by itself allows for a correct assessment of 84% of patients in shock. Thus, in most patients, a quick, commonly 4 minutes or less, evaluation of subcostal views before induction of anesthesia can define the hemodynamic phenotype of each patient with septic shock and tailor treatment accordingly (**Fig. 1**, Videos 1 and 2).[18,19]

The FOCUS examination is not accurate for detecting fluid responsiveness, whereas it performs as a diagnostic tool for severe hypovolemia (a combination of end-expiratory IVC diameter of <1 cm and hyperdynamic ventricular function).[20] Additionally, IVC size and collapsibility can noninvasively and accurately estimate central venous pressure (CVP) in patients who are spontaneously breathing and have been used extensively by cardiologists during echocardiography evaluation. FOCUS-estimated CVP may be used as a substitute for central venous catheter–transduced CVP and avoids placing invasive lines for the sole purpose of CVP measurement, particularly given notoriously clinically inaccurate estimates of CVP.[21]

Current literature suggests that patients with septic shock can exhibit five echo-defined clusters: (1) hyperdynamic (23.3%), (2) persistent hypovolemia (19.4%), (3) well-resuscitated (16.9%), (4) LV systolic dysfunction (17.7%), and (5) RV failure (22.5%).[22] This clustering used transesophageal echocardiography evaluation, in addition to quantitation of LV systolic and diastolic function, RV function, fluid responsiveness, and fluid tolerance. Furthermore, the following parameters comprised the quantification of fluid responsiveness and fluid tolerance: LVEF, fractional area change, mitral Doppler E and A-wave velocity, maximal tissue Doppler velocity of the lateral aspect of the mitral annulus at early diastole, RV/LV end-diastolic area, superior vena cava collapsibility index, velocity-time integral in the LVOT, and the diameter of the aortic annulus to calculate LV stroke volume and cardiac index. Such quantitative assessment requires incremental provider training, and consumes additional time, making this type of assessment inaccessible to frontline providers providing care to these patients. Additionally, in the previously mentioned report patients with preexisting cardiac disease were excluded from the described clustering scheme (12.2% of the initial cohort). Finally, the proposed scheme does not account for fluid tolerance, the increasingly important concept, which was conceptualized in the FALLS protocol.[23]

To equip the provider with a rapid patient assessment tool before the induction of anesthesia, we developed an abbreviated heart and lung ultrasound protocol. This entire protocol can be performed rapidly in the operating room before induction, after a short training, similar to the training of residents. Our protocol relies on pattern recognition from the subcostal four-chamber and IVC views alongside the lung ultrasonography evaluation (EASy-ALS).[24] Thus, we describe a qualitative characterization of central circulatory phenotypes. These phenotypes encompass acute pathophysiologic changes and preexisting cardiac disease and are based on an assessment of myocardial performance, fluid responsiveness, and fluid tolerance (each phenotype can be described in those terms). As a result, we identify a total of seven phenotypes, which are further grouped into three clusters based on similar management of patients within the cluster (see **Fig. 1**).

In this classification scheme, qualitative analysis of LV function is performed by assessing ventricular size and function, the longitudinal motion of mitral valve and approximation, and thickening of the myocardial walls during systole. Patients with phenotypes 1, 3, 6, and 7 demonstrate apparent normal LV function. Patients with phenotype 3 have findings of thick LV walls and interventricular septum and commonly left atrial dilation, which are visual surrogates for diastolic dysfunction. Patients with phenotype 4 and 5 who are identified by LV dilation and systolic dysfunction can benefit from inotropic agents.

Initial and subsequent EASY phenotypes for septic shock patients

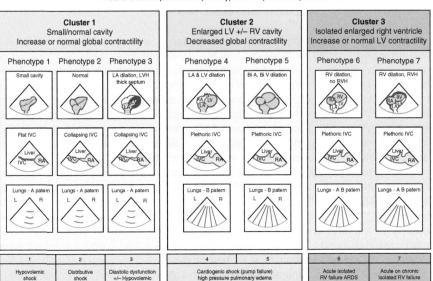

Fig. 1. EASy phenotypes are based on the subcostal four-chamber view (*top row*), subcostal IVC view (*middle row*), and lung evaluation in the upper lung fields (*bottom row*). Phenotypes 1 to 3 are grouped within cluster 1, phenotypes 4 and 5 are part of cluster 2, and phenotypes 6 and 7 are part of cluster 3. In general, cardiac assessment assesses myocardial performance, IVC evaluation provides the estimate of fluid responsiveness, and lung examination defines fluid tolerance (A-profile) and intolerance (B-profile). Phenotype 1 describes the patient with hypovolemic shock with small diastolic ventricular chamber size, collapsed IVC with significant variability in its diameter throughout the respiratory cycle, and A-profile on lung examination. Phenotype 2 is consistent with distributive shock in adequately fluid-resuscitated patient with good cardiac filling, normal IVC size, and A-profile on lung examination. Phenotype 3 describes patient with hypertrophic LV, commonly dilated left atrium, small and collapsible IVC, and A-profile on lung examination. Phenotypes 4 and 5 describe patient with isolated LV (phenotype 4) and biventricular (phenotype 5) dysfunction, usually plethoric IVC and B-profile on lung examination. Phenotype 6 most commonly describes patient with ARDS complicated by RV dysfunction. These patients demonstrate enlarged RV, plethoric IVC, and B-profile on lung examination more commonly reflecting nonhydrostatic edema. Phenotype 7 includes patients with underlying pulmonary hypertension and RV hypertrophy who develop acute on chronic RV failure. These patients have enlarged and hypertrophic RV, plethoric IVC, and variable lung profile (B-profile shown here). Bi A, Bi atrial; Bi V, Bi ventricular; HTN, hypertension; LA, left atrium; LVH, left ventricular hypertrophy; RA, right atrium; RVH, right ventricular hypertrophy. (*Courtesy of* N. Bughrara, MD, Albany, NY.)

Qualitative analysis of RV consists of assessing RV size relative to LV, RV/LV end-diastolic area, and RV free wall thickness during diastole. RV/LR end-diastolic area ratio of more than 1 indicates severe RV dilation. RV wall thickness during diastole greater than 1 cm indicates severe RV hypertrophy and differentiates between phenotypes 6 and 7, both of which have dilated RV.

The complementary echocardiographic evaluation includes color-flow Doppler imaging of the mitral, tricuspid, and aortic valves. Indeed, it is a useful application as a screening tool for severe valvular disease (regurgitation and stenosis). Last, atrial collapse during systole and/or ventricular collapse during diastole facilitates the characterization of cardiac tamponade in patients with pericardial effusion.

Lung assessment adds exponential value to cardiac ultrasound and IVC assessment, with the presence of B-lines in the upper lung fields indicating an increase in lung water and the relative decrease in lung aeration, consistent with pulmonary edema. As a rule of thumb, the presence of three or more B-lines in both lung fields (Video 3) together with plethoric IVC (Video 4) indicates fluid intolerance. However, the presence of A-lines (Video 5) in both upper lung fields suggests that pulmonary capillary wedge pressure is less than 18 and consistent with fluid tolerance. The presence of sizable pleural effusion (Video 6) is easily detected by applying an ultrasound probe in the flanks. Occasionally, large pleural effusions can contribute to obstructive shock, especially if there is a concomitant pericardial effusion.

Once anesthesia induction and initiation of mechanical ventilation takes place, volume responsiveness evaluation are screened with pulse pressure variation. A pulse pressure variation higher than 12% correlates with an appropriate increase in stroke volume and cardiac output (fluid bolus). However, the patient must be passively ventilated (no efforts) with tidal volume more than 8 mL/kg, respiratory rate less than 30 breaths/min, in sinus rhythm, and has no RV failure. EASy examination before induction can help to assess the RV size and function and rule out RV failure because this phenotype can produce false-positive pulse pressure variation.

ANESTHETIC MANAGEMENT BASED ON FOCUS-DRIVEN HEMODYNAMIC PHENOTYPES

We identify three distinct major hemodynamic clusters and a total of seven phenotypes based on a three-step EASy-ALS examination:

1. Subcostal four-chamber view
2. IVC view
3. Abbreviated lung views

Additional distinct phenotypes are described separately using the same approach (valvular disease, tamponade). The described EASy-ALS assessment of patients with septic shock (see **Fig. 1**) can guide anesthesiologists in tailoring perioperative hemodynamic management (**Fig. 2**).

CLUSTER 1: PATIENT WITH NORMAL OR HYPERACTIVE CARDIAC SYSTOLIC FUNCTION
Phenotype 1: Small Left Ventricular/Right Ventricular Cavity

This phenotype describes absolute or relative hypovolemia (Video 7). Findings include hypercontractile (collapsible) ventricles with flat or markedly collapsible IVC (**Fig. 3**, Video 8). Most patients with sepsis at hospital admission fall into this category. These patients are at risk for cardiac arrest because of the alteration in cardiopulmonary interactions with the initiation of positive pressure ventilation.[25] The goal for this phenotype is to provide initial aggressive fluid administration, alongside vasoactive agents if the patient remains in shock despite the rapid infusion of volume. Vasopressor agents of choice include norepinephrine, vasopressin, and occasionally phenylephrine (eg, if dysrhythmias, particularly atrial fibrillation).

Phenotype 2: Normal Left Ventricular/Right Ventricular Cavity

This phenotype is consistent with the vasodilatory state (Video 9). Findings include hypercontractile LV and RV with collapsible IVC and average end-diastolic cavity

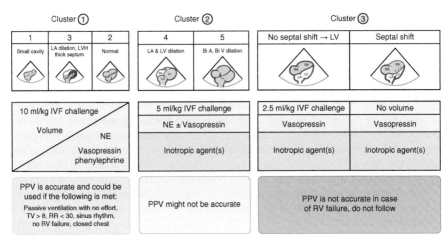

Fig. 2. Organization of ultrasound findings into phenotypes and clusters allows providers to develop a systematic approach to patient optimization immediately before induction of anesthesia. The mainstay therapy for patients in cluster 1 includes fluid resuscitation, and as the inferior vena cava becomes fuller and interstitial B-line pattern appears on lung examination the therapy shifts toward vasoactive medications. These patients could be followed in the operating room using serial EASy examination and pulse pressure variation. Depending on IVC evaluation and lung examination patients in cluster 2 may benefit from small titrated fluid boluses 2.5 to 5 mL/kg (under conditions of collapsible IVC, A-profile on lung examination); however, the mainstay therapy usually consists of using vasoactive medications and occasionally inotropic agents when end-organ perfusion is not restored. In these patients, pulse pressure variation is of value, and additional evaluation of LV diastolic function if appropriate expert is available. Patients in cluster 3 present particular challenges, and assessment of septal shift is required to establish whether RV function is compensated (septum does not bow into the LV during diastole allowing for adequate LV filling) or not. Gentle fluid loading on a scale of 2.5 mL/kg can be provided when function is compensated, and such measures as diuresis or renal-replacement therapy undertaken when RV function is decompensated. The mainstay therapy includes maintenance of systemic blood pressure with vasoactive medications and inotropic support and minimizing increases in pulmonary pressures by avoiding hypoxemia/hypercapnea and through the use of pulmonary vasodilators. IVF, intravenous fluid; NE, norepinephrine. (*Courtesy of* N. Bughrara, MD, Albany, NY.)

size (see **Fig. 3**). This cardiovascular profile is most likely represented by patients who have received volume resuscitation and lack ventricular systolic dysfunction. The primary mechanism of persistent hypotension is inappropriate systemic vasodilation. This phenotype corresponds to the previously described high cardiac output circulatory shock. In these patients, volume responsiveness should be assessed using fluid challenge. B-line ultrasound pattern in the upper lungs can indicate fluid intolerance. In this phenotype, vasopressor support should be the mainstem therapy (norepinephrine, ± vasopressin, ± phenylephrine). Initiation of vasopressor support can unmask LV/RV dysfunction, and the patient's phenotype could be transformed into phenotype 4 (see **Fig. 3**). Patients resistant to traditional vasopressors can benefit from an infusion of methylene blue and/or angiotensin II, which can be used only if the cardiac index is high or normal.

Phenotype 3: Small Cavity, Thick Hypertrophic Left Ventricle

This phenotype requires special considerations in perioperative care (Video 10). These patients commonly demonstrate diastolic dysfunction and hypotension

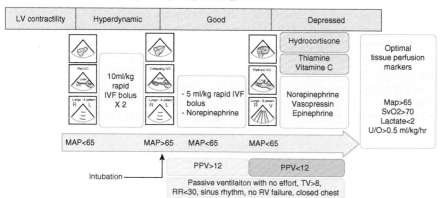

Fig. 3. Example of progressive resuscitation and serial evaluation of a patient with septic shock who presented to the operating room initially demonstrating phenotype 1. Accordingly, the patient received fluid boluses 10 mL/kg at a time until he demonstrated phenotype 2 and systemic mean arterial pressure was greater than 65 mm Hg. After intubation and initiation of positive pressure ventilation, pulse pressure variation was used to guide further fluid therapy in addition to serial EASy examinations. Norepinephrine was added because of persistent hypotension. When patient developed left ventricular dysfunction, plethoric inferior vena cava, and interstitial edema pattern on lung examination (phenotype 4), fluid was halted and epinephrine added; additional metabolic support with hydrocortisone, vitamin C, and thiamine was offered. In accordance with Surviving Sepsis Guidelines tissue perfusion markers were followed throughout the case, and goals of resuscitation are stated in the *box* on the far right. MAP, mean arterial pressure; OR, operating room; PPV, pulse pressure variation; RR, respiratory rate; TV, tidal volume. (*Courtesy of* N. Bughrara, MD, Albany, NY.)

because of systolic anterior movement of the mitral valve with dynamic obstruction of the LVOT. Underlying LV hypertrophy is usually secondary to long-standing significant hypertension or significant aortic stenosis. Thus, they require higher pressures to fill the LV appropriately, while also being at risk for pulmonary edema. It is essential to optimize their fluid status before induction of anesthesia because if the IVC is collapsible, precipitous hypotension results. In addition to cautious fluid loading concomitant vasopressor should be used during induction to counteract vasodilation caused by the anesthetics. These patients have a higher mortality rate.[26]

CLUSTER 2: ENLARGED LEFT VENTRICULAR ± RIGHT VENTRICULAR CAVITY WITH DECREASED GLOBAL CONTRACTILITY
Dilated Left Atrium and Left Ventricle (Phenotype 4) and Concomitantly Dilated Right Atrium and Right Ventricle (Phenotype 5)

This cluster is represented by individuals with underlying chronic LV dysfunction (multiple etiologies), or those who develop myocardial dysfunction after initiation of vasopressor support (unmasking effect), or those who develop stress cardiomyopathy (Videos 11 and 12). Patients with LV dysfunction are predisposed to having a normal to increased central blood volume. Hence, they might not tolerate aggressive fluid resuscitation, so echocardiographic assessment of fluid responsiveness and ventricular contractility is warranted. Moreover, other modalities to assess fluid responsiveness, including pulse pressure variation (screening), and LVOT variability with Doppler, straight leg raising test, or small intravenous fluid bolus challenge-response can better characterize their need for fluid resuscitation. Also, vasopressors with inotropic properties (norepinephrine ± dobutamine, ± epinephrine) are preferred choices in this scenario. The agent should be titrated up to reach a goal mean arterial pressure of 65 to 70 mm Hg before the induction of general anesthesia. General anesthetics should be titrated by using the lowest effective dose, and the patient should receive additional doses of norepinephrine during induction. Assessment of fluid responsiveness, including pulse pressure variation (screening), and LVOT variability with Doppler is limited with RV dysfunction because it represents inconsistent RV stroke volume rather than central hypovolemia. Of note, straight leg raising test or smaller intravenous bolus challenge-response with the reassessment of RV morphology (interventricular septum and cavity enlargement) can gauge volume administration in this challenging clinical setting.

CLUSTER 3: ISOLATED RIGHT ATRIUM AND RIGHT VENTRICLE DILATION WITH NORMAL OR HYPERACTIVE LEFT VENTRICLE FUNCTION
Isolated Right Ventricle Dilation (Phenotype 6) and Isolated Right Atrium and Right Ventricle Dilation + Right Ventricle Hypertrophy (Phenotype 7)

These phenotypes describe RV dysfunction (Video 13). These patients are at risk of developing RV failure, characterized by elevated CVP, and in the most severe form resulting in low cardiac output and worsening systemic hypotension. Severe RV dilation or dysfunction leads to RV geometry change and interventricular septal shift toward the LV, thus reducing LV preload with ensuring hypotension. In turn, hypotension reduces coronary perfusion and leads to RV free wall ischemia, even more decreasing RV free wall contractility. This sequence of progressive changes leads to a quick deadly downward spiral to cardiac arrest within minutes. The initial goal is to convert RV failure with hypotension to RV failure without hypotension (mean arterial pressure >65 mm Hg) by using vasopressor to maintain RV myocardial perfusion. Vasopressin is a vasopressor of choice because it causes an increase in systemic vascular resistance without an increase in PVR. Phenylephrine and Norepinephrine could be used cautiously because they also increase PVR and can worsen the RV dilation. The second goal is to improve RV loading conditions by preventing further increase in PVR (avoiding and treating hypoxia, acidemia, hypercarbia), optimizing intrathoracic pressure (ie, positive end-expiratory pressure) and initiation of pulmonary vasodilators, that is, inhaled prostacyclin and inhaled nitric oxide. Inodilators (dobutamine, levosimendan, or milrinone) also optimize RV loading conditions and contractility. Finally, diuresis and renal-replacement therapy improve the RV geometry and system compliance through optimization of preload (Fig. 4). Dysrhythmias should be treated aggressively, with amiodarone being the drug of choice for atrial fibrillation.

Last, in phenotype 7, the presence of RV hypertrophy (RV free wall thickness >0.8 cm) represents long-standing pulmonary hypertension, The clinical management is similar to those patients with dilated RV because of acute RV failure. Awake intubation should be considered with keeping the patient breathing spontaneously, the positive end-expiratory pressure level is then started at zero and slowly dialed up, because these patients are at high risk of developing cardiac arrest on induction.

DISTINCT AND LESS PREVALENT PHENOTYPES
Phenotype 8: Pericardial Effusion ± Pleural Effusion Leading to Obstructive Shock

Findings include pericardial effusion with or without tamponade physiology (atrial collapse during systole and/or ventricular collapse during diastole) (see Video 6;

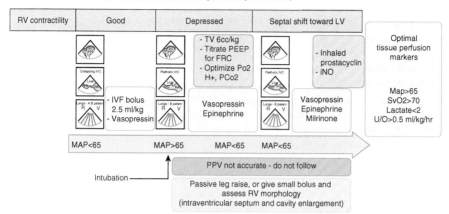

Phenotype 7 (Septic shock/preexisting pulmonary HTN/ARDS)

Fig. 4. Example of resuscitation of a patient with preexisting pulmonary hypertension with RV hypertrophy who developed ARDS and septic shock (phenotype 7). Initially, small fluid boluses 2.5 mL/kg at a time were provided until inferior vena cava became fuller and systemic mean arterial pressure improved to greater than 65 mm Hg. On induction of anesthesia, intubation, and initiation of positive-pressure ventilation using protective strategy with low tidal volumes and titrated positive end-expiratory pressure and fraction of inspired oxygen, RV function became decompensated with bowing of interventricular septum through cardiac cycle toward the left ventricle. At this point vasoactive medications (vasopressin) and inotropic (epinephrine and milrinone) were added and patient was started on pulmonary vasodilator (inhaled prostacyclin). Pulse pressure variation readings are inaccurate in a patient with decompensated RV function and was not followed. In accordance with Surviving Sepsis Guidelines tissue perfusion markers were followed throughout the case, and goals of resuscitation are stated in the *box* on the far right. FRC, functional residual capacity; PEEP, positive end-expiratory pressure. (*Courtesy of N. Bughrara, MD, Albany, NY.*)

Video 14). In patients with septic shock, acute kidney injury and hyperuricemia could precipitate pericardial effusion.

In case of the presence of concomitant large pleural effusion pleural fluid should be drained first before anesthetizing patients for placement of pericardial window. Tamponade physiology causes obstructive shock, which leads to plethoric IVC. In this situation fluid should be given despite plethoric IVC to keep the patients "full, fast and tight." When IVC is collapsible then shock cannot be explained by obstruction physiology only and is probably caused by hypovolemia. Under these circumstances optimizing volume status by giving rapid volume boluses is necessary before making diagnosis of obstructive shock secondary to tamponade (**Fig. 5**).

Phenotype 9: Gross Valvular Heart Disease

The use of two-dimensional echocardiography and color flow Doppler imaging facilitates recognition of confirmatory signs of possible infectious endocarditis when there is reasonable clinical suspicion of this condition (Video 15). Indeed, early identification of heart systolic failure caused by severe valvular dysfunction, large mobile vegetations, and the presence of abscess are crucial in the characterization of patient's hemodynamics and ventricular function in the setting of possible infectious endocarditis. Of note, in patients with low clinical suspicion for infectious endocarditis, a negative, high-quality, transthoracic echocardiography is sufficient for excluding infection,

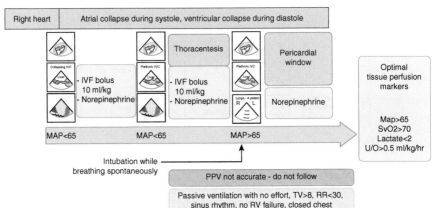

Fig. 5. Although not included in this classification of hemodynamic phenotypes, obstructive physiology is occasionally present in patients with septic shock, and large pleural effusions confound clinical presentation of these patients. In this example, patient presented with pericardial and large pleural effusion; however, still flat and collapsible IVC. He received titrated 10 mL/kg fluid boluses and vasoactive support with norepinephrine until IVC became fuller and systemic mean arterial pressure improved to greater than 65 mm Hg. Thoracentesis was performed and pleural effusion evacuated resulting in A-profile on lung examination. Subsequently, the patient was intubated while breathing spontaneously and pericardial window was performed. In accordance with Surviving Sepsis Guidelines tissue perfusion markers were followed throughout the case, and goals of resuscitation are stated in the *box* on the far right. (*Courtesy of* N. Bughrara, MD, Albany, NY.)

whereas an initial negative transthoracic echocardiography warrants a transesophageal echocardiography examination in situations of high clinical suspicion for infectious endocarditis (including presence of *Staphylococcus aureus* bacteremia, previous heart valve surgery).

DISCLOSURE

N. Bughrara has nothing to disclose. J.L. Diaz-Gomez is a consultant for Philips Healthcare. A. Pustavoitau is an advisor and part-owner of Coaptech, LLC.

SUPPLEMENTARY DATA

Supplementary data related to this article can be found online at https://doi.org/10.1016/j.anclin.2019.11.001.

REFERENCES

1. Vieillard-Baron A, Cecconi M. Understanding cardiac failure in sepsis. Intensive Care Med 2014;40:1560–3.
2. Bouhemad B, Nicolas-Robin A, Arbelot C, et al. Isolated and reversible impairment of ventricular relaxation in patients with septic shock*. Crit Care Med 2008;36(3):766–74.
3. Beesley SJ, Weber G, Sarge T, et al. Septic cardiomyopathy. Crit Care Med 2018; 46(4):625–34.

4. Berrios RAS, O'Horo JC, Velagapudi V, et al. Correlation of left ventricular systolic dysfunction determined by low ejection fraction and 30-day mortality in patients with severe sepsis and septic shock: a systematic review and meta-analysis. J Crit Care 2014;29(4):495–9.

5. Stanton T, Leano R, Marwick TH. Prediction of all-cause mortality from global longitudinal speckle strain: comparison with ejection fraction and wall motion scoring. Circ Cardiovasc Imaging 2009;2:356–64.

6. Lanspa MJ, Pittman JE, Hirshberg EL, et al. Association of left ventricular longitudinal strain with central venous oxygen saturation and serum lactate in patients with early severe sepsis and septic shock. Crit Care 2015;19:304.

7. Palmieri V, Innocenti F, Guzzo A, et al. Left ventricular systolic longitudinal function as predictor of outcome in patients with sepsis. Circ Cardiovasc Imaging 2015;8:e003865.

8. Bessière F, Khenifer S, Dubourg J, et al. Prognostic value of troponins in sepsis: a meta-analysis. Intensive Care Med 2013;39(7):1181–9.

9. Morelli A, Donati A, Ertmer C, et al. Microvascular effects of heart rate control with esmolol in patients with septic shock. Crit Care Med 2013;41(9):2162–8.

10. Pinto BB, Rehberg S, Ertmer C, et al. Role of levosimendan in sepsis and septic shock. Curr Opin Anaesthesiol 2008;21(2):168–77.

11. Sanfilippo F, Corredor C, Landesberg G, et al. Tissue Doppler assessment of diastolic function and relationship with mortality in critically ill septic patients: systematic review and meta-analysis. Br J Anaesth 2017;119:583–94.

12. Chan CM, Klinger JR. The right ventricle in sepsis. Clin Chest Med 2008;29(4): 661–76.

13. Dhainaut JF, Lanore JJ, Gournay JMD, et al. Right ventricular dysfunction in patients with septic shock. Intensive Care Med 1988;14(S1):488–91.

14. Liu D, Du B, Long Y, et al. Right ventricular function of patients with septic shock: clinical significance. Zhonghua Wai Ke Za Zhi 2000;38(7):488–92.

15. Klein Klouwenberg PMCK, Frencken JF, Kuipers S, et al. Incidence, predictors, and outcomes of new-onset atrial fibrillation in critically ill patients with sepsis: a cohort study. Am J Respir Crit Care Med 2017;195(2):205–11.

16. Walkey AJ, Evans SR, Winter MR, et al. Practice patterns and outcomes of treatments for atrial fibrillation during sepsis: a propensity-matched cohort study. Chest 2016;149(1):74–83.

17. Jensen MB, Sloth E, Larsen KM, et al. Transthoracic echocardiography for cardiopulmonary monitoring in intensive care. Eur J Anesthesiol 2004;21(9):700–7.

18. Bughrara NF, Emr KS, Renew JR, et al. Echocardiographic Assessment Using Subxiphoid-only View (EASY) Compared to Focused Transthoracic Echocardiography (FOTE): a multicenter prospective study [abstract], in Anesthesiology Annual Meeting-American Society of Anesthesiologists. San Francisco, October 15, 2018. Abstract no. A3089.

19. Bughrara NF, Meuli M, Renew JR, et al. Is Four Days of Extensive Training in Focused Transthoracic Echocardiography (FOTE) During Post Anesthesia Care Unit (PACU) rotation [abstract], in Anesthesiology Annual Meeting-American Society of Anesthesiologists. San Francisco, October 14, 2018. Abstract no. A2130.

20. Feissel M, Michard FDR, Faller J-P, et al. The respiratory variation in inferior vena cava diameter as a guide to fluid therapy. Intensive Care Med 2004;30(9):834–7.

21. Figg KK, Nemergut EC. Error in central venous pressure measurement. Anesth Analg 2009;108(4):1209–11.

22. Geri G, Vignon P, Aubry A, et al. Cardiovascular clusters in septic shock combining clinical and echocardiographic parameters: a post hoc analysis. Intensive Care Med 2019;45(5):657–67.
23. Lichtenstein D. Fluid administration limited by lung sonography: the place of lung ultrasound in assessment of acute circulatory failure (the FALLS-protocol). Expert Rev Respir Med 2012;6(2):155–62.
24. Bughrara N, Cha S, Pustavoitau A. Focused point of care ultrasound in cardiac arrest. In: Diaz-Gomez J, Nikravan S, Conlon T, editors. Comprehensive critical care ultrasound. 2nd edition. Society of Critical Care Medicine, in press.
25. Jaber S, Amraoui J, Lefrant JY, et al. Clinical practice and risk factors for immediate complications of endotracheal intubation in the intensive care unit: a prospective, multiple-center study. Crit Care Med 2006;34(9):2355–61.
26. Chauvet JL, El-Dash S, Delastre O, et al. Early dynamic left intraventricular obstruction is associated with hypovolemia and high mortality in septic shock patients. Crit Care 2015;19:262.

Anesthesia for Patients with Extensive Trauma

Alexander C. Fort, MD[a],*, Richard A. Zack-Guasp, MD[b]

KEYWORDS

- Trauma anesthesiology • Trauma anesthesia • Emergency airway management
- Hemorrhagic shock • Hypotensive resuscitation • Permissive hypotension
- Massive transfusion protocol

KEY POINTS

- Initial management of severely injured patients with trauma requires coordinated efforts among multiple specialists and hospitals in a protocolized approach that follows Advanced Trauma Life Support guidelines.
- Hemorrhagic shock is one of the leading causes of preventable injury and mortality; early stratification of patients based on the degree of hemorrhage aids in timely and adequate resuscitation.
- Resuscitative efforts must be closely coordinated with surgical control of bleeding for definitive management of hemorrhage.
- After acute injuries are addressed and stabilized, late resuscitation continues in an attempt to optimize and improve long-term patient outcomes.

INTRODUCTION

Acute injuries provide a major challenge for health care teams given the need for a swift, comprehensive, and coordinated response from multispecialty and multidisciplinary teams. In the United States, between the ages of 1 and 44 years, injuries account for 59% of all deaths.[1,2] Among trauma populations, one of the leading causes of morbidity and mortality is hemorrhagic shock, a major source of global morbidity and mortality accounting for nearly 2 million deaths worldwide per year.[3] In the United States alone, nearly 60,000 patients per year die of hemorrhagic shock, and hemorrhage following trauma accounts for 30% to 40% of deaths in the first 24 hours after injury.[3,4] Understanding the early management of traumatically injured

[a] Department of Anesthesiology, Perioperative Medicine and Pain Management, University of Miami Miller School of Medicine, University of Miami, 1611 Northwest 12th Avenue, Suite C300, Miami, FL 33136, USA; [b] Department of Anesthesiology, Bruce W. Carter Medical Center, Department of Veteran's Health Administration, 1201 Northwest 16th Street, Room B333, Miami, FL 33136, USA
* Corresponding author.
E-mail address: acfort@med.miami.edu

Anesthesiology Clin 38 (2020) 135–148
https://doi.org/10.1016/j.anclin.2019.10.012
anesthesiology.theclinics.com
1932-2275/20/© 2019 Elsevier Inc. All rights reserved.

patients along with the physiologic compensatory mechanisms that ensue in response to trauma is crucial in the development of strategies to improve patient outcomes. Management of patients with trauma begins in the prehospital setting and may continue for days after initial stabilization. Adequate stratification of patients and timely management has been seen to improve outcomes in the trauma population.

Early Management

The in-hospital initial management of severely injured patients with trauma starts in the trauma bay. The Advanced Trauma Life Support (ATLS) course, developed by the Committee on Trauma of the American College of Surgeons, provides an algorithmic approach to the initial evaluation of patients with trauma. The ATLS model is essential for all personnel, including surgeons, anesthesiologists, nurse anesthetists, and nurses, in order to understand the priorities when facing a traumatically injured patient. The emphasis of ATLS is the primary survey, which uses the ABCDE mnemonic (**Table 1**) to provide the care team with a prioritized road map in initial care. As part of the early assessment, calculation of a Glasgow Coma Scale (GCS) score (**Table 2**) is valuable in making decisions on intubation and establishing initial neurologic function in patients with traumatic brain injury (TBI).[5]

The initial stabilization efforts in patients with extensive trauma use the military concept of damage control resuscitation (DCR). The anesthesia team plays an integral role in DCR given its continuum from the emergency room to the operating room to the

Table 1 Advanced Trauma Life Support primary survey	
Airway	Evaluate vocal response Inspect for airway obstruction Inspect for facial or laryngeal fractures Suction oropharyngeal contents
Breathing	Auscultation Inspect and palpate chest wall Percuss thorax Place pulse oximeter Provide oxygen
Circulation	Assess level of consciousness, skin perfusion, and pulse Direct manual pressure Tourniquets Chest radiograph Pelvic radiograph FAST Diagnostic peritoneal lavage Intravenous access Laboratory studies Fluid resuscitation and blood products
Disability	Rapid neurologic evaluation using Glasgow Coma Scale score
Exposure and Environmental Control	Expose patient for thorough examination Warm intravenous fluids Warm room and blankets

Abbreviation: FAST, focused assessment with sonography in trauma.

The goal of the primary survey to is identify life-threatening conditions and begin to address those conditions simultaneously.

Data from 10th Edition of the Advanced Trauma Life Support® (ATLS®) Student Course Manual, 2018. American College of Surgeons Chicago, IL.

Table 2 Glasgow Coma Scale		
Category	**Best Response**	**Score**
Eye opening	Spontaneous	4
	To speech	3
	To pain	2
	None	1
Verbal	Oriented	5
	Confused	4
	Inappropriate speech	3
	Incomprehensible sounds	2
	None	1
Motor	Obeys commands	6
	Localizes to painful stimuli	5
	Withdraws from painful stimuli	4
	Abnormal flexion (decorticate posturing)	3
	Abnormal extension (decerebrate posturing)	2
	None	1

The GCS score is the sum of the best response in each category. Patients who are intubated are automatically given a verbal score of 1.

Data from Teasdale G, Maas A, Lecky F, et al. The Glasgow Coma Scale at 40 years: standing the test of time. Lancet Neurol 2014;13(8):844-854.

intensive care unit. DCR was developed from the earlier concept of damage control surgery (DCS). DCS was described in the early 1980s whereby the abdominal compartment was quickly packed and injuries formally repaired later in an effort to avoid coagulopathy.[6] The contemporary elements of DCS include controlling surgical bleeding, containing gastrointestinal spillage, placing surgical packing (sponges), and applying a temporary abdominal closure.[7,8] The critical goals of DCR are outlined in **Box 1**.

Unique Trauma Populations

Although the early management of patients with trauma follows a specific algorithm, several different trauma populations exist, each with its own considerations that may affect anesthetic management (**Fig. 1**). The wide spectrum of disorders that accompanies patients with polytrauma may require the care of specialists such as

Box 1 Damage control resuscitation
DCS
Early initiation of blood product transfusions
Reduced crystalloid fluid administration
Permissive hypotension (hypotensive resuscitation) in select populations
Avoidance or reversal of hypothermia
Avoidance or reversal of acidosis
Correction of coagulopathy
Data from Ball CG. Damage control resuscitation: history, theory and technique. Can J Surg 2014;57(1):55-60.

neurosurgeons, cardiothoracic surgeons, or orthopedic surgeons. This possibility also means that trauma anesthesiologists must be capable of managing several complex anesthetic issues that may otherwise be managed by anesthesia subspecialists. These unique issues may include thoracic trauma requiring initiation of extracorporeal membrane oxygenation or lung isolation, neurotrauma requiring management of increased intracranial pressures, and trauma in pregnancy. When faced with challenging scenarios, the anesthesiologist is an integral part of the multispecialty trauma team.

Airway Management

Decisions to intubate should involve both the anesthesiologist and traumatologist. Major trauma societies, including the Eastern Association for the Surgery of Trauma and ATLS, have published indications for endotracheal intubation in patients with trauma.[9,10] Although the American Society of Anesthesiologist (ASA) difficult airway algorithm is an excellent guide for trauma anesthesiologists, often direct trauma to the airway or patient factors such as combativeness necessitate a unique approach to the trauma airway (**Fig. 2**).[11–13] If laryngoscopy is challenging, alternative airway management devices must be available. These devices include supraglottic airways, video laryngoscopes, endotracheal tube introducers (ie, bougie), and fiberoptic endoscopes. Regardless of the algorithm used, trauma personnel must be immediately available to intervene with a cricothyroidotomy in the event of an inability to intubate or rescue with ventilation.

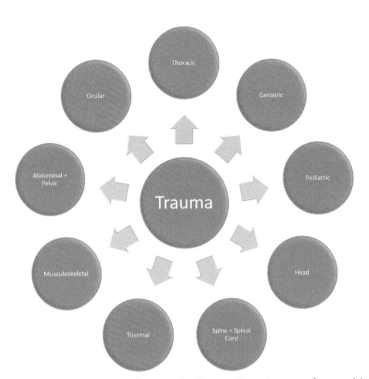

Fig. 1. Several unique trauma populations exist that require unique care from multispecialty teams. Although the initial care of patients with trauma remains similar between patient groups, further care diverges.

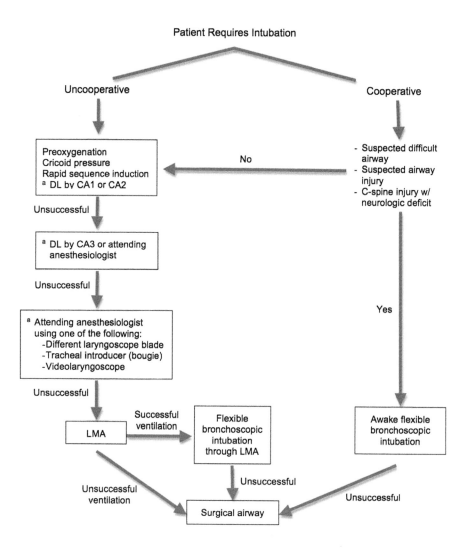

Fig. 2. Ryder Trauma Center emergency airway algorithm. CA1, clinical anesthesia 1 resident (postgraduate year 2); CA2, clinical anesthesia 2 resident (postgraduate year 3); CA3, clinical anesthesia 3 resident (postgraduate year 4); DL, direct laryngoscopy; LMA, laryngeal mask airway. (*From* Diez C, Varon AJ. Airway Management. In: Varon AJ, Smith CE, editors. Essentials of Trauma Anesthesia. Cambridge: Cambridge University Press; 2012; with permission.)

Vascular Access: Venous and Arterial

One of the most important, and sometimes vital, early interventions needed in patients with trauma is establishing peripheral intravenous (IV) access. It is recommended to obtain at least 2 large-bore (at least 18 gauge) peripheral venous catheters, ideally in the forearm or antecubital region.[10] Central venous or intraosseous access should be obtained in cases in which vascular access is challenging or the use of high-risk medications such as vasopressors or inotropes is expected. Central venous catheters (CVCs) can also be used to obtain a central venous pressure, which is an additional tool to track resuscitation efforts.

The main CVC insertion sites include the internal jugular vein, subclavian vein, and femoral vein. The site should be chosen based on site accessibility, patient anatomy, and trauma location. The subclavian approach is often favored given its patency during hypotension, ability to access without ultrasonography, and low rate of infection. The presence of a thick tunica reinforcing the walls of the vessel and attaching it to surrounding ligaments, fascia, and periosteum helps maintain the lumen patency.

There are several different types of common vascular access devices (**Table 3**) used in the trauma setting. These devices differ in their caliber, length, and number of lumens.

Aside from central access, arterial blood pressure monitoring is critically important in patients with hemodynamic instability. The indications for arterial access in patients with trauma include:

- Close hemodynamic monitoring (beat-to-beat data acquisition)
- Frequent blood sampling
- Continuous cardiac output monitoring (if using a noninvasive continuous cardiac output device)

Patients with trauma with severe injuries tend to present with significant hemodynamic lability and are at increased risk of arrhythmias, which makes blood pressure monitoring via a traditional inflatable cuff less reliable. For this reason, in patients with extensive trauma, arterial line placement should be attempted before induction of general anesthesia if time permits. Sites for arterial cannulation include radial, brachial, axillary, femoral, and dorsalis pedis. Of these, the radial artery is the most commonly used given its superficial location and accessibility to anesthesiologists. Radial arterial line placement is also recommended in cases of abdominal or chest trauma, in which aortic cross-clamping may be required. In cases of hemodynamic instability and lack of a palpable pulse, the femoral approach may be preferred because of its larger caliber.

Table 3 Venous access devices			
Device Type	Size	Length	Lumens
Peripheral intravenous line	14–18 G	>1″	1
Rapid infusion catheter	7 or 8.5 Fr	5.08 or 6.35 cm (2″ or 2.5″)	1
Intraosseous line	15 G	15, 25 or 45 mm	1
Central venous catheter	7–9 Fr	16, 20, 24 cm	3–4
Percutaneous sheath introducer	4–8 Fr	7.5–11 cm	1
Multiaccess catheter	9 Fr + 12 G	11.5 cm	2

Data from Teleflex. Vascular Access Products. Available at: teleflex.com/usa/product-areas/vascular-access/products. Accessed Sept 5 2019.

Induction of Anesthesia

Agents used during induction of anesthesia should be chosen based on their pharmacologic properties and the patient's clinical condition. The emergence of airway management and the presence of hemodynamic instability or head injuries should be considered when choosing induction techniques and medications. The primary goal of induction should be to maintain hemodynamic stability while providing an adequate level of pain control, amnesia, and securing the airway promptly in order to avoid secondary injuries related to hypoxia and aspiration. Importantly, regardless of the induction agent used, intravenous anesthetics may precipitate profound shock or even cardiac arrest via the inhibition of circulating catecholamines. As such, the multidisciplinary trauma team must be immediately available during the period of induction.

The most commonly used method for induction of anesthesia in patients with trauma is rapid sequence intubation (RSI). Patients with traumatic injuries are generally considered to have a full stomach and to be at high risk of aspiration given that the last oral intake cannot be confirmed, blood from oropharyngeal injuries can be swallowed, and sympathetic stimulation may result in decreased gastric emptying.[14,15]

Although propofol has been widely used as an induction drug of choice for general anesthesia, hypotension associated with induction doses make the use of etomidate (0.2–0.3 mg/kg IV) and ketamine (1–4.5 mg/kg IV) preferred agents in most emergency trauma settings. Under normal circumstances, the use of these two agents is associated with less cardiovascular depression. However, in the setting of critical illness, their use may lead to cardiovascular compromise given associated conditions such as hypothermia, alcohol or drug intoxication, hemorrhagic shock, and metabolic disturbances.[16,17]

Amnestic agents should be strongly considered before or following induction of anesthesia should the clinical scenario permit. Patients with trauma are at high risk for surgical recall under general anesthesia given lower doses of anesthetics in the setting of hemodynamic instability and are also at risk for significant pain given their injuries.[18] Therefore, the use of a benzodiazepine, such as midazolam (0.1 mg/kg IV) for its amnestic properties and an opioid for pain control should be strongly considered. In addition, alternative agents such as scopolamine (tertiary ammonium vagolytic) can be considered as an alternative or adjunct to benzodiazepines in order to prevent recall.[19] Commonly used intravenous anesthetics with agent-specific considerations in trauma are listed in **Table 4**.

Paralytics

Administration of induction agents is followed by use of neuromuscular blocking agents that allow optimal intubating conditions. The neuromuscular agent of choice in trauma is succinylcholine (1–2 mg/kg IV) given its quick onset of action (<1 minute) and short duration of action (5–10 minutes), the latter characteristic making it more suitable for cases of difficult intubation. The use of succinylcholine is contraindicated in certain circumstances (**Box 2**), in which case the neuromuscular agent of choice becomes rocuronium (1.2 mg/kg for RSI) given its quick onset of action at this higher dose. Rocuronium has a longer duration of action but does have a specific reversal agent (sugammadex). If rocuronium is used in the setting of a nonreassuring airway, then sugammadex should be immediately available for reversal. Regardless of the paralytic used, a trauma team should be ready for potential airway compromise and the need for emergent cricothyrotomy.

Table 4
Intravenous anesthetics

Drug Name	Mechanism of Action	Induction Dose (mg/kg IV)	Physiologic Response	Trauma Considerations
Midazolam	Binds to $GABA_A$ receptor complex prolonging chloride ion channel opening	0.2–0.4	• Dose-dependent anxiolytic • Anterograde amnestic • Hypnotic • Sedative • Anticonvulsant • Spinally mediated muscle relaxant	• Given the high incidence of recall in emergency trauma cases (up to 40%), its use is highly recommended when hemodynamics may tolerate
Thiopental	Mimics the action of GABA by directly activating chloride ion channels and prolonging opening	3–5	• Direct myocardial depression • Peripheral vasodilation • Decrease in $CMRO_2$, CBF, and ICP	• Not commonly used as primary induction agent • Useful in the management of TBI
Propofol	• Enhances activity of GABA-activated chloride ion channels • Ion channel blocking effects in the cerebral cortex and nicotinic acetylcholine receptors	1.5–2.5	• Decreases $CMRO_2$, CBF, and ICP • Dose-dependent respiratory and cardiovascular depression	• Less commonly used in trauma given potential hypotension with induction doses
Etomidate	• Augments GABA-gated chloride currents • Associated with direct activation of GABA receptors at high doses	0.2–0.3	• Decreases $CMRO_2$, CBF, and ICP • Minimal cardiorespiratory depression • Associated with adrenal suppression and cortisol synthesis inhibition	• Useful for induction of patients with hemodynamic instability • Not recommended as prolonged infusion as adrenal suppression may lead to further hypotension
Ketamine	• Primary antagonistic activity at NMDA receptors • Binds to non-NMDA glutamate, nicotinic, muscarinic, monoaminergic, and kappa-opioid receptors	1–2	• Produces functional dissociation between the thalamocortical and limbic systems • Minimal respiratory depression • Potent bronchodilator • Profound analgesia and amnesia • May potentially increase heart rate and blood pressure	• Given its favorable hemodynamic and analgesic/amnesic profile it is a common induction agent in hemodynamically unstable patients

Abbreviations: CBF, cerebral blood flow; $CMRO_2$, cerebral metabolic rate of oxygen; GABA, gamma-aminobutyric acid; ICP, intracranial pressure; NMDA, *N*-methyl-D-aspartate.

Data from White PF, Eng MR. Intravenous anesthetics. In: Barash PG, Cullen BF, Stoelting RK, et al, eds. Clinical Anesthesia, 6th edition. Philadelphia: Lippincott Williams & Wilkins; 2009.

Box 2
Succinylcholine contraindications in trauma populations

- Hyperkalemia (K>5.5 mEq/L)
- 48 to 72 hours (peak 7–10 days) after major burn, crush injury, or polytrauma
- Increased intracranial pressure
- Increased intraocular pressure
- History of malignant hyperthermia
- Chronic myopathies
- Denervating neuromuscular diseases

Data from Martyn JA, Richtsfeld M. Succinylcholine-induced hyperkalemia in acquired pathologic states: etiologic factors and molecular mechanisms. Anesthesiology 2006;104(1):158-69.

Maintenance of Anesthesia

As in most cases of general anesthesia, maintenance of anesthesia is most frequently achieved with the use of inhaled anesthetics. Achieving an adequate depth of anesthesia in a hemodynamically unstable trauma patient requires several considerations. There are many factors that potentially decrease the minimum alveolar concentration (MAC); common examples in a trauma population include hemorrhagic shock, which can be associated with a 25% decrease in MAC, and alcohol intoxication, which can result in a variable decreases in MAC.[20] Inhaled anesthetics, including sevoflurane, isoflurane, and desflurane, are associated with decreases in arterial blood pressure via a decreased cardiac output and increased peripheral vasodilation. Given these effects, achieving an adequate MAC may be challenging in unstable patients with trauma.

Nitrous oxide is another commonly used inhaled anesthetic that results in stimulation of the sympathetic nervous system, leading to tachycardia and hypertension in healthy patients. Patients with trauma are unique in their profound sympathetic stimulation; this may unmask the direct myocardial depressive effects of nitrous oxide, leading to hemodynamic instability. In addition, nitrous oxide may result in an increased incidence of arrhythmias. In the setting of a known pneumothorax or chest trauma, nitrous oxide is contraindicated because of expansion of air-containing cavities. In addition, nitrous oxide decreases the fraction of inspired oxygen, leading to hypoxemia and secondary injuries in certain patient populations.

Initial Resuscitation

The lethal triad of trauma (hypothermia, acidosis, and coagulopathy) can cause profound morbidity and mortality in severely injured patients with trauma. Roughly 25% of patients with trauma present to the hospital with a coagulopathy.[21] Administration of large -volume crystalloid resuscitation may be appropriate in most critically ill patients with hemodynamic compromise; however, in patients with severe hemorrhage caused by trauma, this approach has been found to increase mortality.[22] The definition of a large volume of crystalloid is generally considered to be greater than 1.5 L during the initial bolus or 3 L within the first 6 hours.[10,23] Aggressive crystalloid resuscitation has been associated with increased hydrostatic pressure destabilizing formed clots, dilution of clotting factors, decreased oxygen carrying capacity of blood, and further blood loss.[24–26]

Hypotensive resuscitation or permissive hypotension refers to maintaining a lower than normal blood pressure, adequate to provide essential organ perfusion but low enough to limit bleeding and allow surgical control of hemorrhage. Several studies have shown benefit with this technique in the setting of active hemorrhage; however, positive results have not been replicated consistently.[27–29] A landmark study described this concept in patients with penetrating torso injury, in which fluid restriction conferred a survival benefit if delayed until the time of definitive hemostasis.[30] Several recent systematic reviews support the concept of permissive hypotension, with 1 study showing a survival benefit in penetrating or blunt hemorrhagic injury with systolic blood pressure (SBP) goals between 50 and 70 mm Hg or mean arterial pressure (MAP) targets greater than 50 mm Hg.[31,32] Official guidelines from major societies do not clearly identify an optimal SBP or MAP in early resuscitation.[10] ATLS suggests the strategy may be a bridge to definitive therapy in the setting of penetrating trauma with hemorrhage; no specific hemodynamic goals are recommended. European practice guidelines and recent review provide more defined recommendations, specifically a target SBP of 80 to 90 mm Hg until major bleeding has been stopped, with higher goals (MAP $\geq$ 80 mm Hg) in the setting of TBI.[33,34]

Massive Transfusion

Under normal conditions, physiologic compensatory mechanisms maintain adequate end-organ perfusion when blood loss is less than 30% of the total blood volume.[35] When blood loss exceeds this threshold, hypoperfusion usually ensues and clinical signs of shock become apparent. Mild to moderate blood loss can be managed with infusion of crystalloids or colloids and tolerated well, but, once blood loss becomes more significant and the amount of volume administered exceeds 1.5 L, dilution of coagulation factors ensues, leading to worsening coagulopathy and further blood loss.[36] At this point, blood product administration should begin and be guided by laboratory values, as long as the patient remains hemodynamically stable. As blood loss progresses, products must be administered based on clinical findings, at which point a massive transfusion protocol (MTP) is useful in the management and rapid correction of coagulopathy. The main goal of instituting an MTP is to rapidly (up to 500 mL/min) provide warmed blood component therapy in a balanced ratio.[34]

Although several definitions have been used to describe massive transfusion in the trauma literature, the most common definition is the transfusion of at least 10 units of packed red blood cells (PRBCs) in a 24-hour period.[37,38] The more dynamic definitions of MTP, such as the replacement of greater than 50% of total blood volume in 3 hours or the transfusion of at least 4 units of blood within an hour (when the administration of more products is expected), may be more useful in daily practice.[39,40] Rapid identification of the degree of blood loss has been shown to affect patient outcomes, because delays in initiation of massive transfusion have been associated with an increase in the odds of mortality by 5% for every minute in delay.[41]

Blood Component Therapy, Factor Replacement, and Hemostatic Agents

Although some literature suggests that whole-blood transfusion seems ideal in bleeding patients, given limited health care resources, logistical concerns, and the need for the efficient use of blood product reservoirs, blood component transfusion is almost universally used in the modern health care environment.[42] There is no consensus recommendation on the correct ratio of product administration; however, a balanced approach to transfusion of PRBCs, fresh frozen plasma (FFP), platelets, and cryoprecipitate is a widely accepted practice. Several studies suggest a ratio of 1:1:1 (ratio of PRBCs to FFP to platelets) reduces mortality from hemorrhage.[43–45]

In addition to the typical blood products administered as part of an MTP, other hemostatic products that may be used in severely coagulopathic patients with clinical evidence of significant blood loss. Factor VII, prothrombin complex concentrate, cell salvage techniques, and antifibrinolytics are among these products; if given in the correct clinical scenario, they are important adjuncts in the control of ongoing bleeding. Of these, the antifibrinolytic tranexamic acid (TXA) has been shown to reduce the need for transfusions and mortality when administered within 3 hours of injury, but it is associated with an increased risk of mortality if administered after this period.[46,47] TXA is being incorporated more frequently into MTPs because it has been shown to decrease the number of products administered in order to achieve hemostasis, avoiding potential adverse effects of massive blood product transfusion.[48] The specific indications for TXA vary; however, experts suggest dosing the medication whenever an MTP is activated.[49] Risks versus benefits must be weighed and individualized based on specific patient factors, including the possibility of thrombotic complications when administering TXA.[50,51]

Coagulation Monitoring

Although coagulation testing using traditional laboratory tests such as prothrombin time, partial thromboplastin time, platelet count, and fibrinogen level remains useful in the care of patients with trauma, newer real-time tests are becoming more widespread. These viscoelastic assays, the 2 most common being rotational thromboelastometry and rapid thromboelastography, provide information on clot formation and coagulation abnormalities that are less evident or even masked by traditional testing.[52] By identifying specific abnormalities in coagulation, anesthesiologists are able to provide a more tailored blood component or antifibrinolytic. The use of these assays requires close coordination with laboratory and information technology personnel in order to run the test rapidly and have a means, generally a monitor in an operating room or procedure suite, to monitor the results in real time.

Late Resuscitation

Late resuscitation begins once the source of bleeding has been controlled; this period allows time for a more controlled resuscitation guided by laboratory data and more advanced monitoring techniques. During this stage, additional blood products are administered as needed to correct laboratory value derangements or obvious clinical findings. Intravenous fluids may be administered in attempts to optimize fluid status and tissue perfusion using traditional and contemporary clinical tools, including urinary output, clearance of serum lactate levels, continuous cardiac output monitoring, and bedside echocardiography. The goal of late resuscitation is optimization of the patient and minimization of complications in order to achieve long-term recovery.

SUMMARY

Patients with extensive trauma require multidisciplinary and coordinated care in order to address issues in a protocolized, stepwise fashion. The trauma anesthesiologist is a critical member of this team from the moment the patient enters the trauma bay. Unique characteristics in the care of traumatically injured patients require an understanding of pathophysiology, pharmacology, and airway issues that may be unique to certain trauma populations. Trauma anesthesiologists have a great responsibility in understanding these complex and dynamic issues but also a great opportunity to provide an excellent result for the patient.

DISCLOSURE

The authors have nothing to disclose.

REFERENCES

1. Centers for Disease Control and Prevention. Ten leading causes of death and injury. 2017. Available at: https://www.cdc.gov/injury/wisqars/LeadingCauses.html. Accessed September 1, 2019.
2. Centers for Disease Control and Prevention. Key injury and violence data. 2017. Available at: https://www.cdc.gov/injury/wisqars/overview/key_data.html. Accessed September 1, 2019.
3. Lozano R, Naghavi M, Foreman K, et al. Global and regional mortality from 235 causes of death for 20 age groups in 1990 and 2010: a systematic analysis for the Global Burden of Disease Study 2010. Lancet 2012;380(9859):2095–128.
4. Kauvar DS, Lefering R, Wade CE. Impact of hemorrhage on trauma outcome: an overview of epidemiology, clinical presentations, and therapeutic considerations. J Trauma 2006;60(6 Suppl):S3–11.
5. Teasdale G, Maas A, Lecky F, et al. The Glasgow Coma Scale at 40 years: standing the test of time. Lancet Neurol 2014;13(8):844–54.
6. Stone HH, Strom PR, Mullins RJ. Management of the major coagulopathy with onset during laparotomy. Ann Surg 1983;197(5):532–5.
7. Ball CG. Damage control resuscitation: history, theory and technique. Can J Surg 2014;57(1):55–60.
8. Rotondo MF, Schwab CW, McGonigal MD, et al. 'Damage control': an approach for improved survival in exsanguinating penetrating abdominal injury. J Trauma 1993;35(3):375–82 [discussion: 382–3].
9. Mayglothling J, Duane TM, Gibbs M, et al. Emergency tracheal intubation immediately following traumatic injury: an Eastern Association for the Surgery of Trauma practice management guideline. J Trauma Acute Care Surg 2012;73(5 Suppl 4):S333–40.
10. American College of Surgeons' Committee on Trauma. Advanced trauma life support®. 10th edition. Chicago: American College of Surgeons; 2018.
11. Apfelbaum JL, Hagberg CA, Caplan RA, et al. Practice guidelines for management of the difficult airway: an updated report by the American Society of Anesthesiologists Task Force on Management of the Difficult Airway. Anesthesiology 2013;118(2):251–70.
12. Diez C, Varon AJ. Airway management and initial resuscitation of the trauma patient. Curr Opin Crit Care 2009;15(6):542–7.
13. Diez C, Varon AJ. Airway management. In: Varon AJ, Smith C, editors. Essentials of trauma anesthesia. Cambridge (United Kingdom): Cambridge University Press; 2012. p. 28–42.
14. Kao CH, ChangLai SP, Chieng PU, et al. Gastric emptying in head-injured patients. Am J Gastroenterol 1998;93(7):1108–12.
15. Browning KN, Travagli RA. Central nervous system control of gastrointestinal motility and secretion and modulation of gastrointestinal functions. Compr Physiol 2014;4(4):1339–68.
16. Dewhirst E, Frazier WJ, Leder M, et al. Cardiac arrest following ketamine administration for rapid sequence intubation. J Intensive Care Med 2013;28(6):375–9.
17. Cotton BA, Guillamondegui OD, Fleming SB, et al. Increased risk of adrenal insufficiency following etomidate exposure in critically injured patients. Arch Surg 2008;143(1):62–7 [discussion : 67].

18. Domino KB, Posner KL, Caplan RA, et al. Awareness during anesthesia: a closed claims analysis. Anesthesiology 1999;90(4):1053–61.

19. Hartmannsgruber MW, Gabrielli A, Layon AJ, et al. The traumatic airway: the anesthesiologist's role in the emergency room. Int Anesthesiol Clin 2000;38(4): 87–104.

20. Wolfson B, Freed B. Influence of alcohol on anesthetic requirements and acute toxicity. Anesth Analg 1980;59(11):826–30.

21. Brohi K, Singh J, Heron M, et al. Acute traumatic coagulopathy. J Trauma 2003; 54(6):1127–30.

22. Jones DG, Nantais J, Rezende-Neto JB, et al. Crystalloid resuscitation in trauma patients: deleterious effect of 5L or more in the first 24h. BMC Surg 2018;18(1):93.

23. Shafi S, Collinsworth AW, Richter KM, et al. Bundles of care for resuscitation from hemorrhagic shock and severe brain injury in trauma patients-Translating knowledge into practice. J Trauma Acute Care Surg 2016;81(4):780–94.

24. Hardy JF, de Moerloose P, Samama CM. The coagulopathy of massive transfusion. Vox Sang 2005;89(3):123–7.

25. Cosgriff N, Moore EE, Sauaia A, et al. Predicting life-threatening coagulopathy in the massively transfused trauma patient: hypothermia and acidoses revisited. J Trauma 1997;42(5):857–61 [discussion: 861–2].

26. Cotton BA, Guy JS, Morris JA Jr, et al. The cellular, metabolic, and systemic consequences of aggressive fluid resuscitation strategies. Shock 2006;26(2): 115–21.

27. Dutton RP, Mackenzie CF, Scalea TM. Hypotensive resuscitation during active hemorrhage: impact on in-hospital mortality. J Trauma 2002;52(6):1141–6.

28. Li T, Zhu Y, Hu Y, et al. Ideal permissive hypotension to resuscitate uncontrolled hemorrhagic shock and the tolerance time in rats. Anesthesiology 2011;114(1): 111–9.

29. Morrison CA, Carrick MM, Norman MA, et al. Hypotensive resuscitation strategy reduces transfusion requirements and severe postoperative coagulopathy in trauma patients with hemorrhagic shock: preliminary results of a randomized controlled trial. J Trauma 2011;70(3):652–63.

30. Bickell WH, Wall MJ Jr, Pepe PE, et al. Immediate versus delayed fluid resuscitation for hypotensive patients with penetrating torso injuries. N Engl J Med 1994; 331(17):1105–9.

31. Tran A, Yates J, Lau A, et al. Permissive hypotension versus conventional resuscitation strategies in adult trauma patients with hemorrhagic shock: A systematic review and meta-analysis of randomized controlled trials. J Trauma Acute Care Surg 2018;84(5):802–8.

32. Albreiki M, Voegeli D. Permissive hypotensive resuscitation in adult patients with traumatic haemorrhagic shock: a systematic review. Eur J Trauma Emerg Surg 2018;44(2):191–202.

33. Spahn DR, Bouillon B, Cerny V, et al. The European guideline on management of major bleeding and coagulopathy following trauma: fifth edition. Crit Care 2019; 23(1):98.

34. King DR. Initial care of the severely injured patient. N Engl J Med 2019;380(8): 763–70.

35. Mutschler M, Nienaber U, Brockamp T, et al. A critical reappraisal of the ATLS® classification of hypovolaemic shock: does it really reflect clinical reality? Resuscitation 2013;84(3):309–13.

36. Ley EJ, Clond MA, Srour MK, et al. Emergency department crystalloid resuscitation of 1.5 L or more is associated with increased mortality in elderly and nonelderly trauma patients. J Trauma 2011;70(2):398–400.
37. Lim RC Jr, Olcott CT, Robinson AJ, et al. Platelet response and coagulation changes following massive blood replacement. J Trauma 1973;13(7):577–82.
38. Malone DL, Hess JR, Fingerhut A. Massive transfusion practices around the globe and a suggestion for a common massive transfusion protocol. J Trauma 2006;60(6 Suppl):S91–6.
39. Fakhry SM, Sheldon GF. Massive transfusion in the surgical patient. In: Jeffries LC, Brecher ME, editors. Massive Transfusion. Bethesda (MD): American Association of Blood Banks; 1994.
40. Moltzan CJ, Anderson DA, Callum J, et al. The evidence for the use of recombinant factor VIIa in massive bleeding: development of a transfusion policy framework. Transfus Med 2008;18(2):112–20.
41. Meyer DE, Vincent LE, Fox EE, et al. Every minute counts: Time to delivery of initial massive transfusion cooler and its impact on mortality. J Trauma Acute Care Surg 2017;83(1):19–24.
42. Repine TB, Perkins JG, Kauvar DS, et al. The use of fresh whole blood in massive transfusion. J Trauma 2006;60(6 Suppl):S59–69.
43. Cannon JW, Khan MA, Raja AS, et al. Damage control resuscitation in patients with severe traumatic hemorrhage: a practice management guideline from the Eastern Association for the Surgery of Trauma. J Trauma Acute Care Surg 2017;82(3):605–17.
44. Holcomb JB, Tilley BC, Baraniuk S, et al. Transfusion of plasma, platelets, and red blood cells in a 1:1:1 vs a 1:1:2 ratio and mortality in patients with severe trauma: the PROPPR randomized clinical trial. JAMA 2015;313(5):471–82.
45. Holcomb JB, del Junco DJ, Fox EE, et al. The prospective, observational, multicenter, major trauma transfusion (PROMMTT) study: comparative effectiveness of a time-varying treatment with competing risks. JAMA Surg 2013;148(2):127–36.
46. Crash collaborators, Roberts I, Shakur H, Afolabi A, et al. The importance of early treatment with tranexamic acid in bleeding trauma patients: an exploratory analysis of the CRASH-2 randomised controlled trial. Lancet 2011;377(9771): 1096–101, 1101.e1-2.
47. Crash trial collaborators, Shakur H, Roberts I, Bautista R, et al. Effects of tranexamic acid on death, vascular occlusive events, and blood transfusion in trauma patients with significant haemorrhage (CRASH-2): a randomised, placebo-controlled trial. Lancet 2010;376(9734):23–32.
48. Godbey EA, Schwartz J. 'Massive transfusion protocols and the use of tranexamic acid'. Curr Opin Hematol 2018;25(6):482–5.
49. Cannon JW. Hemorrhagic Shock. N Engl J Med 2018;378(4):370–9.
50. Nishida T, Kinoshita T, Yamakawa K. Tranexamic acid and trauma-induced coagulopathy. J Intensive Care 2017;5:5.
51. Myers SP, Kutcher ME, Rosengart MR, et al. Tranexamic acid administration is associated with an increased risk of posttraumatic venous thromboembolism. J Trauma Acute Care Surg 2019;86(1):20–7.
52. Theusinger OM, Levy JH. Point of care devices for assessing bleeding and coagulation in the trauma patient. Anesthesiol Clin 2013;31(1):55–65.

Anesthesia for Endocrine Emergencies

Dasun Peramunage, MD[a], Sara Nikravan, MD[b,c],*

KEYWORDS

- Pheochromocytoma • Paraganglioma • Insulinoma • Hyperthyroidism
- Thyrotoxicosis • Hypothyroidism • Hypoglycemia • Myxedema coma

KEY POINTS

- Pheochromocytomas, although rare, have significant risk for morbidity and mortality, requiring diligent preoperative preparation, intraoperative management, and postoperative monitoring for successful resection.
- Both thyrotoxicosis and myxedema coma, although opposite on the spectrum of thyroid disease, have a high mortality rate if left untreated prior to surgical intervention. Slow and careful achievement of euthyroidism preoperatively is optimal when possible.
- Adrenal insufficiency is encountered most often intraoperatively when caring for patients on chronic steroid therapy. Anesthesiologists should have a low threshold for stress-dose steroid administration, keeping in mind the mineralocorticoid effects of their treatment choice.
- Carcinoid syndrome often manifests with hemodynamic perturbations from the secretion of vasoactive peptide as well as the ramifications of carcinoid heart disease from their chronic exposure. Right-sided heart disease is most common.
- Although insulinomas are rare, when encountered, a thorough evaluation for malignancy must be undertaken secondary to their association with multiple endocrine neoplasia type 1. The mainstay of anesthetic management requires balancing hypoglycemia during exposure and manipulation with the risk for postresection hyperglycemia.

PHEOCHROMOCYTOMAS AND PARAGANGLIOMAS

Introduction

Pheochromocytomas and paragangliomas are rare catecholamine-secreting neuroendocrine tumors derived from chromaffin cells located in the adrenal medulla and adjacent to sympathetic ganglia. Pheochromocytoma refers to tumors that arise

[a] Department of Anesthesiology, Virginia Mason Medical Center, 1100 Ninth Avenue, B2-AN, Seattle, WA 98101, USA; [b] Division of Cardiothoracic Anesthesiology, Department of Anesthesiology, Virginia Mason Medical Center, 1100 Ninth Avenue, B2-AN, Seattle, WA 98101, USA; [c] Division of Critical Care Medicine, Virginia Mason Medical Center, 1100 Ninth Avenue, B2-AN, Seattle, WA 98101, USA
* Corresponding author.
E-mail address: nikravan@uw.edu
Twitter: @Nikradoc (S.N.)

Anesthesiology Clin 38 (2020) 149–163
https://doi.org/10.1016/j.anclin.2019.10.006
1932-2275/20/© 2019 Elsevier Inc. All rights reserved.
anesthesiology.theclinics.com

from within the adrenal medulla, whereas extra-adrenal catecholamine-secreting tumors are referred to as paragangliomas. Approximately 80% to 85% of catecholamine-secreting neuroendocrine tumors originate from the adrenal medulla whereas 15% to 20% occur in extra-adrenal tissue.[1] A majority of paragangliomas are nonfunctioning and found in the head and neck. Most functional paragangliomas are found in the abdomen.[2] Hereditary syndromes, such as multiple endocrine neoplasia type 2, von Hippel-Lindau syndrome, and neurofibromatosis type 1, have an association with pheochromocytomas. It is estimated there are approximately 500 to 1600 of these cases per year in the United States.[3] Approximately 0.05% to 0.1% of patients with sustained hypertension carry a pheochromocytoma diagnosis, but this may not capture the full incidence because more than half of patients present with paroxysmal hypertension or normotension.[1]

Signs and Symptoms, Diagnosis, and Surgical Treatment

The classic triad of symptoms is headache, palpitations, and diaphoresis; these symptoms are secondary to the intermittent or sustained release of catecholamines (namely norepinephrine, epinephrine, and dopamine) from tumor cells. Additionally, other nonspecific symptoms, such as flushing, weight loss, trembling, orthostatic hypotension, hyperglycemia, pallor, and anxiety, are reported. A diagnosis of suspected pheochromocytomas and paragangliomas relies on serum and urine measurement of metanephrine and normetanephrine, which are metabolites of epinephrine and norepinephrine respectively. A 4-fold increase in these metabolites has a high specificity and sensitivity in both adults and children. To reduce false-positive results, patients must abstain from caffeine, strenuous physical exercise, and smoking 8 hours to 12 hour prior to testing, and venous samples should be drawn while the patient is supine. If metanephrine levels are elevated above the reference range but below the 4-fold threshold, then a clonidine suppression test prior to serum measurement of catecholamines and metanephrines can be performed.[4] If serum levels do not decrease after the suppression test, then either computed tomography (CT) or magnetic resonance imaging (MRI) can be used for tumor localization. If metastatic disease is suspected, then functional imaging with 123I-metaiodobenzylguanidine, a radiolabeled norepinephrine analog, can help localized other tumor sites.[4]

Surgery remains the definitive treatment of pheochromocytomas and paragangliomas that have been diagnosed and localized. Although once thought to be exquisitely risky given the need for abdominal insufflation, laparoscopic surgery now is the preferred technique for tumor resection. Certain cases may still require open procedures. Laparoscopic resections can be performed in either a transabdominal or retroperitoneal approach.

Preoperative Evaluation and Preparation

It is critical to perform thorough preoperative evaluation and optimization prior to surgical resection. The morbidity and mortality of patients undergoing resection increases significantly if patients are not adequately optimized prior to surgery.[5] The focus of the preoperative period should be to control hypertension, reverse chronic intravascular volume depletion, treat cardiac arrhythmias, evaluate cardiac function, and address electrolyte disturbances and hyperglycemia.

Preoperative α-blockade has been the primary pharmacologic therapy for blood pressure control prior to surgical resection. It often is initiated 10 days to 14 days prior to the day of surgery and has the benefit of both normalizing blood pressure and allowing for expansion of intravascular volume. Phenoxybenzamine, an irreversible nonselective α-receptor antagonist, often is used as a preoperative antihypertensive. Short-acting α_1-antagonists, such as prazosin and doxazosin, also may be used. Given the nonselective nature and expense of phenoxybenzamine, investigators are looking to directly compare selective versus nonselective α-blockers. Currently, there is a clinical trial under way comparing phenoxybenzamine to doxazosin and their respective morbidity, mortality, hemodynamic instability, cost, and quality-of-life measures in patients prior to pheochromocytoma resection, which may yield some interesting results (NCT03176693).

The adequacy of preoperative α-blockade is defined by the Roizen[6] criteria. These criteria include in-hospital blood pressure less than 160/90 mm Hg 24 hours prior to surgery; no orthostatic hypotension with blood pressure less than 80/45 mm Hg; no ST or T wave changes prior to surgery; and no more than 5 premature ventricular contractions in a minute.[6] Long-acting α-antagonists are withheld 12 hours to 24 hours prior to surgery. Calcium channel blockers also can be used as adjuncts to α-blockade therapy. β-Blockers also may be considered preoperatively but only after an adequate duration of α-blockade has been initiated. This is done to avoid the hypertensive complications of unopposed α-stimulation.

A preoperative cardiac evaluation is essential prior to surgery. A 12-lead electrocardiogram can be helpful in identifying evidence of ischemia, bundle branch block, and left ventricular hypertrophy. Furthermore, echocardiography is useful in identifying the various structural cardiac changes associated with chronically elevated circulating catecholamines. Cardiac manifestations of pheochromocytomas are varied and may include catecholamine-induced cardiomyopathy, Takotsubo cardiomyopathy, left ventricular hypertrophy with diastolic dysfunction, and dilated cardiomyopathy.[7,8] Although rare, patients with pheochromocytoma can develop myocarditis, making troponin evaluations and assessment for leukocytosis in addition to electrocardiography and echocardiography also important. Echocardiography is also useful in diagnosing cardiac paragangliomas.[8]

Perioperative Management

The primary anesthetic goal for pheochromocytoma resection is to maintain stable hemodynamics intraoperatively. Catecholamine surges can occur with noxious stimuli, such as during laryngoscopy, surgical stimulation, and abdominal insufflation. The most profound surge in catecholamines occurs during surgical manipulation of the tumor itself. This can be followed by profound hypotension once the tumor is devascularized. Preinduction anxiolysis may be helpful because anxiety may provoke a catecholamine surge as well.

Medications that inhibit the reuptake of catecholamines, promote the release of catecholamines, or are associated with histamine release should be avoided. These include medications, such as desflurane, ketamine, morphine, atracurium, pancuronium, ephedrine, and metoclopramide.[9,10] It is the authors' recommendation to list metoclopramide as an allergy preoperatively once there is suspicion for a pheochromocytoma to ensure avoidance of administration. Direct vasodilators, such as nicardipine and sodium nitroprusside, can be used to treat intraoperative hypertension whereas esmolol can be used to treat tachycardia. These medications should be readily available for use during induction, insufflation, and surgical resection. Propofol, short-acting opioids, and midazolam can be safely used for induction, and anesthesia can be maintained with sevoflurane or isoflurane.[9] Magnesium sulfate, remifentanil, and dexmedetomidine infusions also can be used to blunt sympathetic surges associated with direct laryngoscopy and surgical manipulation.[10] Norepinephrine often is used to treat hypotension after tumor resection and vasopressin is also considered to treat refractory hypotension. Intraoperative hyperglycemia should be managed with an insulin infusion, although close postoperative monitoring is necessary because glucose levels can decrease spuriously once the tumor has been resected.

Invasive hemodynamic monitoring is essential for pheochromocytoma surgery. All patients should have an arterial line placed prior to the induction of anesthesia for hemodynamic monitoring. A transesophageal echocardiogram should be considered to guide intraoperative fluid management and diagnose myocardial ischemia. Obtaining central venous access is essential for infusion of vasoactive medications and monitoring right atrial pressure, placement of which also should be considered preinduction. Pulmonary artery catheterization may be useful in patients with existing cardiac dysfunction.[9,10]

Postoperatively, patients require close monitoring of their hemodynamics, electrolytes, and glucose in the intensive care unit. If patients are unresponsive or drowsy, hypoglycemia and hyponatremia must be ruled out. Postoperative hypertension can be the result of inadequate analgesia, fluid overload, urinary retention, ligation of the renal artery, underlying primary hypertension, or undiagnosed metastatic disease/incomplete tumor resection. Persistent postoperative hypotension may be due to residual vasodilation from anesthetics or inadequate intravascular volume.

Despite being rare, pheochromocytomas and their ability to secrete vasoactive catecholamines with potential for catastrophic morbidity and mortality have captivated the attention of anesthesiologists for decades. Understanding of the disease process and careful preoperative preparation can set the stage for successful resection, intraoperative course, and postoperative recovery.

THYROTOXICOSIS/THYROID STORM
Introduction

Thyrotoxicosis is a clinical condition where inappropriately elevated tissue thyroid hormone levels, as in hyperthyroidism, cause a hypermetabolic physiologic state. The prevalence of hyperthyroidism in the United States is approximately 1.2%, with 0.5% having overt disease leaving the remaining 0.7% with subclinical disease.[11] Subclinical disease, which can present with the same signs and symptoms as overt disease, is defined as both thyroxine (T4) and triiodothyronine (T3) levels within the normal reference range with low or undetectable serum thyroid-stimulating hormone (TSH). Common causes for hyperthyroidism are Graves disease, toxic multinodular goiter, and toxic adenoma.

Signs and Symptoms

The symptoms of thyrotoxicosis are mediated by the hypermetabolic state induced by T3, the active form of thyroid hormone, which can affect almost all organ systems. Patients may present with hyperactive neurologic symptoms, such as anxiety, insomnia, agitation, and hyperactivity. Heat intolerance and increased perspiration, goiter formation, weight loss despite increased appetite, muscle weakness and wasting, and eyelid retraction with periorbital edema and ophthalmoplegia are other common signs and symptoms of thyrotoxicosis. The cardiovascular manifestations of thyrotoxicosis include palpitations, atrial fibrillation, tachycardia, exercise intolerance, dyspnea on exertion, and widened pulse pressure. Patients often present with a high cardiac output state secondary to elevated thyroid hormone, reducing peripheral vascular resistance and activating the renin-angiotensin-aldosterone system to increase plasma volume and preload while directly increasing myocardial contractility and resting heart rate.[12] Paradoxically, patients may present with symptoms of heart failure due to preexisting cardiomyopathies, rate-related left ventricular dysfunction due to tachycardia or atrial fibrillation, or right heart failure from pulmonary hypertension. Approximately 65% of patients with Graves disease have pulmonary hypertension.[12]

Diagnosis

Measurements of serum TSH and free T4 are used to diagnose suspected hyperthyroidism, with TSH measurements having the highest sensitivity. A diagnosis is confirmed when TSH levels are below normal reference ranges while T4 levels are normal or elevated. A normal serum TSH, with the absence of a pituitary adenoma or thyroid hormone resistance, precludes hyperthyroidism as a diagnosis. Euthyroid hyperthyroxinemia is a condition where total serum T4 concentrations are elevated but serum TSH levels are normal. This can be secondary to thyroid hormone–binding protein disorders or medications, such as propranolol, amiodarone, or amphetamine abuse, that can lead to inhibition of T4 to T3 conversion.[11] A clinical diagnosis of Graves disease can be made with the presence of a symmetrically enlarged thyroid gland, ophthalmopathy, and moderate to severe hyperthyroidism. Imaging of radioactive iodine uptake is performed when the clinical diagnosis of Graves disease is unclear. Depending on the etiology of the hyperthyroidism, treatment options include radioactive iodine, antithyroid drug therapies, and surgery. Thyroidectomy is indicated for suspected thyroid malignancy, goiters with obstructive symptoms or retrosternal extension, recurrent hyperthyroidism, or failure to respond to medical management.

Perioperative Evaluation and Treatment

In untreated or undertreated thyrotoxicosis, stress from surgery or trauma can precipitate thyroid storm, which has a high mortality. Therefore, it is recommended that patients with thyrotoxicosis should be euthyroid prior to either elective surgery or a thyroidectomy. Antithyroid medications, such as methimazole and propylthiouracil, which directly inhibit synthesis of thyroid hormone, are first-line therapies but can take 6 weeks to 8 weeks to achieve a euthyroid state. Common major side effects of both medications are agranulocytosis, thrombocytopenia, and aplastic anemia; propylthiouracil is additionally associated with fulminant liver failure and antineutrophil cytoplasmic antibody–positive vasculitis.[11,13] A β-adrenergic blocker should be started in the elderly, patients with a resting heart rate over 90 beats per minutes, or patients with coexisting cardiovascular disease. In patients where β-blockade is contraindicated, calcium channel blockers, such as verapamil or diltiazem, may be indicated to control heart rates.[11] Prior to a thyroidectomy for Graves disease, it is recommended that preoperative oral iodine solutions be given because they have been shown to decrease intraoperative blood loss by decreasing thyroid vascularity and blood flow.[11,14] Preoperative evaluation should include an investigation of symptoms associated with thyrotoxicosis with particular attention to cardiopulmonary functions. Routine TSH levels should not be drawn preoperatively unless thyrotoxicosis is suspected or a patient is on antithyroid therapy. The etiology of thyrotoxicosis should be considered because medullary thyroid cancer often is associated with concurrent pheochromocytomas. A thorough airway evaluation should be performed and any imaging of the airway should be reviewed because goiters can compromise the airway or mediastinal structures if there is substernal extension of the mass. Endotracheal intubation is preferred over laryngeal mask airway placement due to risk of displacement or laryngospasm with surgical manipulation.[15] Common postoperative complications of a thyroidectomy include hypocalcemia, airway compromise from laryngeal edema, tracheomalacia, recurrent laryngeal nerve damage, and hematoma.[15]

Thyroid storm or thyrotoxic crisis is a severe form of thyrotoxicosis that is acutely life threatening, with a mortality of 10% to 20%; the pathophysiology of thyroid storm is likely due to the increased catecholamine levels during states of stress that stimulate up-regulated β_1-adrenergic receptors secondary to thyrotoxicosis.[16] Symptoms include hyperthermia, tachycardia/atrial fibrillation, congestive heart failure, jaundice, and central nervous system manifestations ranging in severity from agitation and delirium to seizures and coma. Under general anesthesia, the symptoms of thyroid storm can be difficult to differentiate from malignant hyperthermia. Biochemical assessment of thyroid function should not delay treatment because TSH and T4 levels are not noticeably different from other thyrotoxic states.[16] Treatment involves aggressive pharmacologic inhibition of thyroid hormone synthesis and function along with supportive care. Blockade of T4-T3 conversion and new hormone synthesis is managed with propylthiouracil; methimazole also can be used but the onset of action is delayed in comparison to propylthiouracil. Tachyarrhythmias are managed promptly with β-blockade. Propranolol has the added benefit of blocking conversion of T4 to T3 at higher doses. Unstable tachyarrhythmias should be treated with cardioversion. After initiation of propylthiouracil or methimazole therapy, high doses of oral iodine (saturated solution of potassium iodide or Lugol solution) or iopanoic acid, a radiocontrast agent, are used to block new hormone synthesis and thyroid hormone release via the Wolff–Chaikoff effect. High-dose steroids, such as hydrocortisone or dexamethasone, are used as prophylaxis against relative adrenal insufficiency and also provide the added benefit of reducing T4 to T3 conversion. Cholestyramine can be used as an adjuvant therapy because it prevents enterohepatic recirculation of thyroid hormone by binding to it in the gut.[14] Supportive management of fever with acetaminophen and cooling blankets along with adequate fluid resuscitation and electrolyte repletion is initiated as well. Vasopressors should be administered in the setting of circulatory shock. Once treatment of thyroid storm is initiated, hemodynamic, thermoregulatory, and neurologic stability can be seen in 24 hours to 72 hours.[16]

HYPOTHYROIDISM/MYXEDEMA COMA
Introduction

Hypothyroidism is defined as a pathologic deficiency in thyroid hormone. Diagnosis is based on biochemical markers that subdivide the condition into overt and subclinical hypothyroidism. Overt disease is defined by TSH concentrations above the clinical reference range and free T4 concentrations below the reference range; subclinical hypothyroidism is defined by TSH concentrations above the reference range and free T4 concentrations within the normal range. In the United States, the incidence of overt hypothyroidism is approximately 0.3% to 3.7% and frequently is seen in women and the elderly.[17] Hypothyroidism is commonly found in patients with other autoimmune conditions like type 1 diabetes mellitus or celiac disease and in patients with Down syndrome or Turner syndrome. A vast majority of hypothyroidism cases are due to a primary deficiency in thyroid hormone; fewer than 1% of cases are due to central or peripheral hypothyroidism.[17] Hashimoto disease, a chronic autoimmune thyroiditis, is the most common cause of primary hypothyroidism in areas with sufficient dietary iodine intake, whereas iodine poor diets can lead to primary hypothyroidism as well. Medications, such as amiodarone or lithium, can decrease both thyroid hormone synthesis and release. Primary hypothyroidism also is seen after radioiodine therapy and thyroidectomy for thyrotoxicosis.

Signs and Symptoms

The clinical presentation of hypothyroidism is variable and can range from asymptomatic to myxedema coma, which is life threatening. Owing to the wide systemic effects of thyroid hormone, symptoms of hypothyroidism can be broad and classically include fatigue, lethargy, impaired cognitive function, hoarseness, cold intolerance, weight gain despite loss of appetite, constipation, dry skin, and hair loss. A clinical diagnosis is difficult because symptoms often are nonspecific and populations at risk, such as the elderly, present with fewer and nonclassic signs and symptoms. Hypothyroidism can have a profound effect on cardiac physiology including elevation in diastolic pressures, narrow pulse pressures, bradycardia, QTc prolongation, and a decrease in cardiac contractility; in comparison to euthyroid patients, cardiac output may decrease as much as 30% to 50% in patients with hypothyroidism.[18] A decrease in circulating thyroid hormone leads to an increase in catecholamines and systemic vascular resistance, which leads to diastolic hypertension. A degree of diastolic impairment also is present in these patients. In severe hypothyroidism, myocardial depression can be refractory to inotropes, likely due to down-regulation of β-adrenergic receptors.[19] Coronary artery disease and the risk of ischemic stroke are increased in chronic hypothyroidism, likely secondary the hyperlipidemia and hypertension. Subclinical hypothyroidism has been associated with an increased risk of heart failure. Furthermore, there is an increased incidence of pericardial effusion. Surfactant production and ventilatory response to hypoxia and hypercapnia is reduced. In addition, pleural effusions can be associated with severe hypothyroidism.[19]

Perioperative Evaluation and Treatment

It is recommended that prior to proceeding with elective surgery, patients with hypothyroidism be euthyroid, based on laboratory data (TSH in the normal reference range) and clinical evidence. Patients typically are treated with levothyroxine and, rarely, liothyronine; these medications generally are continued in the perioperative period. In those patients with symptoms of severe chronic hypothyroidism or myxedema coma, there is a substantial perioperative risk of complications. These patients present with a high risk of cardiovascular collapse due to catecholamine resistant cardiac depression. Additionally, generalized edema presents a challenge to securing the airway. Patients also are at risk of aspiration due to delayed gastric emptying and altered mental status. Patients are exquisitely sensitive to sedating medications due to changes in ventilatory response to hypoxia and hypercapnia along with depressed mental status. Anemia and electrolyte abnormalities are common findings; in particular, hyponatremia can be precipitated by increases in circulating antidiuretic hormone. Furthermore, volume status should be assessed carefully because hypothyroidism leads to fluid shifts into the extravascular space due to increases in capillary permeability, leaving patients with decreased intravascular volume. In the setting of emergent surgery, it is recommended that thyroid hormones be normalized as rapidly as possible. In a subset of patients with hypothyroidism and anginal symptoms requiring revascularization, there is a growing body of evidence that their cardiac ischemia may worsen with replacement of thyroid hormone and may benefit more with revascularization prior to beginning thyroid hormone replacement therapy.[18] In cases of severe hypothyroidism, the risk of cardiovascular ischemia must be weighed against the risk of coma and/or cardiovascular collapse from surgical intervention, making close monitoring and careful management of great importance while determining the best route of intervention.

The mortality rate of myxedema coma can be as high as 40%; initial symptoms include lethargy, altered mental status, hypothermia, and bradycardia, quickly progressing to multiorgan failure and death if not promptly recognized and treated.[17] The initial therapy for patients with myxedema coma is intravenous levothyroxine administration, starting with a loading dose and followed by a daily maintenance dose until clinical improvement is noticed, which can take up to week. In severe cases, the addition of intravenous liothyronine may be considered because conversion of T4 to T3 often is decreased in myxedema coma; liothyronine should be used cautiously because high doses have been associated with an increase in mortality.[20] Improvements in mental status, cardiac, and pulmonary function are the clinical endpoints for therapy. Empiric glucocorticoid therapy is recommended along with supportive therapy.

ADRENAL INSUFFICIENCY
Introduction

Adrenal insufficiency is caused by a cortisol production deficiency in the adrenal cortex. In conditions of acute stress, such as surgery, trauma, or infection, adrenal suppression prevents the increase in endogenous cortisol production, a normal physiologic response to stress, and may lead to adrenal crisis, a life-threatening state of acute adrenal insufficiency with a high mortality. The causes of adrenal insufficiency can be broadly categorized into primary, secondary, and tertiary. Autoimmune destruction of the adrenal cortex, such as in Addison disease, makes up approximately 80% to 90% of primary adrenal insufficiency diagnoses.[21] Secondary adrenal insufficiency involves the suppression of corticotropin release by the pituitary, such as in the case of space-occupying lesions, or, as in cases of pituitary apoplexy or pituitary surgery, necrosis or damage to the pituitary itself. In the perioperative setting, tertiary adrenal insufficiency due to suppression of the hypothalamus-pituitary-adrenal axis (HPAA) with high-dose steroid therapy and sudden withdrawal of these medications is the most likely cause of adrenal insufficiency to be encountered by an anesthesia provider. The use of exogenous glucocorticoids of 5-mg prednisolone equivalents or higher, regardless of the route of delivery, for longer than 4 weeks suppresses the HPAA.[22] Adrenal insufficiency also is common in the critically ill population but often is reversible. Furthermore, medications, such as etomidate, can cause adrenal suppression.

Signs, Symptoms, and Perioperative Management

Adrenal insufficiency presents insidiously with nonspecific symptoms, and often the diagnosis is made during a hospitalization for adrenal crisis. Signs and symptoms for adrenal insufficiency include fatigue (84%–95% of patients), weight loss (66%–76%), appetite loss (53%–67%), gastrointestinal symptoms (nausea, vomiting, and abdominal pain) (49%–62%), myalgias (46%–40%), and hyponatremia (70%–80%); in primary adrenal insufficiency, skin hyperpigmentation (41%–74%), salt craving (38%–64%), hyperkalemia (30%–40%), and postural hypotension (55%–68%) are seen.[22] The adrenocorticotropic hormone (ACTH) stimulation test is used for diagnosis of adrenal insufficiency. Baseline ACTH levels and serum cortisol levels are measured before and after stimulation with 250 µg of parenteral ACTH (at 30 minutes and 60 minutes after injection). A peak cortisol below 18 µg/dL to 20 µg/dL supports the diagnosis of adrenal insufficiency with ACTH levels differentiating between primary and the other forms. Once the diagnosis is confirmed, hydrocortisone therapy is started, with dosing titrated based on clinical judgment and perception of symptom resolution.

In adrenal crisis, patients present with hypotension and hypovolemic shock that is refractory to fluids and inotropes. Cortisol modulates catecholamine activity and regulates β-adrenergic receptor synthesis and activity. Approximately 50% of patients with adrenal insufficiency are at risk of developing adrenal crisis, and those with previous episodes of adrenal crisis are likely to have repeat crisis episodes.[23]

Management of adrenal crisis involves fluid resuscitation and steroid replacement. To correct for concurrent hyponatremia, isotonic saline is the preferred crystalloid, with a liter bolus given over an hour and subsequent boluses given as needed and based on frequent assessments of serum electrolytes.[23] Hypoglycemia is corrected by adding dextrose to the solution. Cortisol replacement therapy is started without delay; parenteral hydrocortisone, 100 mg, is given followed by a 100-mg to 300-mg daily dose of hydrocortisone given as a continuous infusion or divided bolus every 6 hours; careful monitoring of serum sodium concentrations is necessary in secondary adrenal insufficiency because cortisol replacement can cause rapid correcting of hyponatremia, which can lead to osmotic demyelination syndrome.[23] Supplemental mineralocorticoid therapy is unnecessary when doses of hydrocortisone exceed 50 mg/d. Treatment of adrenal crisis should not be delayed to perform the ACTH stimulation test, but baseline ACTH and cortisol levels may be drawn prior to starting steroid therapy.

Perioperative management of adrenal insufficiency with stress-dose steroids is a challenge to the anesthesia provider. On one hand, withholding steroids may precipitate a life-threatening adrenal crisis triggered by surgical stress. Glucocorticoid therapy, on the other hand, can also cause immunosuppression with increased risk of infection, hyperglycemia, and poor wound healing. Unfortunately, the literature as a whole does not provide robust evidence regarding perioperative stress-dose steroids because most studies are insufficiently powered and lack consistency in study inclusion criteria. Perioperative stress-dose steroids should be based on surgical stress risk (**Table 1**) and whether a patient has adrenal insufficiency based on ACTH stimulation testing or is at high risk of HPAA suppression (taking at least 20 mg/d prednisolone equivalents for more than 3 weeks or having signs of Cushing syndrome); patients at low risk for HPAA suppression, such as those taking less than 5 mg/d of prednisone equivalents without evidence of HPAA suppression, do not need perioperative stress-dose steroids.[24] Further evaluation is warranted for patients at intermediate risk for HPAA suppression. For an elective surgery, these patients should be referred to a specialist to evaluate their HPAA integrity. If testing is unavailable or the timing of

Table 1		
Surgical stress by procedure and recommended steroid dosing		
Surgery Type	**Examples**	**Recommended Steroid Dosing**
Superficial	Dental surgery, biopsy	Usual daily dose
Minor	Inguinal hernia repair, colonoscopy, uterine curettage, hand surgery	Usual daily dose + hydrocortisone, 50 mg, intravenous; preincision + hydrocortisone, 25 mg, intravenous, every 8 h × 24 h
Moderate	Lower extremity revascularization, total joint replacement, cholecystectomy, colon resection	Usual daily dose + hydrocortisone, 50 mg, intravenous; preincision + hydrocortisone, 25 mg, intravenous, every 8 h × 24 h
Major	Thoracic surgery, cardiovascular surgery, trauma, Whipple, cesarean section	Usual daily dose + hydrocortisone, 100 mg, intravenous; preincision, followed by hydrocortisone, 200 mg/d, infusion for more than 24 h, or hydrocortisone, 50 mg, intravenous, bolus every 8 h × 24 h

Adapted from Liu MM, Reidy AB, Saatee S, et al. Perioperative Steroid Management: Approaches Based on Current Evidence. Anesthesiology 2017;127(1):168; with permission.

surgery does not permit it, then perioperative stress-dose steroids may be deferred if the patient is otherwise healthy and does not exhibit signs of Cushing syndrome, but the anesthesia provider should have a low threshold for rescue-dose steroids in the event of unexplained perioperative hypotension.[24] Additionally, when dosing perioperative stress-dose steroids, the mineralocorticoid properties of the medication should be taken into account because they can cause dose-dependent edema and hypokalemia based on their mineralocorticoid activity.

CARCINOID SYNDROME
Introduction

Carcinoid tumors are slow-growing neoplasms that arise from neuroendocrine cells. The overall incidence of carcinoid tumors is rare, with an estimated 1 case to 2 cases per 100,000 people in the United States.[25] In autopsy examinations, however, the rate of incidentally found carcinoid tumors may be as high as 8%, which suggests under-diagnosis of this condition.[26,27] A majority of tumors are found the gastrointestinal tract, primarily in the appendix, rectum, and ilium, and the respiratory tract, such as in the lungs, trachea, and bronchi. It has been reported that the 5-year survival after diagnosis can be as high as 72% to 78% as for localized or regional disease and 72% for regional disease.[27] These tumors can release hormones and vasoactive peptides, such as serotonin, histamines, dopamine, substance P, prostaglandins, and kallikreins.

Signs and Symptoms

Carcinoid syndrome can arise when vasoactive peptides secreted from tumor cells enter the systemic circulation and classically manifest as episodic flushing, wheezing, and diarrhea. Other clinical manifestations, however, include hypertension, hypotension, and carcinoid heart disease. In patients with carcinoid tumors, approximately 15% to 18% develop carcinoid syndrome.[26] Carcinoid syndrome is rare because most tumors are gastrointestinal in origin and any physiologically active peptides released by the tumors are metabolized by the liver before they can enter systemic circulation. Metastatic disease, especially into the liver, allows these vasoactive substances to bypass hepatic metabolization and manifest as carcinoid syndrome.

Prolonged exposure to vasogenic peptides secreted by metastatic carcinoid tumors lead to carcinoid heart disease. Approximately 50% of patients who develop carcinoid syndrome go on to develop carcinoid heart disease.[28] Presence of carcinoid heart disease is in itself an independent negative prognostic factor in advanced carcinoid disease with a 3-year survival rate of 31% if left untreated.[29] With chronic exposure to vasoactive peptides, fibrinous tissue plaques form on the endocardium and lead to remodeling of the surface of valve leaflets, chordae, papillary muscle, and chambers. In carcinoid heart disease, the structures of the right heart are disproportionately affected as the pulmonary circulation metabolizes these vasogenic substrates, which minimizes the exposure of the left heart to these peptides. Approximately 10% of carcinoid heart disease involves the left heart, often as a result of shunting of vasoactive peptides through a patent foramen ovale, bronchial carcinoid tumors, or high circulating levels of peptides that overwhelm the capacity for hepatic and pulmonary metabolism of these compounds.[29] In the right heart, valvular abnormalities, such as tricuspid regurgitation and pulmonary valvular stenosis or regurgitation, predominate. In patients with severe cardiac disease and well-controlled systemic carcinoid disease, valvular surgery can improve long-term outcomes.[28,30] A diagnosis of carcinoid heart disease based solely on clinical signs of right heart failure can be challenging because most patients with severe valvular pathology show mild symptoms or are asymptomatic. Early and routine echocardiography is recommended for patients with carcinoid syndrome because clinical decompensation from carcinoid heart disease can be rapid.

Diagnosis and Treatment

If carcinoid-like symptoms are present, diagnosis is confirmed with the measurement of urinary 5-hydroxyindoleacetic acid (5-HIAA) and serum chromogranin A. 5-HIAA is a metabolite of serotonin and levels are measured by collecting urinary samples over 24 hours. Chromogranin A is a protein secreted by neuroendocrine tumors. In diagnosis of carcinoid tumors, urine 5-HIAA has 73% sensitivity and 100% specificity, and chromogranin A has 80% sensitivity and 95% specificity.[31] In addition to diagnosing carcinoid tumors, urine 5-HIAA levels also are used to monitor tumor activity and therapy. Once a diagnosis is confirmed, CR, MRI, endoscopy, and somatostatin receptor scintigraphy can be used to localize tumors.

Long-acting somatostatin analog therapy is the cornerstone of medical management for carcinoid syndrome. Carcinoid tumors have an up-regulation of type 2 somatostatin receptors, which are the site of action for somatostatin and its analogs, octreotide and lanreotide.[26] Somatostatin analog doses are titrated to maintain a target 5-HIAA level less than 300 mmol/d. When tumors have metastasized to the liver, transarterial embolization of the hepatic artery is a treatment modality that can reduce the serum vasoactive peptide burden. For localized disease or metastatic disease, especially the liver, surgical intervention potentially is curative or can greatly decrease serum vasoactive peptide levels. In patients with advance carcinoid heart disease, valve replacement has been shown to increase 2-year survival rates to 40% as opposed to only 8% with medical management only.[29]

Perioperative Evaluation and Management

Perioperative evaluation for carcinoid syndrome should primarily focus on identifying signs of carcinoid cardiac disease and symptoms of excessive neuropeptide activity indicative of uncontrolled carcinoid syndrome or crisis. An increased risk of postoperative complications has been reported with patients who have carcinoid heart disease or high levels of urinary 5-HIAA.[26] Preoperative echocardiography should be reviewed for evidence of cardiac dysfunction or structural cardiac abnormalities. Exercise intolerance or evidence of heart failure on history or physical examination warrants immediate cardiac reevaluation prior to surgery. In the setting of diarrhea and high gastric output, careful evaluation of preoperative electrolytes and fluid intravascular volume is necessary.

In the perioperative period, the primary anesthetic management goal is to avoid triggers that may precipitate a carcinoid crisis. This includes the use of anxiolytic medications in the preoperative setting because emotional stress may trigger a crisis. Octreotide is the therapeutic agent of choice for managing intraoperative carcinoid crisis involving bronchospasm or severe hypotension/hypertension. Due to the unpredictable onset of an intraoperative carcinoid crisis and rarity of the condition, intraoperative therapy regimens are based on expert recommendations. Generally, it is recommended that intravenous octreotide therapy should be initiated prior to surgery (from 2 weeks to 24 hours prior to surgery) and maintained with a continuous intraoperative infusion with additional supplemental administration when carcinoid syndrome is suspected.[26,29,31,32] Octreotide doses, up to 500 μg/h, reportedly have been used intraoperatively without major side effects.[32] Aprotinin, a kallikrein inhibitor, can be considered if hypotension is refractory to octreotide.[26] A bolus of octreotide prior to mechanical manipulation of the tumor either during the presurgical prepping or during intraoperative handling of the tumor should be considered because these actions can trigger a crisis. Frequent intraoperative blood glucose monitoring is necessary because octreotide can cause hyperglycemia. Intraoperative medications that are associated with histamine release (such as thiopental, morphine, and meperidine) should be avoided because they can trigger a carcinoid crisis, and succinylcholine should be avoided because fasciculations theoretically can stimulate tumor activity. Induction of anesthesia with propofol or etomidate and maintenance with volatile agents generally is considered safe.[31,32] Increased levels of serum serotonin can delay emergence from anesthesia.[26] It is recommended that routine monitoring for facial flushing or elevated airway pressures be used as surrogate marker for carcinoid crisis–related hypotension and that phenylephrine, vasopressin, calcium, or methylene blue be used to treat octreotide refractory hypotension.[33]

Given the sudden hemodynamic instability and need for rapid intervention during a carcinoid crisis, invasive hemodynamic monitors, such as an arterial line, central venous, and pulmonary artery catheter, are recommended. Additionally, transesophageal echocardiography should be considered, especially in the setting of hepatic metastasis of carcinoid heart disease. Although β-agonists (ephedrine, epinephrine, norepinephrine, dopamine, and isoproterenol) can trigger the release of vasoactive peptides from carcinoid tumors, they may be warranted in the setting of hypotension due to cardiac dysfunction.

Postoperatively, patients require hemodynamic monitoring in the intensive care unit. Residual tumor or metastatic disease can cause persistent release of vasoactive neuropeptides in the postoperative period and lead to hemodynamic instability. It is, therefore, recommended that patients continue octreotide therapy into the postoperative period.

INSULINOMA
Introduction

Insulinomas are rare insulin-secreting intrapancreatic neuroendocrine tumors. Most insulinomas are benign in nature and present in the fourth or fifth decade of life, with 90% being less than 2 cm solitary lesions.[34] Multiple endocrine neoplasia type 1 is associated with approximately 5% to 10% of patients diagnosed with insulinomas and this cohort carries a higher risk for malignancy.[35]

Signs and Symptoms

Patients with insulinomas present with symptoms of hypoglycemia associated with the unregulated secretion of insulin by tumor cells. Hypoglycemia may lead to seizures, fatigue, confusion, behavioral changes, loss of consciousness, and even death. Hypoglycemia also stimulates discharge of the sympathetic nervous system, leading to palpitations, sweating, tremors, and anxiety. Because these symptoms are nonspecific, endogenous hyperinsulinemia may be considered only in the presence of Whipple triad: the symptoms associated with hypoglycemia, low plasma glucose levels, and resolution of symptoms after the administration of glucose. Furthermore, factitious hyperinsulinemia must be ruled out as antidiabetic medications, such as insulin and sulfonylureas, can lead to hypoglycemia.

Diagnosis and Perioperative Management

The gold standard for diagnosis of an insulinoma is a supervised 72-hour fasting test. After the diagnosis, localization is performed using modalities, such as CT, somatostatin receptor scintigraphy, endoscopic ultrasound, and intra-arterial calcium stimulation.[34] Because most tumors are small and benign, surgical resection is potentially curative with techniques, such as enucleation, for clearly localized small lesions and larger resections for more involved tumors. Surgical resection in 1 cohort of patients led to a 100% 5-year disease-free survival rate and 96% 10-year disease-free survival rate.[35]

Anesthetic management during surgical resection involves balancing hypoglycemia during the exposure and manipulation of the tumor and hyperglycemia after the resection is completed. Preoperative hypoglycemia is avoided with oral and intravenous administration of glucose and frequent monitoring of blood glucose levels.[36,37] After tumor excision, some surgeons use intraoperative elevations of plasma glucose levels, which can be expected 30 minutes to 90 minutes after tumor removal, to determine if the resection was complete.[36,38] Iatrogenic changes in plasma glucose, such as with corticosteroid therapy or dextrose infusions, can pose a challenge in making this assessment. The development of rapid insulin assays allows the timely measurement of plasma insulin levels after tumor resection and may provide a means to assess the adequacy of surgery without exposing the patient to prolonged periods of hypoglycemia.[38]

DISCLOSURE

The authors have nothing to disclose.

REFERENCES

1. Lenders JW, Eisenhofer G, Mannelli M, et al. Phaeochromocytoma. Lancet 2005; 366(9486):665–75.
2. Erickson D, Kudva YC, Ebersold MJ, et al. Benign paragangliomas: clinical presentation and treatment outcomes in 236 patients. J Clin Endocrinol Metab 2001; 86(11):5210–6.
3. Chen H, Sippel RS, Pacak K. The NANETS consensus guideline for the diagnosis and management of neuroendocrine tumors: pheochromocytoma, paraganglioma & medullary thyroid cancer. Pancreas 2010;39(6):775–83.
4. Eisenhofer G, Goldstein DS, Walther MM, et al. Biochemical diagnosis of pheochromocytoma: how to distinguish true- from false-positive test results. J Clin Endocrinol Metab 2003;88(6):2656–66.
5. Kinney MA, Warner ME, vanHeerden JA, et al. Perianesthetic risks and outcomes of pheochromocytoma and paraganglioma resection. Anesth Analg 2000;91(5): 1118–23.
6. Roizen MF, Horrigan RW, Koike M, et al. A prospective randomized trial of four anesthetic techniques for resection of pheochromocytoma. Anesthesiology 1982;57:A43.
7. Prejbisz A, Lenders JWM, Eisenhofer G, et al. Cardiovascular manifestations of phaeochromocytoma. J Hypertens 2011;29(11):2049–60.
8. Gu YW, Poste J, Kunal M, et al. Cardiovascular manifestations of pheochromocytoma. Cardiol Rev 2017;25(5):215.
9. Ramakrishna H. Pheochromocytoma resection: current concepts in anesthetic management. J Anaesthesiol Clin Pharmacol 2015;31(3):317–23.
10. Perioperative care of phaeochromocytoma - BJA Education. (n.d.). Available at: https://bjaed.org/article/S2058-5349(17)30072-0/fulltext. Accessed May 4, 2019.
11. Burch H, Cooper D, Garber J, et al. Hyperthyroidism and other causes of thyrotoxicosis: management guidelines of the American Thyroid Association and

American Association of clinical endocrinoloigists. Endocr Pract 2011;17(3): 456–520.

12. Klein I, Danzi S. Thyroid disease and the heart. Circulation 2007;116(15): 1725–35.

13. Franklyn JA, Boelaert K. Thyrotoxicosis. Lancet 2012;379(9821):1155–66.

14. Ross DS, Burch HB, Cooper DS, et al. 2016 American Thyroid Association guidelines for diagnosis and management of hyperthyroidism and other causes of thyrotoxicosis. Thyroid 2016;26(10):1343–421.

15. Farling PA. Thyroid disease. Br J Anaesth 2000;85(1):15–28.

16. Carroll R, Matfin G. Endocrine and metabolic emergencies: thyroid storm. Ther Adv Endocrinol Metab 2010;1(3):139–45.

17. Chaker L, Bianco AC, Jonklaas J, et al. Hypothyroidism. Lancet 2017;390(10101): 1550–62.

18. Palace MR. Perioperative management of thyroid dysfunction. Health Serv Insights 2017;10. https://doi.org/10.1177/1178632916689677.

19. Bennett-Guerrero E, Kramer DC, Schwinn DA. Effect of chronic and acute thyroid hormone reduction on perioperative outcome. Anesth Analg 1997;85(1):30–6.

20. Jonklaas J, Bianco AC, Bauer AJ, et al. Guidelines for the treatment of hypothyroidism: prepared by the American Thyroid Association task force on thyroid hormone replacement. Thyroid 2014;24(12):1670–751.

21. Charmandari E, Nicolaides NC, Chrousos GP. Adrenal insufficiency. Lancet 2014; 383(9935):2152–67.

22. Bancos I, Hahner S, Tomlinson J, et al. Diagnosis and management of adrenal insufficiency. Lancet Diabetes Endocrinol 2015;3(3):216–26.

23. Puar THK, Stikkelbroeck NMML, Smans LCCJ, et al. Adrenal crisis: still a deadly event in the 21st century. Am J Med 2016;129(3):339.e1-9.

24. Liu MM, Reidy AB, Saatee S, et al. Perioperative steroid management approaches based on current evidence. Anesthesiology 2017;127(1):166–72.

25. Kulke MH, Mayer RJ. Carcinoid tumors. N Engl J Med 1999;340(11):858–68.

26. Dierdorf SF. Carcinoid tumor and carcinoid syndrome. Curr Opin Anaesthesiol 2003;16(3):343–7.

27. Modlin IM, Lye KD, Kidd M. A 5-decade analysis of 13,715 carcinoid tumors. Cancer 2003;97(4):934–59.

28. Patel C, Mathur M, Escarcega RO, et al. Carcinoid heart disease: current understanding and future directions. Am Heart J 2014;167(6):789–95.

29. Davar J, Connolly HM, Caplin ME, et al. Diagnosing and managing carcinoid heart disease in patients with neuroendocrine tumors: an expert statement. J Am Coll Cardiol 2017;69(10):1288–304.

30. Bernheim AM, Connolly HM, Hobday TJ, et al. Carcinoid heart disease. Prog Cardiovasc Dis 2007;49(6):439–51.

31. Powell B, Al Mukhtar A, Mills GH. Carcinoid: the disease and its implications for anaesthesia. Contin Educ Anaesth Crit Care Pain 2011;11(1):9–13.

32. Mancuso K, Kaye AD, Boudreaux JP, et al. Carcinoid syndrome and perioperative anesthetic considerations. J Clin Anesth 2011;23(4):329–41.

33. Castillo J, Silvay G, Weiner M. Anesthetic management of patients with carcinoid syndrome and carcinoid heart disease: the Mount Sinai algorithm. J Cardiothorac Vasc Anesth 2018;32(2):1023–31.

34. Tucker ON, Crotty PL, Conlon KC. The management of insulinoma. Br J Surg 2006;93:264–75.

35. Crippa S, Zerbi A, Boninsegna L, et al. Surgical management of insulinomas: short- and long-term outcomes after enucleations and pancreatic resections. Arch Surg 2012;147(3):261–6.
36. Lamont ASM, Jones D. Anaesthetic management of insulinoma. Anaesth Intensive Care 1978;6(3):261–2.
37. Chari P, Pandit SK, Kataria RN, et al. Anaesthetic management of insulinoma. Anaesthesia 1977;32:261–4.
38. Carneiro DM, Levi JU, Irvin GL. Rapid insulin assay for intraoperative confirmation of complete resection of insulinomas. Surgery 2002;132(6):937–43.

Malignant Hyperthermia Update

Herodotos Ellinas, MD*, Meredith A. Albrecht, MD, PhD

KEYWORDS

- Malignant hyperthermia • Dantrolene • MHAUS
- Caffeine-halothane contracture test • Charcoal filters

KEY POINTS

- Malignant hyperthermia (MH) is an autosomal dominant disorder with variable penetration; most individuals susceptible to this disease have a genetic defect in the ryanodine receptor type 1 (RyR1) gene.
- It invariably presents with hypercarbia despite adequate ventilation, mixed respiratory-metabolic acidosis, tachycardia, and hyperpyrexia.
- If untreated or diagnosed late, MH progresses to a multiorgan system failure that includes cardiac dysrhythmias (cardiac arrest), renal insufficiency (renal failure, hyperkalemia), and disseminated intravascular coagulation.
- The contracture test is the gold standard in ruling out MH; fresh muscle tissue must be obtained at a certified muscle biopsy center.
- Key MH-associated disorders include central core disease ; King-Denborough syndrome; multiminicore disease; Native American myopathy; and myopathies associated with RYR1, CACNA1S, and STAC3 mutations.

INTRODUCTION
Timeline

After many years of uncertainty, malignant hyperthermia (MH) was eventually confirmed as a human disease in 3 descendants by in vitro muscle biopsy. A 21-year-old engineering student at the University of Melbourne presented at the Royal Melbourne Hospital in Australia in April of 1960 after sustaining an open leg fracture during a pedestrian–motor vehicle collision. He was anxious and afraid to undergo anesthesia because 10 of his close relatives died perioperatively after having a general anesthetic for minor procedures. He was told not to worry because ether was thought to be the culprit for those anesthetics, but a new anesthetic called halothane was available, one that was safer. Within 10 minutes of general anesthesia, the student

Department of Anesthesiology, Medical College of Wisconsin, 9200 West Wisconsin Avenue, Milwaukee, WI 53226, USA
* Corresponding author.
E-mail address: hellinas@mcw.edu
Twitter: @herodotosE (H.E.)

Anesthesiology Clin 38 (2020) 165–181
https://doi.org/10.1016/j.anclin.2019.10.010
1932-2275/20/© 2019 Elsevier Inc. All rights reserved.

anesthesiology.theclinics.com

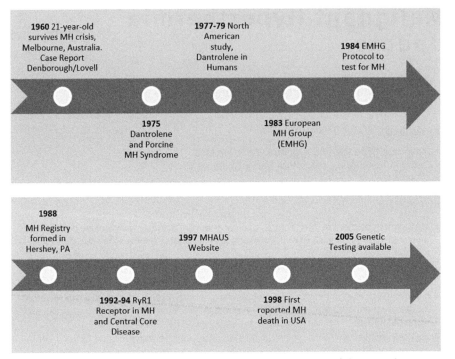

Fig. 1. MH timeline. MHAUS, Malignant Hyperthermia Association of the United States.

developed hypotension, tachycardia, and hyperthermia, the procedure was quickly completed, and he was cooled down, surviving the incident. A year later, he underwent an uneventful spinal anesthetic for treatment of ureteral stones (**Fig. 1**).[1]

In 2005, a University of Wisconsin La Crosse student underwent shoulder surgery at a local hospital and died of multiorgan failure 3 days later, with symptoms related to MH.[2]

In the 1960 to 1970s, 80% of patients diagnosed with MH died. Forty years later, mortality has been reduced to less than 5%. This significant reduction has been attributed to the introduction of dantrolene, education, end-tidal CO_2 ($ETco_2$) universal detection, and patient counseling and testing.[3]

Susceptibility

MH is a rare but potentially lethal skeletal muscle disorder affecting calcium release channels. The incidence is reported as an estimate between 1 in 10,000 to 30,000 and 1 in 100,000 to 250,000 depending on geographic location and age.[4–6] However, genetic mutation prevalence is reported as 1 in 2000 to 3000 with individuals not manifesting an MH event until multiple anesthetics have been administered.[6] MH affects all ethnic groups, occurs more frequently in men than in women, and has a higher incidence in the younger population.[4]

MH is inherited in a mendelian autosomal dominant pattern with variable penetration. Most individuals susceptible to MH have a defect in the ryanodine receptor type 1 (*RYR1*) gene (MHS1 form) on chromosome 19, a gene that regulates the synthesis of the ryanodine receptor 1 protein. There are more than 400 mutations associated with this gene, 34 of them linked to MH.[4] Less than 1% of susceptible persons have a mutation in the calcium voltage-gated channel subunit alpha 1S (*CAC-NA1S*) gene (*MHS5* form), a gene that instructs the synthesis of calcium channels in addition to activating the *RYR1* channel.[7] Defects in these genes cause abnormal excitation-contraction coupling, the process by which a chemical signal is converted to the mechanical act of contraction via calcium ion release.

Clinical Findings

The initial manifestations of a hypermetabolic state cause fast depletion of ATP, leading to the clinical picture of increased CO_2 production, respiratory acidosis, increased temperature, and increased oxygen demands. The secondary manifestations result from the anaerobic state created after the ATP is depleted; metabolic acidosis and lactate formation ensue.

If diagnosed late, MH progresses to a multiorgan system failure that includes cardiac dysrhythmias (cardiac arrest), renal insufficiency (renal failure, hyperkalemia), and disseminated intravascular coagulation (DIC).

Although the disorder leads to certain death if untreated or diagnosed late, the introduction of dantrolene, a muscle relaxant, has improved mortalities from 80% to less than 5% in 2006.[4] In a study by Larach and colleagues,[8] cardiac arrest and death still occurred in young, healthy individuals undergoing low-risk to intermediate-risk procedures despite the use of dantrolene. Risk factors associated with high mortality include muscular build and development of DIC.

Risk Assessment/Testing

Who should get tested? Malignant hyperthermia clinical grading scale

To avoid MH complications, all genetically susceptible individuals must be identified (**Fig. 2, Table 1**). However, the testing for MH can be complex and expensive, so it is vitally important to narrow in on high-risk individuals. The first screen is personal and family anesthetic history investigating prior adverse reactions. Approximately one-half of patients who develop acute MH have 1 or 2 uneventful prior exposures to triggering agents.[9] Some patients who develop MH have had multiple uneventful prior triggering anesthetics.[6,10]

When a patient reports a personal or family history of an adverse reaction to anesthesia, the patient's anesthetic and hospital records should be reviewed and assessed for the likelihood of MH. If details are unavailable, it is better to treat the patient as MH susceptible (MHS) until further testing is pursued. A clinical grading scale has been

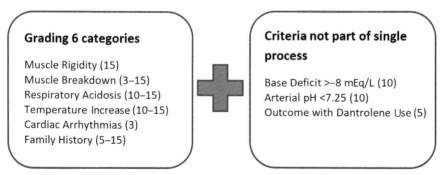

Grading 6 categories

Muscle Rigidity (15)
Muscle Breakdown (3–15)
Respiratory Acidosis (10–15)
Temperature Increase (10–15)
Cardiac Arrhythmias (3)
Family History (5–15)

Criteria not part of single process

Base Deficit >–8 mEq/L (10)
Arterial pH <7.25 (10)
Outcome with Dantrolene Use (5)

Fig. 2. MH risk grading. Numbers in parentheses are the points designated per category. (*Data from* Larach MG, Localio AR, Allen GC, et al. A clinical grading scale to predict malignant hyperthermia susceptibility. Anesthesiology 1994;80(4):771-779.)

Table 1
Scoring rules for the malignant hyperthermia (MH) clinical grading scale

MH indicators
>   Review the list of clinical indicators. If any indicator is present, add the points applicable for each indicator while observing the double-counting rule below, which applies to multiple indicators representing a single process.
>   If no indicator is present, the patient's MH score is zero.

Double-counting
>   If more than one indicator represents a single process, *count only the indicator with the highest score*. Application of this rule prevents double-counting when one clinical process has more than one clinical manifestation.
>   Exception: the score for any relevant indicators in the final category of **Table 2** ("other indicators") *should* be added to the total score without regard to double-counting.

MH susceptibility indicators
>   The italicized indicators listed below apply only to MH susceptibility. Do not use these indicators to score an MH event. To calculate the score for MH susceptibility, add the score of the italicized indicators below to the score for the highest ranking MH event.
>   *Positive family history of MH in relative of first degree*
>   *Positive family history of MH in relative not of first degree*
>   *Resting elevated serum creatinine kinase*
>   *Positive family history of MH together with another indicator from the patient's own anesthetic experience other than elevated serum creatine kinase*

Interpreting the raw score: MH rank and qualitative likelihood

Raw Score Range	MH Rank	Description of Likelihood
0	1	Almost never
3–9	2	Unlikely
10–19	3	Somewhat less than likely
20–34	4	Somewhat greater than likely
35–49	5	Very likely
50+	6	Almost certain

From Larach MG, Localio AR, Allen GC, et al. A clinical grading scale to predict malignant hyperthermia susceptibility. Anesthesiology 1994;80(4):774; with permission.

developed to help determine the likelihood that a prior event represents true MH.[11] This scale was developed by a consensus of experts and has not been validated by either genetic or contracture testing, but it is commonly used to counsel patients and make recommendations for testing (see **Table 1**).

Any patient or family member who had a past episode with a clinical grading score greater than or equal to 20 should be tested.

Of note, there are several case reports of patients with fevers and/or muscle cramping in response to hot environments, strenuous exercise, or both found to be MHS. These events are referred to as awake MH[12] and should be treated with caution with nontriggering anesthetics.

Testing Options

The most sensitive test for MHS is the contracture test, which is considered the gold standard to rule out MH. Contracture testing involves an in vitro muscle bioassay that is available only at specialized testing centers and may not be paid for by insurance. The test is highly sensitive so negative results generally rule out a diagnosis of MHS. However, there is up to a 20% false-positive rate. Patients with a positive contracture test should also undergo genetic testing for a causative

---

Box 1
Indications for testing for malignant hyperthermia

Contracture test indications

1. Family history of MH or known MHS relative.

2. Adverse reaction to a general anesthetic that included a triggering agent. Patients and family members with an MH grading score greater than or equal to 20 should be tested. The test should be performed 3 to 6 months after the event (depending on the degree of rhabdomyolysis).

3. Patients with severe masseter muscle rigidity (or generalized rigidity) during a triggering anesthetic who also have muscle breakdown with a creatine kinase level greater than 10,000 IU/L.

4. Family history of unexplained perioperative death when the records are unable to be obtained.

5. Could be helpful if a patient has a history of rhabdomyolysis following anesthesia after the clinical exclusion of other myopathies.

6. Could be helpful if a patient has a history of severe or recurrent inexplicable exercise-induced or heat-induced rhabdomyolysis (awake MH) or exertional heat stroke requiring hospitalization with no predisposing factors being present.

7. Could be helpful in patients with a suspicious history of MH who are entering military service.

Genetic testing indications

1. Patients with a confirmed or highly suspicious clinical episode of MH

2. Patients with a positive contracture test

3. Patients with an MHS relative determined by a positive contracture test

4. Patients with an MHS relative determined by a confirmed or highly suspicious clinical episode of MH

5. Patients with relatives with known causal *RYR1* mutation

MH mutation, which can then be assessed in family members to determine malignant hyperthermia susceptibility. However, not all mutations that cause MH have been identified, so genetic testing has a very high false-negative rate, with sensitivity of less than 50%.[13,14] Positive genetic tests in patients with negative contracture tests have rarely occurred.[15]

Despite the high false-negative rate with genetic testing, most patients undergo genetic testing first instead of a muscle biopsy both because of cost (procedure and center selection) and to avoid an invasive procedure (the muscle biopsy). Some patients choose not to get tested, thus rendering themselves and their entire families MHS, which not only results in changing future anesthetic plans but also affects military eligibility, occupation choices, and insurance implications.

Contracture Test

Indications for testing are listed in **Box 1**.

Protocols

Contracture tests evaluate the in vitro response of the patient's skeletal muscle (using a 75–100-mm [3–4-inch] biopsy from the thigh) to RYR1 agonists (caffeine and halothane). The testing needs to be performed using fresh tissue obtained under a nontriggering anesthetic at an MH muscle biopsy center. If abnormally high levels of contractile force are found with agonist exposure, the testing is positive. Two different protocols have been developed independently:

- The caffeine-halothane contracture test (CHCT) is administered by the North American Malignant Hyperthermia Group with a sensitivity of 97% and a specificity of 78%.[16] There are 5 sites in North America that perform the test, with 1 of the sites located in Canada (California, Maryland, Minnesota, North Carolina, and Toronto).
- The in vitro contracture test (IVCT) was developed by the European Malignant Hyperthermia Group and has a sensitivity of 99% and a specificity of 94%. There are 15 sites accredited worldwide that perform the IVCT. A listing is on the European Malignant Hyperthermia Group Web site.[17]

Both protocols use slightly different methodologies but there are no appreciable differences in test accuracy. Because these is no gold standard for definitive diagnosis, the true rates of false-positives and false-negatives are unknown. If the contracture test is negative because there is such a low false-negative rate, the patients are not considered MHS and may receive triggering anesthetics. There have been case reports of patients with known MH mutations who have received negative contracture test results,[18] but that is a very rare finding. If the contracture test is positive, the patient should be considered MHS and should not receive triggering anesthetics. About 1 in 5 patients with a positive CHCT (North America) have a false-positive result. Despite that high rate, most MH experts think that patients with a positive test should be considered MHS because of the high mortality of an MH crisis. All patients with a positive contracture test should also get genetic testing (if not already done) to guide further testing for family members. Because most mutations have not been identified, the genetic results do not change the diagnosis of MHS for the index patient.

The disadvantage of the contracture tests is that it requires fresh muscle tissue, so the patient must travel to one of the designated centers to get the biopsy. The biopsy results in 2 to 7 days of relative disability. The test is approximately $6000 to $10,000 and although in the United States the contracture test is covered by most insurances, lodging and travel expenses are not. It is strongly encouraged that patients obtain insurance carrier approval before the procedure. In Canada, the cost is covered by the patient's provincial health plan.[19]

Genetic Testing

Molecular genetic testing requires a blood sample sent to a testing center. The Malignant Hyperthermia Association of the United States (MHAUS) Web site lists 5 accredited laboratories in the United States.[20] Most centers use next-generation sequencing to study each sample. A genetic panel evaluates the most common *RYR1* mutations on chromosome 19 and mutations associated with *CACNA1S* and *STAC3* genes.[21] There are currently 48 known mutations in the RYR1 and 2 in the dihydropyridine receptor.[22] If a specific mutation is discovered, other family members can be tested at a reduced price. More than 1 mutation may be present within a family so, even if a family member is negative for the proband's mutation, it does not mean that person can be completely ruled out for MH.[23] Genetic testing is generally done on patients with a positive contracture test to determine the MH causative agent, patients with a family member with a known MH event or positive contracture tests, or patients with a suspicious clinical history for an MH episode. Most patients undergo the genetic testing before the contracture test.

Genetic testing costs between $800 to $4000 (larger amount for full gene sequencing). Insurance companies sometimes cover the testing. MHAUS can help argue for insurance to cover genetic testing for possible MHS patients.[19]

Genetic testing results

Test results indicate:

1. A mutation associated with MH, thus identifying the patient as MHS and requiring nontriggering anesthetics.
2. A DNA variation of uncertain significance, which does not rule out MHS. These patients should be treated as MHS unless a negative contracture test is obtained.
3. No known DNA mutation that causes MH. This result does not eliminate the possibility of MH because only a small percentage of possible mutations are known and the overall sensitivity of full RYR1 testing is only about 60%.[13–15,24,25]

Counseling

When patients have a presumed diagnosis of MHS they should avoid all triggering anesthetics and future anesthesia providers should be notified of their MHS status. Methods to alert future clinicians of this high risk include a letter from the anesthesiologist after the initial event, notation on the patient's electronic or paper medical record including allergy to succinylcholine and potent volatile anesthetics, and a MedicAlert bracelet. An MH-specific MedicAlert bracelet is available via MHAUS and the MedicAlert Foundation.[26] These patients should also be informed that they are at an increased risk for heat stroke or MH-like symptoms in hot environments or with strenuous exercise. Patients with muscle cramping and increases in body temperature with exercise or when exposed to a hot environment should immediately attempt surface cooling or immersion in cold water and consider fever reduction medications such as acetaminophen. If these episodes occur frequently, oral dantrolene can be considered. Patients are also strongly advised to receive an influenza vaccination annually because severe influenza has been associated with rhabdomyolysis.

Once a patient is identified as MHS, it is best, if possible, to genetically test the parents to determine which branch of the family the genetic mutation arises from or whether it is spontaneous.

Disorders Associated with Malignant Hyperthermia

There are several reports of concerning MH-like incidences, but the only confirmed predisposing disorders are the following myopathies:

1. Central core disease: first identified in 1973, it is a skeletal muscle disorder with disorganized central areas of muscle fibers (cores). Its clinical presentation includes hypotonia, especially of proximal muscles, and skeletal abnormalities (contractures, scoliosis, hip dislocation).[27]
2. King-Denborough syndrome: identified in 1970 after a survey in Australia and New Zealand, this congenital myopathy usually affects male children and has the clinical features of short stature, dysmorphic facial features, hypotonia, and skeletal anomalies.[28]
3. Multiminicore disease: skeletal muscle weakness in 4 different forms with the histology of disorganized so-called minicore fibers.[29] Classic presentation is in infancy

or early childhood with predominant muscle weakness of the muscles of trunk and neck.[23,30,31]

4. Native American myopathy: first reported in the Lumbee Indians of North Carolina, this rare disorder presents with congenital weakness and arthrogryposis.[32]
5. Myopathies that have an association with *RYR1*, *CACNA1S*, and *STAC3*[23,30] mutations.

Mitochondrial disorders are not associated with MH, and nontriggering anesthetics are not required to manage such patients during general anesthesia.

Muscular dystrophies such as Duchenne and Becker are also not associated with MH but, because of the high risk of rhabdomyolysis and hyperkalemia, succinylcholine should be avoided.

Management

Scenario 1

A 14-year-old boy with no significant past medical history presents after a motor vehicle accident for exploratory laparotomy. His symptoms include abdominal tenderness, nausea and vomiting, and increased temperature to 37.5°C. He undergoes general anesthetic with rapid sequence induction with succinylcholine and maintained on sevoflurane. Twenty minutes into his anesthetic, his $ETco_2$ remains increased at 65 mm Hg despite hyperventilation, his heart rate ranges In the 130 to 140 beats/min, his systolic blood pressure is in the mid-70s, and his temperature is up to 39.3°C.

Differential diagnosis
1. Sepsis with peritonitis
2. MH
3. Anaphylaxis
4. Inadequate anesthesia and/or analgesia
5. Anesthesia machine dysfunction
6. Other disorders to consider in all cases with a hypermetabolic state presentation (tachycardia, hyperthermia, hypercarbia, hemodynamic instability) include:
   a. Thyrotoxicosis
   b. Pheochromocytoma
   c. Neuroleptic malignant syndrome
   d. Serotonin syndrome
   e. Intoxication (illicit drugs such as cocaine)
   f. Heat stroke
   g. Iatrogenic overheating

You ensure adequate anesthesia and analgesia, you provide broad-spectrum antibiotics, but you are still concerned about an MH event. How should you procced?

MHAUS has an active Web site[33] where professionals and patients can get important information regarding MH. Here are their recommendations for managing an MH crisis:

- Discontinue triggering agents (such as succinylcholine and potent volatile anesthetics: desflurane, isoflurane, sevoflurane)
- Notify surgeon
- Stop the procedure or continue with nontriggering anesthetic agents if patient stable and emergent procedure
- Call for help
- Call MHAUS hotline 1-800-MH-HYPER (644-9737)
- Hyperventilate with 100% oxygen, flows 10 L/min

- Insert activated charcoal filters to both inspiratory and expiratory limbs of the anesthesia machine; may need to replace hourly if saturated
- Administer dantrolene[34] 2.5 mg/kg and continue every 4 to 6 hours or continuous infusion until hypermetabolic state resolves and hemodynamic stability occurs for at least 24 hours; monitoring for recrudescence in intensive care setting
  - The older formulation 20 mg/60 mL sterile water required use of 9 vials to treat a 70-kg adult and was cumbersome to reconstitute
  - The newer formulation 250 mg/5 mL sterile water has a quicker reconstitution rate and requires only 1 vial to treat an average adult of 70 kg
- Monitor arterial blood gases for pH, base excess, and serum potassium level; check serial creatine kinase (CK) concentrations and a coagulation panel
- Treat acidosis with sodium bicarbonate
- Treat hyperkalemia with Ca^{2+}, glucose, and insulin
- Place Foley catheter and maintain diuresis with furosemide or mannitol
- Institute core body cooling if temperature greater than 39°C with ice packs, cold saline lavage of body cavities and the surgical site; stop when temperature less than 38°C
- Consider cardiopulmonary bypass
- Report event to MHAUS by completing the North American Malignant Hyperthermia Registry (NAMHR) form[35]
- Provide counseling for testing and future anesthetics

Algorithms such as the one outlined earlier have also been created by the American College of Surgeons[36] and the Society for Pediatric Anesthesia to guide providers in managing an MH crisis. A summary of recommended medications, doses, and side effects is included in **Table 2**.

Scenario 2

A 10-year-old girl with no prior anesthetic history presents with a tibial fracture for open reduction and internal fixation. Her family history is significant for the death of her maternal grandfather after an anesthetic and a 7-day intensive care unit admission of her maternal aunt after appendectomy. Additional information reveals no parental general anesthetics (other than maternal spinal anesthetic for cesarean section) and a comment of "My sister [maternal aunt] had to be cooled off during anesthesia and was given a special medication but survived."

What should be your anesthetic plan? Based on this information, you may consider this girl as MHS and proceed with a nontriggering anesthetic (no succinylcholine or volatile anesthetics: desflurane, isoflurane, sevoflurane). Medications considered safe when faced with such a scenario include the ones outlined in **Box 2**. Counseling for genetic testing/muscle biopsy should also be considered.

Malignant Hyperthermia Clinical Controversies

A recent consensus statement published by MHAUS[37] discusses 6 clinical questions regarding optimal care of patients with MH. This particular consensus statement was published in both *Anesthesia and Analgesia* and on the MHAUS Web site, where these recommendations join other MHAUS recommendations derived in a similar fashion.[38] This 2-year process produced recommendations that are not standards, guidelines, practice parameters, or clinical requirements, as clearly stated on the MHAUS Web site. Their recommendations do not guarantee any particular clinical outcome and are subject to revision based on the clinical situation.[39]

Table 2
Malignant hyperthermia management medications

Medications	Dosing	Instructions	Side Effects	Maximum Dose
Dantrolene 250 mg, powder (newer preparation)	2.5 mg/kg IV q 5 min	Reconstitute 250 mg in 5 mL of sterile water until clear	Muscle weakness, especially hand grip and leg muscles	10 mg/kg
	—	Includes 0.125 g of mannitol/250-mg vial	Thrombophlebitis with extravasation caused by high pH	—
	1 mg/kg IV q 4–6 h	Maintenance	—	—
	0.25 mg/kg/h	Infusion for maintenance	—	—
Dantrolene 20 mg, powder (older preparation)	2.5 mg/kg IV q 5 min	Reconstitute in 60 mL of sterile water until clear	Hepatotoxicity	—
	—	Includes 3 g of mannitol/20 mg	—	—
Sodium bicarbonate 1 mEq/m	1–2 mEq/kg IV	For BE >−8 or hyperkalemia (K>5.9)	—	50 mEq
	1 mEq/kg/h	For increased creatinine kinase level or persistent hyperkalemia	—	—
Hyperkalemia	—	K>5.9 and/or ECG changes	—	—
Calcium chloride	10 mg/kg IV	—	—	2 g
Calcium gluconate	30 mg/kg IV	—	—	3 g
Regular insulin	0.1 U/kg IV	—	Hypoglycemia, monitor blood glucose q 30 min	10 U
Dextrose D50/25 g amp	50 mL IV	Adult dose	—	—
	0.5–1 g/kg	Pediatric dose	—	50 g
Albuterol	4–10 puffs ETT	—	—	—
Furosemide	0.5–1 mg/kg IV	—	Overdiuresis and electrolyte derangement	—
	—	—	Monitor urinary output	—

Abbreviations: BE, base excess; ECG, electrocardiogram; ETT, endotracheal tube; IV, intravenous; q, every.

Box 2
Malignant hyperthermia–safe medications

Anxiolytics
  Diazepam
  Lorazepam
  Midazolam

Barbiturates
  Methohexital

Intravenous anesthetics
  Dexmedetomidine
  Etomidate
  Ketamine
  Propofol

Local anesthetics
  Bupivacaine
  Lidocaine
  Ropivacaine

Muscle relaxants (nondepolarizing)
  Cisatracurium
  Rocuronium
  Vecuronium

Nitrous oxide

Opioids

How much dantrolene should be available at sites that may only use a depolarizing agent but no potent volatile anesthetic?

Should dantrolene be stocked in clinical facilities where volatile agents are not available or administered and succinylcholine is only available for emergency airway rescue? The controversy is based on the cost of having a full dose of dantrolene available versus the rarity of an MH event and the effect of dantrolene on MH crisis outcome. Many outpatient ambulatory centers and associations think that it is not cost-effective to stock dantrolene at each ambulatory anesthesia site, especially because the incidence of MH in the general population is very low and the incidence of an acute MH episode triggered by succinylcholine alone is also low. The likelihood of both events occurring is rare. Aderibigbe and colleagues[40] did an analysis of maintaining 720 mg of dantrolene (36 × 20-mg vials, MHAUS recommendation at the time) at ambulatory surgery centers in the United States and found that practice to be cost-effective. The Multicenter Perioperative Outcomes Group (MPOG) investigated the incidence of solo use of succinylcholine (no potent volatile use) for triggering MH episodes[41] and found 24 cases (literature review, North American MH Registry, MPOG database, and anesthesia closed claims project database). In the NAMHR, MH events triggered by succinylcholine alone are at a rate of 1.4%.[9,42] In Europe, 1% of biopsy-proven MH events were triggered by succinylcholine alone.[43] The MPOG publication also showed that succinylcholine was used by 46% of clinicians encountering a grade IV mask ventilation (impossible mask ventilation),[41] a situation that might be encountered in an office-based anesthesia situation. Therefore, there is a risk of an acute MH attack at an ambulatory surgical center that only stocks succinylcholine for airway rescue.

Because complications caused by an MH event increase by a factor of 1.6 for every 30-minute delay in the administration of dantrolene,[9] MHAUS recommends that dantrolene (up to 10 mg/kg) should be present at any anesthesia site that uses MH triggering agents (including succinylcholine). MHAUS thought that the incidence of possible MH and the consequences of an acute episode of MH without dantrolene treatment are greater than the expense of stocking dantrolene at each site.[37]

What is the definition of malignant hyperthermia masseter muscle rigidity, its association with malignant hyperthermia, and its clinical management?

There can be confusion in diagnosing masseter muscle rigidity (MMR) caused by an MH event versus the normal effects from succinylcholine administration. To differentiate between these 2 options, it is necessary to assess for severe masseter rigidity looking for so-called jaws of steel.[44] When severe MMR is present, other clinical and laboratory signs of acute MH should be assessed, such as tachycardia, hypercarbia, other muscle rigidity, hyperthermia, myoglobinuria, metabolic acidosis, and hyperkalemia. MMR does not predict an MH episode with complete accuracy and there can be a delay before the start of the acute MH episode. Patients with myotonic muscle disorders after succinylcholine often have severe MMR and no MH episodes.[45,46]

MHAUS recommends that severe MMR can be the first sign of an acute MH event, but there are no hard data to determine the likelihood of developing MH after the occurrence of such an event. If no other signs of MH occur, the patient should still be assessed for rhabdomyolysis, which in the absence of MH should cause suspicion of an undiagnosed myopathic disorder.[37]

MHAUS recommends that if an anesthetic is necessary in a patient that has experienced MMR during prior anesthetics but has not had a full evaluation for MHS or myopathy, a nontriggering anesthetic should be used. If MMR occurs during a current anesthetic, all triggering agents should be stopped and the patient should be observed closely for other signs of MH. If MMR occurs during an elective procedure, it should be postponed until further critical analysis of the patient and the risk of MH can be assessed. Severe MMR is less likely to be from an MH attack in the setting of temporomandibular joint disorder.[37]

What is the association of malignant hyperthermia heat-related and exercise-related rhabdomyolysis?

MHS patients can develop a nonanesthetic MH-like sickness during conditions of heat, exercise, stress, or viral illness. This MH-like illness may involve hyperthermia, muscle rigidity, rhabdomyolysis, and hyperkalemia.[47,48] There are multiple published case reports of patients with a history of heat-induced or exercise-induced rhabdomyolysis who have either subsequently developed MH after exposure to triggering agents or who have tested positive on an MH contracture biopsy.[49–52] In addition, case reports exist showing heat stroke being effectively treated with dantrolene.[53] It has been estimated that about 20% to 30% of cases of heat-induced or exercise-induced rhabdomyolysis are the result of MH-related RYR1 variants.[54]

Definitive criteria for MH susceptibility have not been determined in patients who have developed an MH-like illness after heat, exercise, stress, or illness. MHAUS considers that certain clinical characteristics of the MH-like illness place patients at high risk for MH susceptibility, including:

1. Greater than 1-week delayed muscle function return to baseline
2. Persistent increase in CK level greater than 5 times normal for 2 weeks
3. Rhabdomyolysis with acute kidney injury that persists for 2 weeks
4. Personal or family history of rhabdomyolysis

5. Personal or family history of recurrent muscle cramps interfering with normal activities
6. Personal or family history of rhabdomyolysis after a statin
7. CK peak level greater than 100,000 U/L

If multiple other people experienced exercise-related heat stroke or rhabdomyolysis at the same time as the patient, then the MH-like illness is most likely unrelated to MH.[37]

Patients should engage in physical activity as tolerated if they are identified as MHS. If these patients do develop adverse effects during exercise or heat, then they should restrict their activity.[37]

What should the management be for hyperthermia following a malignant hyperthermia crisis?

Treatment of an acute MH episode should focus on discontinuing triggering agents, hyperventilation, timely dantrolene administration, treatment of the patient's metabolic abnormalities, and reduction of hyperthermia. Prolonged hyperthermia is associated with worsened outcomes, so the focus should be on cooling once dantrolene is administered. Primary categories for cooling include pharmacologic, noninvasive, and invasive. Pharmacologic cooling effectiveness with acetaminophen and nonsteroidal antiinflammatory agents in the treatment of MH hyperthermia has not been determined.[37,42]

Noninvasive cooling techniques are preferred to invasive ones, with the most common being ice packing, forced air cooling, circulating cool water blankets, cold intravenous (IV) fluids, and ice-water immersion. In healthy volunteers, 40 mL/kg infusion of 4°C fluid decreased the core temperature by about 2.5°C and an infusion of 20°C fluid decreased the core temperature by about 1.4°C.[55] The cold fluid infusion method is limited by the amount of IV fluid that can be safely administered to the patient. Ice packing (typically neck, groin, axillae) is effective but direct ice-to-skin contact can cause tissue damage. Convection cooling (or merely removing all covers on the patient and allowing radiant heat loss) is easy and risk free but has limited ability to cool. To improve radiant heat loss and convection cooling, the room temperature should be decreased as much as possible. Circulating cool water blankets, nowadays more prevalent in most US operating rooms, when set to 4°C provide an effective cooling method. Ice-water immersion is very effective but generally impractical.[56,57]

Invasive cooling methods include lavages (rectal, bladder, gastric, or peritoneal), esophageal heat exchangers, intravascular heat exchange devices, and cardiopulmonary bypass.[57] Gastric, bladder, and rectal lavage are ineffective because of the small contact surface area. Peritoneal lavage is effective but requires special equipment and skills that most anesthesiologists do not possess. Esophageal heat exchanges are of limited use and are not commonly available.[58] Cardiopulmonary bypass is effective and frequently available but, because of the level of invasiveness, it is infrequently used.

MHAUS recommends that cooling should never distract from dantrolene administration and hyperventilation. If both dantrolene and hyperventilation are started promptly, dangerous levels of hyperthermia generally do not occur so active cooling may not be necessary. If the patient's temperature is persistently more than 38°C, then active cooling should be started first with noninvasive cooling methods such as ice packs and circulating water blankets. If necessary, the patient should receive IV infusion of refrigerated fluids starting at 20 mL/kg. Other invasive techniques of cooling are rarely needed.[37]

After treatment of an acute malignant hyperthermia episode, what should be the subsequent administration of dantrolene?

What is the risk of MH reoccurrence, recrudescence, or relapse? About 20% of patients have an acute MH reoccurrence. This reoccurrence generally happens within 9 hours of the initial event, and 80% of reoccurrences happen within 16 hours. Clinical signs of a reoccurrence are muscle rigidity, worsening rhabdomyolysis, respiratory acidosis, and hyperthermia.[59] MHAUS recommends that after the initial dantrolene bolus to treat the acute MH event, the patient should receive a 1 mg/kg redosage of dantrolene every 4 to 6 hours for at least 24 hours (see **Table 2**). This maintenance dose can be given as either an infusion or a bolus dose. The dantrolene redosage can be stopped or the interval between doses increased to 8 to 12 hours if core temperature is less than 38°C, CK level is decreasing, no myoglobinuria in present, muscle rigidity is decreasing, and there is metabolic stability for 24 hours.[37]

Can patients with personal or family history of malignant hyperthermia be anesthetized safely before any diagnostic testing has occurred?

Patients with known or a suspected personal or family history of MH have been denied access to general anesthesia until MH susceptibility testing has been performed. These patients have also been told that their surgery must occur in a hospital setting instead of an outpatient facility. However, this situation (MHS patient desiring surgery before MH testing) can be common.[60] Some MHS patients refuse to undergo diagnostic testing because of the geographic distance to the nearest test center and lack of insurance coverage for the testing.

MHAUS advises that MHS patients who have not yet been tested should be allowed to receive non–MH-triggering general anesthesia. These patients can also get surgery at ambulatory surgical centers if the center is prepared to recognize and treat an MH crisis per MHAUS guidelines.[30,37,61,62]

DISCLOSURE

The authors have nothing to disclose.

REFERENCES

1. Denborough MA. Malignant hyperthermia. 1962. Anesthesiology 2008;108(1): 156–7.
2. Schott K. UW-L student dies from rare condition triggered by anesthesia La Crosse Tribune. 2005. Available at: https://lacrossetribune.com/news/uw-l-student-dies-from-rare-condition-triggered-by-anesthesia/article_587543bd-0613-52d0-954e-0d0ebd961d68.html. Accessed July 29, 2019.
3. Rosenberg H, Rothstein A. Malignant hyperthermia death holds many lessons. In: Anesthesia patient safety foundation newsletter, vol. 21. Anesthesia Patient Safety Foundation; 2006. p. 32–4. Available at: https://www.apsf.org/article/malignant-hyperthermia-death-holds-many-lessons.
4. Rosenberg H, Pollock N, Schiemann A, et al. Malignant hyperthermia: a review. Orphanet J Rare Dis 2015;10:93.
5. Rosenberg H. Malignant hyperthermia syndrome. MHAUS Website 2010.
6. Riazi S, Kraeva N, Hopkins PM. Updated guide for the management of malignant hyperthermia. Can J Anaesth 2018;65(6):709–21.
7. Rosenberg H, Sambuughin N, Riazi S, et al. Malignant Hyperthermia Susceptibility. In: Adam MP, Ardinger HH, Pagon RA, et al, editors. GeneReviews® [Internet]. Seattle (WA): University of Washington, Seattle; 1993-2019.

8. Larach MG, Brandom BW, Allen GC, et al. Cardiac arrests and deaths associated with malignant hyperthermia in north america from 1987 to 2006: a report from the north american malignant hyperthermia registry of the malignant hyperthermia association of the United States. Anesthesiology 2008;108(4):603–11.
9. Larach MG, Gronert GA, Allen GC, et al. Clinical presentation, treatment, and complications of malignant hyperthermia in North America from 1987 to 2006. Anesth Analg 2010;110(2):498–507.
10. Strazis KP, Fox AW. Malignant hyperthermia: a review of published cases. Anesth Analg 1993;77(2):297–304.
11. Larach MG, Localio AR, Allen GC, et al. A clinical grading scale to predict malignant hyperthermia susceptibility. Anesthesiology 1994;80(4):771–9.
12. Zvaritch E, Gillies R, Kraeva N, et al. Fatal awake malignant hyperthermia episodes in a family with malignant hyperthermia susceptibility: a case series. Can J Anaesth 2019;66(5):540–5.
13. Sei Y, Sambuughin N, Muldoon S. Malignant hyperthermia genetic testing in North America Working group Meeting. Bethesda Maryland. September 4-5, 2002. Anesthesiology 2004;100(2):464–5.
14. Sei Y, Sambuughin NN, Davis EJ, et al. Malignant hyperthermia in North America: genetic screening of the three hot spots in the type I ryanodine receptor gene. Anesthesiology 2004;101(4):824–30.
15. Robinson RL, Anetseder MJ, Brancadoro V, et al. Recent advances in the diagnosis of malignant hyperthermia susceptibility: how confident can we be of genetic testing? Eur J Hum Genet 2003;11(4):342–8.
16. Allen GC, Larach MG, Kunselman AR. The sensitivity and specificity of the caffeine-halothane contracture test: a report from the North American Malignant Hyperthermia Registry. The North American Malignant Hyperthermia Registry of MHAUS. Anesthesiology 1998;88(3):579–88.
17. EMHG. European Malignant hyperthermia group Accredited Labs. Available at: https://www.emhg.org/accredited. Accessed July 29, 2019.
18. Brandt A, Schleithoff L, Jurkat-Rott K, et al. Screening of the ryanodine receptor gene in 105 malignant hyperthermia families: novel mutations and concordance with the in vitro contracture test. Hum Mol Genet 1999;8(11):2055–62.
19. MHAUS. Malignant Hyperthermia Association of the United States: Testing for malignant hyperthermia susceptibility: How do I counsel my patients. Available at: https://www.mhaus.org/testing/introduction-to-mh-testing/testing-for-malignant-hyperthermia-mh-susceptibility-how-do-i-counsel-my-patients/. Accessed July 29, 2019.
20. MHAUS. Malignant hyperthermia association of the United States: malignant hyperthermia - testing: genetic testing. Available at: https://www.mhaus.org/testing/genetic-testing/. Accessed July 29, 2019.
21. McCarthy TV, Healy JM, Heffron JJ, et al. Localization of the malignant hyperthermia susceptibility locus to human chromosome 19q12-13.2. Nature 1990; 343(6258):562–4.
22. EMHG. European Malignant Hyperthermia Group: Diagnostic MH Mutations. Available at: https://www.emhg.org/diagnostic-mutations. Accessed July 29, 2019.
23. Litman RS. Susceptibility to malignant hyperthermia: evaluation and management. UpToDate; 2019.
24. Girard T, Treves S, Voronkov E, et al. Molecular genetic testing for malignant hyperthermia susceptibility. Anesthesiology 2004;100(5):1076–80.

25. Brandom BW, Bina S, Wong CA, et al. Ryanodine receptor type 1 gene variants in the malignant hyperthermia-susceptible population of the United States. Anesth Analg 2013;116(5):1078–86.
26. MHAUS. Malignant hyperthermia association of the United States: Identification Tag Program. Available at: https://www.mhaus.org/patients-and-families/identification-tag-program/. Accessed July 29, 2019.
27. NIH. National Institutes of Health: US National Library of medicine: central core disease. Genetics Home reference Web site. 2019. Available at: https://www.ncbi.nlm.nih.gov/pubmed/. Accessed June 29, 2019.
28. King JO, Denborough MA. Anesthetic-induced malignant hyperpyrexia in children. J Pediatr 1973;83(1):37–40.
29. Guis S, Figarella-Branger D, Monnier N, et al. Multiminicore disease in a family susceptible to malignant hyperthermia: histology, in vitro contracture tests, and genetic characterization. Arch Neurol 2004;61(1):106–13.
30. Litman RS. Malignant hyperthermia: clinical diagnosis and management of an acute crisis. UpToDate; 2019.
31. NIH. National Institutes of Health: US National Library of Medicine: Multiminicore Disease. Genetics Home Reference Web site. Available at: https://ghr.nlm.nih.gov/condition/multiminicore-disease. Accessed June 29, 2019.
32. Stamm DS, Aylsworth AS, Stajich JM, et al. Native American myopathy: congenital myopathy with cleft palate, skeletal anomalies, and susceptibility to malignant hyperthermia. Am J Med Genet A 2008;146A(14):1832–41.
33. MHAUS. Home - malignant hyperthermia association of the United States (MHAUS). Available at: https://www.mhaus.org/. Accessed June 29, 2019.
34. Krause T, Gerbershagen MU, Fiege M, et al. Dantrolene–a review of its pharmacology, therapeutic use and new developments. Anaesthesia 2004;59(4):364–73.
35. NAMHR. North American MH Registry (NAMHR) maintained by the University of Florida Department of Anesthesiology. Available at: https://anest.ufl.edu/namhr/. Accessed June 29, 2019.
36. Ziewacz JE, Arriaga AF, Bader AM, et al. Crisis checklists for the operating room: development and pilot testing. J Am Coll Surg 2011;213(2):212–7.e10.
37. Litman RS, Smith VI, Larach MG, et al. Consensus Statement of the Malignant Hyperthermia Association of the United States on Unresolved Clinical Questions Concerning the Management of Patients With Malignant Hyperthermia. Anesth Analg 2019;128(4):652–9.
38. MHAUS. Malignant hyperthermia association of the United States recommendations. Available at: https://www.mhaus.org/healthcare-professionals/mhaus-recommendations/. Accessed July 29, 2019.
39. MHAUS. Malignant hyperthermia association of the United States: the MHAUS recommendation development process. Available at: https://www.mhaus.org/healthcare-professionals/mhaus-recommendations/the-mhaus-recommendation-development-process/. Accessed July 29, 2019.
40. Aderibigbe T, Lang BH, Rosenberg H, et al. Cost-effectiveness analysis of stocking dantrolene in ambulatory surgery centers for the treatment of malignant hyperthermia. Anesthesiology 2014;120(6):1333–8.
41. Larach MG, Klumpner TT, Brandom BW, et al. Succinylcholine use and dantrolene availability for malignant hyperthermia treatment: database analyses and systematic review. Anesthesiology 2019;130(1):41–54.
42. Larach MG, Brandom BW, Allen GC, et al. Malignant hyperthermia deaths related to inadequate temperature monitoring, 2007-2012: a report from the North

American malignant hyperthermia registry of the malignant hyperthermia association of the United States. Anesth Analg 2014;119(6):1359–66.

43. Klingler W, Heiderich S, Girard T, et al. Functional and genetic characterization of clinical malignant hyperthermia crises: a multi-centre study. Orphanet J Rare Dis 2014;9:8.

44. Rosenberg H, Davis M, James D, et al. Malignant hyperthermia. Orphanet J Rare Dis 2007;2:21.

45. Parness J, Bandschapp O, Girard T. The myotonias and susceptibility to malignant hyperthermia. Anesth Analg 2009;109(4):1054–64.

46. Parness J. You're "hot" from pumping iron? Anesth Analg 2009;108(3):711–3.

47. Hopkins PM. Is there a link between malignant hyperthermia and exertional heat illness? Br J Sports Med 2007;41(5):283–4 [discussion: 284].

48. Muldoon S, Deuster P, Voelkel M, et al. Exertional heat illness, exertional rhabdomyolysis, and malignant hyperthermia: is there a link? Curr Sports Med Rep 2008; 7(2):74–80.

49. Sagui E, Montigon C, Abriat A, et al. Is there a link between exertional heat stroke and susceptibility to malignant hyperthermia? PLoS One 2015;10(8):e0135496.

50. Hopkins PM, Ellis FR, Halsall PJ. Evidence for related myopathies in exertional heat stroke and malignant hyperthermia. Lancet 1991;338(8781):1491–2.

51. Wappler F, Fiege M, Steinfath M, et al. Evidence for susceptibility to malignant hyperthermia in patients with exercise-induced rhabdomyolysis. Anesthesiology 2001;94(1):95–100.

52. Roux-Buisson N, Monnier N, Sagui E, et al. Identification of variants of the ryanodine receptor type 1 in patients with exertional heat stroke and positive response to the malignant hyperthermia in vitro contracture test. Br J Anaesth 2016;116(4):566–8.

53. Lydiatt JS, Hill GE. Treatment of heat stroke with dantrolene. JAMA 1981; 246(1):41–2.

54. Jungbluth H, Dowling JJ, Ferreiro A, et al. 217th ENMC International Workshop: RYR1-related myopathies, Naarden, The Netherlands, 29-31 January 2016. Neuromuscul Disord 2016;26(9):624–33.

55. Rajek A, Greif R, Sessler DI, et al. Core cooling by central venous infusion of ice-cold (4 degrees C and 20 degrees C) fluid: isolation of core and peripheral thermal compartments. Anesthesiology 2000;93(3):629–37.

56. Taguchi A, Ratnaraj J, Kabon B, et al. Effects of a circulating-water garment and forced-air warming on body heat content and core temperature. Anesthesiology 2004;100(5):1058–64.

57. Plattner O, Kurz A, Sessler DI, et al. Efficacy of intraoperative cooling methods. Anesthesiology 1997;87(5):1089–95.

58. Kalasbail P, Makarova N, Garrett F, et al. Heating and cooling rates with an esophageal heat exchange system. Anesth Analg 2018;126(4):1190–5.

59. Burkman JM, Posner KL, Domino KB. Analysis of the clinical variables associated with recrudescence after malignant hyperthermia reactions. Anesthesiology 2007;106(5):901–6 [quiz: 1077–8].

60. Lu Z, Rosenberg H, Brady JE, et al. Prevalence of malignant hyperthermia diagnosis in new york state ambulatory surgery center discharge records 2002 to 2011. Anesth Analg 2016;122(2):449–53.

61. Litman RS, Joshi GP. Malignant hyperthermia in the ambulatory surgery center: how should we prepare? Anesthesiology 2014;120(6):1306–8.

62. Larach MG, Dirksen SJ, Belani KG, et al. Special article: Creation of a guide for the transfer of care of the malignant hyperthermia patient from ambulatory surgery centers to receiving hospital facilities. Anesth Analg 2012;114(1):94–100.

Anesthesia for Electroconvulsive Therapy

Nikhil Chawla, MBBS

KEYWORDS

- ECT overview • Contraindication for ECT • Induction agents for ECT
- ECT postop complications • Blood pressure management for ECT
- ECT for pregnancy • ECT adjuncts

KEY POINTS

- ECT provides the unique challenge of a non–operating room setting with fast turnover times and time pressure.
- Methohexital along with propofol and etomidate remain the mainstay of induction agents. Succinylcholine is the muscle relaxant of choice.
- Apart from pheochromocytoma, there are no absolute contraindications to ECT. Care should be taken in patients with cardiac disease, cerebral aneurysm, recent stroke, and trauma.
- Hypertension control during treatment is achieved by short-acting intravenous medications such as nitroglycerin and nicardipine. Pretreatment with labetalol and hydralazine should be considered.
- Postprocedure recovery can be challenging, with cognitive impairment and postictal confusion and delirium.

INTRODUCTION

The first described use of electroconvulsive therapy (ECT) dates to the 1930s after the observation of a reduction in schizophrenic symptoms in patients following spontaneous seizure activity.[1] Initially, the seizures were achieved with medications, but subsequently with the application of electric current. The use of ECT therapy has varied significantly since its initial discovery, but has gained in popularity recently. Despite this, the use of ECT remains relatively uncommon.[2]

ECT provides the anesthesia provider with a unique challenge of anesthetizing the patient for a seizure when most intravenous anesthetics are antiepileptics. Usually the treatment location is a non–operating room setting with the possibility of time pressure at a high-volume center. In addition, the physiologic changes the patients undergo are

Department of Anesthesiology, Yale Medicine, Yale University, 333 Cedar Street, TMP-3, New Haven, CT 06510, USA
E-mail address: nikhil.chawla@yale.edu
Twitter: @NChawla10 (N.C.)

Anesthesiology Clin 38 (2020) 183–195
https://doi.org/10.1016/j.anclin.2019.10.007
1932-2275/20/© 2019 Elsevier Inc. All rights reserved.

extreme. All of this makes the delivery of anesthesia nuanced and complicated. This article aims to address the following:

1. ECT overview
2. Indications for ECT
3. Physiologic changes
4. Pretreatment workup
5. Contraindications to ECT
6. Anesthetic considerations
7. Postoperative care

OVERVIEW

ECT usually involves the application of direct current to the scalp of the patient to induce a seizure. The stimulus is generally applied in a pulsed manner with a set amplitude over a period of time to achieve seizures. The energy, width of the pulse, pulse amplitude, total energy, and duration of stimulus can be modified in most modern ECT delivery systems.[3] The variations of these parameters have been studied extensively in the psychiatric literature but are beyond the scope of this article.

The electrodes can be applied in 3 different ways, namely, right unilateral, bitemporal, and bifrontal (**Fig. 1**). The choice of this placement is based on initial symptoms of the patient and response to treatments.[4] The therapeutic benefits do not seem to vary based on the initial technique, although unilateral ECT may be protective against cognitive impairment after treatment.[5] ECT is usually performed multiple times for each patient, and frequency of sessions depends on patient response. The goal of the treatment is to make the patient have a grand mal seizure. Efficacy of therapy is

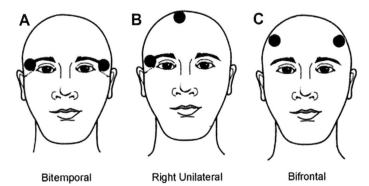

Bitemporal	Right Unilateral	Bifrontal

Fig. 1. Bitemporal, right unilateral, and bifrontal electrode placement. (*A*) Position of stimulating electrodes for bitemporal ECT. Electrodes are positioned symmetrically on either side of the forehead just above the midpoint of a line running from the outer canthus of the eye to the external auditory meatus. (*B*) Position of stimulating electrodes for right unilateral ECT. The right electrode position is same as for bitemporal ECT and the other electrode is placed with the left edge touching a line that runs down the middle of the skull from front to back, just in front of its intersection with a perpendicular line connecting the 2 external auditory canals. (*C*) Position of stimulating electrodes for bifrontal ECT. Electrodes are placed 5 cm above the lateral angle of each orbit on a line parallel to the sagittal plane. (*From* McNally KA, Blumenfeld H. Focal network involvement in generalized seizures: new insights from electroconvulsive therapy. Epilepsy & Behavior 2004;5(1):5; with permission.)

subjectively evaluated based on patient symptoms. However, the following seizure characteristics have been shown to predict success:

- Seizure duration
- Postictal suppression
- Burst suppression

INDICATIONS

Effectiveness of ECT has been repeatedly described in patients with mood disorders. Based on current evidence, ECT is recommended for the following indications[6]:

1. Unipolar major depression
    - Refractory or resistant to antidepressant therapy
    - Need exists for rapid treatment response, such as in pregnancy, persistent suicidal intent, or food refusal leading to dehydration or nutritional compromise
    - Medical comorbidities prevent the use of antidepressant medication
    - Previous response to ECT
    - Psychotic features (eg, delusions or hallucinations)
    - Catatonia
    - Persistent suicidal intent
2. Bipolar depression or mania

PHYSIOLOGIC CHANGES

Inducing a grand mal seizure in patients leads to significant changes, both immediate and long-lasting. The long-lasting effects of ECT are what promote its use. For an anesthesiologist, the significant changes revolve around the cardiovascular system and the central nervous system.

Cardiovascular changes:
- Electrical stimulation necessary to initiate a seizure produces significant cardiovascular changes.
- Initial stimulation is associated with significant parasympathetic outflow, which can present as significant bradycardia or sinus pause. This can be alarming but usually is short-lasting.
- After the initial phase, the sympathetic nervous system takes over, which is characterized by tachycardia, increased systemic vascular resistance, and hypertension. This phase poses the most risk and is poorly tolerated by patients with cardiovascular comorbidities. This phase is self-limited but may last from a few minutes to an hour.

Central nervous system changes:
- ECT can cause a temporary increase in the intracranial pressure, although this is controversial.[7] Increased blood pressure and cerebral blood flow are theorized to be the reason.
- Postictal slowing in the electroencephalogram is well known and has been postulated to be the reason for the success of ECT treatment.[8]
- Post-treatment confusion is commonly seen and has a tendency to lengthen recovery times. Patients can often arouse in a combative fashion.

PRETREATMENT WORKUP

All patients undergoing ECT should undergo a full preanesthetic workup. Obtaining consent for the anesthesia can prove to be problematic given the patient's disease.

Close discussion with the interventional psychiatrist is necessary to ascertain decision-making capabilities. If the patient is deemed incapable, the family needs to be approached for consent for provision of anesthesia care.

The attending anesthesiologist should perform a thorough history taking and physical examination for a general anesthetic. The interview should include a special focus on the following:

- Previous anesthetic history
- Cardiovascular history, especially exercise tolerance, hypertension, coronary artery disease, and valvular abnormalities
- History of seizure disorder
- History of intracranial bleeds, cerebral aneurysm, and neurosurgery
- Pulmonary function
- Chronic anticoagulant status
- History of pacemakers or other implantable cardiac devices
- Medication reconciliation, especially related to antiepileptics and benzodiazepine use

American College of Cardiology/American Heart Association guidelines do not make any recommendations specific to ECT, but based on the cardiovascular strain that is placed on the patients, in the author's opinion it should be regarded as a high-risk procedure for perioperative cardiac events. The patient's exercise tolerance needs to be evaluated and, if unable to assess this, full cardiac risk stratification should be pursued. Evidence of cardiac disease does not necessarily preclude the patient from treatment, but will help plan the hemodynamic monitoring and management during the procedure while enabling a frank discussion with the patient and/or the family regarding the cardiovascular risk from the procedure.

CONTRAINDICATIONS TO ELECTROCONVULSIVE THERAPY

Numerous medical comorbidities can make the delivery of ECT high risk, but there are no absolute contraindications except a known history of pheochromocytoma. Some of the relative contraindications are:

1. *Raised intracranial pressure (ICP) and space-occupying lesions*. Acute or chronic ICP elevation can be worsened by the increase in ICP with ECT. Most of this effect is theorized to be secondary to hypertension, so prevention of acute sustained increases in blood pressure can reduce the risk in these patients.
2. *Recent cerebrovascular accident*. Both hemorrhagic and ischemic causes can be high risk but specifically hemorrhagic owing to the increased risk of rebleeding.
3. *Cerebral aneurysm*. Patients with untreated cerebral aneurysm can be at high risk for an aneurysmal rupture with ECT. There have been cases reports of safe ECT and aneurysmal bleeding with ECT.[9,10] Patients need to evaluated and treated on a case-by-case basis.
4. *Myocardial ischemia*. Ongoing ischemia with angina symptoms needs to be addressed before treatment.
5. *Major unstable orthopedic fractures*. ECT leads to significant generalized clonic movements that can cause failure of alignment.
6. *Cardiovascular conduction defects*. Pacemakers and automatic implantable cardioverter-defibrillators are not considered contraindications for ECT but will require reprogramming before treatment.

ECT has long been considered to be safe during pregnancy,[11,12] despite certain case reports of preterm labor and fetal anomalies. A full consultation with an obstetrician and maternal-fetal medicine specialist should be considered. There should be a multidisciplinary discussion for patients who require ECT during a high-risk pregnancy. Preparation for ECT during pregnancy should include a pelvic examination, discontinuation of nonessential anticholinergic medication, fetal heart rate monitoring, intravenous hydration, and administration of a nonparticulate antacid.[12] During the treatment, the parturient will require general anesthesia with intubation and avoidance of hyperventilation.

ANESTHETIC CONSIDERATIONS

General anesthesia is universally used for ECT. The main objective of the anesthetic for the patients is to provide conditions suitable for a controlled seizure to occur while limiting its consequences. This can be achieved by aiming for the following goals:

- Amnesia
- Immobility for a short duration
- Limiting the injury to self and staff from clonic movements
- Avoidance of hypoxia
- Hemodynamic stability
- Timely recovery from the anesthetic

The anesthetic care for ECT can be divided into four phases in particular:

1. Preprocedure
2. Induction
3. Electrical stimulation and seizure
4. Post seizure

Preprocedure

Most patients receiving ECT have to undergo multiple sessions as part of their therapy.[4,13] The anesthetic care can be titrated on a case-to-case basis. The patient should get an intravenous line placed in the pretreatment area. It is essential for some patients to be pretreated with the following:

1. *Glycopyrrolate*, to reduce secretions and make airway management easier; also for patients who became significantly bradycardic in the previous treatments.
2. *Antihypertensive*. Usually, intravenous labetalol or hydralazine is chosen for quick onset.
3. *Antiemetic*. Ondansetron can be administered preoperatively to reduce postoperative nausea.
4. *Reversal agents*. Patients on ongoing benzodiazepine therapy should be reversed with flumazenil to lower the seizure threshold and obtain appropriate seizure length. Care should be taken to dose appropriately and administer immediately before the treatment to avoid excessive anxiety.
5. *Nonsteroidal anti-inflammatory agents* to help with muscle aches, which is a common complaint after treatment. Usually, intravenous ketorolac is used.

Electroencephalography (EEG) electrodes are placed on the patient to evaluate EEG for seizure activity.

Before induction of anesthesia, a time-out should be performed with the staff involved. After time-out, the patient should receive preoxygenation (denitrogenation) with a handheld mask. Hyperventilation before induction of anesthesia is preferred because it can lead to a decrease in the seizure threshold.[14]

Induction

Induction of anesthesia is commonly achieved with intravenous anesthetics. The choice of the agents is based on the patient's comorbidities and clinical condition. Usually, agents that do not affect the seizure threshold are preferred but not obligatory.

Methohexital, propofol, etomidate, and ketamine are commonly used agents (**Table 1**). The dosing of these agents for ECT varies significantly but needs to be titrated on an individual basis. Dosing also will depend on comorbidities and concomitant medication being used in the patient.

Methohexital

Methohexital is barbiturate with a specific methyl substitution at C-2, which prevents the antiseizure activity while still inducing hypnosis. It is generally considered the "gold standard" for induction of ECT.

The following benefits of methohexital induction are the reasons for the preference for this agent:

- Seizure threshold lowered
- Seizure duration unchanged
- Blunts the sympathetic response to ECT
- Highly lipid soluble, hence relatively short-acting

Adverse effects:
1. Dose-dependent hypotension and myocardial depression like most barbiturates
2. Reflex tachycardia
3. Pain on injection
4. Involuntary movements
5. Allergy and anaphylaxis
6. Acute exacerbation of acute intermittent porphyria

Propofol

Propofol is an antiepileptic, but the use of propofol for ECT is well documented. In comparison with methohexital, it provides better hemodynamics for seizure and better

Table 1 Induction agents for electroconvulsive therapy				
Agent	Effects on Seizure Length	Dose (mg/ kg)	Benefits	Drawbacks
Methohexital	No change	1–1.5	Fast onset, no antiepileptic effect	Involuntary movements, delayed awakening
Etomidate	Increases	0.1–0.3	No hemodynamic changes on induction	Myoclonus, postoperative nausea
Propofol	Decreases	1–2.5	Fast onset, fast awakening, decreased postcognitive decline	Antiepileptic, higher energy required for seizure
Ketamine	No change	1–2	Fast onset, synergistic action in depression	Psychosis, postoperative delirium, exaggerated hypertensive response

cognition after treatment.[15] Despite decreasing the seizure duration, the effects on seizure quality are minimal, and the overall efficacy of ECT seems to be maintained when compared with methohexital.[16]

The following are the benefits of using propofol:
- Short duration of action
- Better recovery after a seizure
- Blood pressure remains lower during treatment
- Seizure quality maintained

Adverse effects:
1. Pain on injection
2. Dose-dependent hypotension and myocardial depression, particularly challenging in patients with cardiac disease or hypovolemia
3. Decreases seizure length
4. Inducing seizure requires a higher voltage and prolonged application

Ketamine

Ketamine is a glutamate antagonist at N-methyl-D-aspartate receptor and has long been known for a variety of central nervous system effects in addition to hypnosis. Chronic and acute pain management are common nonoperating room uses of ketamine. An increasing amount of literature points toward the use of ketamine in mood disorders as a sole therapy.[17–19]

Ketamine is being currently used as therapy in conjunction with ECT to provide a faster response in major depressive episodes,[20] although this is debatable with no large trials available to back this approach. A recent trial investigating the effects of ketamine was able to show no added benefit of using ketamine as an adjunct to ECT, although a small sample size[21] plagued the trial.

The following are the benefits of using ketamine:
- Minimal respiratory depression
- Possible adjunctive effect in treating depression
- Rapid onset and the brief duration of action
- No effect on seizure duration

Adverse effects:
1. Does not blunt sympathetic response to treatment
2. Increased ICP because of cerebral vasodilation
3. Hallucinations and psychosis with induction
4. More severe post-treatment confusion and delirium
5. Increased airway secretions and salivation can make airway management challenging

Etomidate

Etomidate is an imidazole that acts directly on γ-aminobutyric acid receptors to induce hypnosis. It is commonly used in the operating room for patients with a significant hemodynamic compromise for induction of anesthesia. Etomidate prolongs the seizure duration and improves seizure quality in patients in comparison with propofol.[22]

The following are the benefits of using etomidate:
- Improved seizure length and quality
- Flat hemodynamic response to induction, helpful in patients with concurrent cardiac disease
- Short duration of action

Adverse effects:
1. Pain on injection
2. Myoclonic movements after administration
3. Does not blunt sympathetic response
4. Postprocedure nausea and vomiting
5. Can induce cortisol deficiency given the repetitive nature of ECT

Muscle relaxation

Immobility during the seizure is of vital importance in limiting the injury that patients can inflict on themselves and the staff during the clonic phase of grand mal seizure. The muscle relaxation, by the nature of the procedure, has to be induced and should resolve rapidly. The common agents used for this purpose are succinylcholine and rocuronium.

Succinylcholine
Succinylcholine is a depolarizing muscle relaxant that works by initially stimulating the acetylcholine receptors on the neuromuscular junction (NMJ). The success of succinylcholine in ECT is related to its rapid onset of action followed by a rapid reversal. The dosing of succinylcholine needs to be lowered for these patients to prevent prolonged muscle relaxation, as the aim is to achieve relative flaccidity for about 3 to 4 minutes. The dose should be reduced to about 0.5 mg/kg but will need to be titrated based on patient response. The first treatment usually will require the highest dose, and can then be adjusted based on the duration of action. During the first treatment, usually a cuff will be placed on the calf of the patient to prevent succinylcholine block. This assists in identifying the clonic motor activity as electricity is being titrated to induce a seizure with an appropriate length of time.

Advantages of succinylcholine:
• Rapid onset of action
• Rapid recovery
• Predictable response over time
Adverse effects:
1. Can induce bradycardia in younger patients
2. Myalgia secondary to muscle fasciculation
3. Increases airway secretions
4. Prolonged action in patients with pseudocholinesterase deficiency
5. Induces malignant hyperthermia

Rocuronium
Rocuronium is a steroidal nondepolarizing muscle relaxant that causes competitive antagonism at the NMJ acetylcholine receptor. It is widely used to achieve intubating and surgical muscle relaxation in the operating room. Rapid onset of action, when given in high doses, allows for it to be used also in rapid sequence inductions.

In the ECT setting, it is used uncommonly as an alternative to succinylcholine in cases of contraindications. The prolonged duration of action makes it an unsuitable candidate, but with the availability of sugammadex (reversal agent) it can be used successfully in this setting. There are ever-increasing case reports of rocuronium and sugammadex use in ECT patients.

Advantages of rocuronium:
• Rapid onset of action
• Avoids myalgia

- Suitable for patients with contraindications to succinylcholine use
- Predictably reversed with sugammadex

Limitations:

1. Prolonged duration of action in the absence of reversal

Adjuncts

- *Dexmedetomidine* is a centrally acting $\alpha2$-agonist that decreases sympathetic outflow. It does not affect seizure duration, so it is safe to be used for ECT. When used as an adjunct during induction of anesthesia, it can blunt the sympathetic response to the seizure. It does predispose the patient to bradycardia.
- *Lidocaine* should be avoided because it decreases the seizure duration, but sometimes can be used for patient comfort to prevent pain on injection of induction agents.
- Intravenous *theophylline* and *caffeine* have been shown to improve seizure duration in patients with inadequate seizure length.[23]

Airway management

The airway is maintained in patients with bag-mask ventilation after induction of anesthesia. The aim is to maintain appropriate oxygenation and assist with hyperventilation.[14] Usually a dedicated staff member, with experience in airway management, is responsible for mask ventilation. This staff member can be an anesthesia provider or respiratory therapist, based on the setup. Airway carts and adjuncts should be readily available in case of loss of airway patency.

Electrical stimulation will usually cause the clenching of teeth because of masseter activity; hence, the patients will require significant protection with 2 soft bite blocks or full-mouth plastic bite blocks to prevent biting of the tongue. The presence of these adjuncts can make bag-mask ventilation challenging. Airway patency should be confirmed with ventilation attempts before electrical stimulation.

In uncommon circumstances, patients will need endotracheal intubation to secure the airway. Intubation is generally avoided because it adds to the time spent under anesthesia and decreases the efficiency of an ECT suite. The following are some examples of patients' conditions that will require intubation:

- Poorly controlled reflux disease
- History of esophagectomy
- Pregnant patients post 20 weeks gestation
- 48 hours postpartum
- Gastrointestinal obstruction
- Proven difficult airway

Airway support needs to be maintained until the patients recover from the muscle relaxant. This might need patients to receive manually assisted ventilation for up to 5 to 10 minutes. On recovery from the muscle relaxant and hypnosis, the patients tend to obstruct their airways, especially those at high risk for sleep apnea. Airway adjuncts (such as nasal or oral airways), chin lift, and head positioning can all be used to maintain airway patency.

Electrical stimulation and seizure

Electrical stimulation produces immediate widespread muscle activity across the body but more pronounced in the upper body. Appropriate use of bite blocks, manual or physical restraint of the upper extremity, and adequate muscle relaxation will prevent any undue injury to the patient caused by sudden motion with stimulation. A generous amount of conductive gel should be applied to the electrodes to avoid superficial burn injury to the patient. If the patient has an implanted cardiac device, the device should be configured to an acceptable mode by an electrophysiologist before treatment. In case the device is not reprogrammed, a magnet should be available close by for deployment if necessary.

The stimulation usually lasts for 1 to 10 seconds based on prior response to stimulation. First-time treatment will require repeated stimulation to achieve appropriate seizure duration and quality. The charge, pulse width, total energy, and pulse frequency can be altered for each stimulus. This repetitive electrical stimulation might require redosing of induction agents to maintain suitable conditions throughout the therapy.

Successful induction of seizure will lead to an initial tonic phase followed by the clonic phase completing the grand mal nature. A seizure usually lasts from 15 to 70 seconds; the motor activity usually subsides before EEG activity.[24] In the case of short seizures (<15 seconds), patients can be hyperventilated for a brief period of time and restimulated to induce a good seizure. If a seizure lasts beyond 2 minutes, the patient will require an antiepileptic to terminate it. Usually, short-acting benzodiazepine-like midazolam or a small dose of propofol can be attempted first. Patients who were on chronic benzodiazepines and reversed before treatment will need to be redosed with a longer-acting agent such as lorazepam after termination of the seizure.

Hemodynamic instability

ECT can cause significant swings in heart rate and blood pressure of patients. Immediately following the electrical stimulus, the parasympathetic surge follows. Significant bradycardia and sinus pauses are commonly seen but are relatively short-lasting. This effect can be more pronounced in patients chronically on β-blockers. Asystole is uncommon but has been reported. Treatment involves administration of atropine and cardiopulmonary resuscitation for recirculation of the medications. Rarely, patients will require advanced cardiac life support and epinephrine. Patients with a known history of bradycardia with ECT are usually pretreated with anticholinergic agents such as glycopyrrolate before treatment.

A more prolonged sympathetic surge follows the initial parasympathetic activation. This is characterized by an increase in heart rate, myocardial contractility, myocardial oxygen demand, systemic vascular resistance (SVR), and blood pressure. These changes can predispose patients with pre-existing cardiac disease to acute cardiac events. Prompt treatment is essential to prevent any untoward major cardiac events. The following intravenous agents are used frequently.

Labetalol

This intravenous nonselective adrenergic blocker provides both heart rate control and a decrease in SVR and has a rapid onset of action. Labetalol is one of the first-line drugs used in ECT settings to control tachycardia hypertension. Patients with a known history of poorly controlled hypertension in previous treatments can be pretreated with labetalol.

Hydralazine

Hydralazine is a direct-acting vasodilator that acts by decreasing SVR, hence decreasing the blood pressure. The onset of action takes longer and the effect lasts for a longer duration, making it not an ideal choice for ECT.

Nitroglycerin

Nitroglycerin, being a direct smooth muscle relaxant, decreases the blood pressure by decreasing SVR. The onset of action is rapid and the duration of action is very short. It is ideal in patients who will develop hypertension for a very short duration following a seizure. It can be given as intravenous boluses of 40 to 80 μg, titrating to blood pressure. If hypertension persists, nitroglycerin will need to be redosed frequently.

Nicardipine

Nicardipine is a calcium-channel blocker that can be used as an intravenous bolus agent. It reduces SVR while having minimal effect on contractility. Compared with nitroglycerin, it has a similar onset of action and time to hypertension control, but provides better dose response and less tachycardia.[25] It is usually given in boluses of 0.25 to 0.75 mg, titrating to blood pressures. It can be dosed again in the same increments for persistent hypertension.

POST SEIZURE

After regaining consciousness and appropriate respiratory function, the patient's care can be transferred to the postanesthesia care unit. Heart rate, electrocardiography, pulse oximetry, and blood pressure monitoring need to continue for up to an hour after the procedure or until the time that discharge criteria are met. The recovery period is usually complicated by postictal confusion, delirium, and cognitive impairment (which lasts for a few hours). In patients with a documented history of postprocedural confusion, the treatment can be tailored because the use of unilateral ECT can decrease the cognitive impairment in patients,[5] as can the use of propofol instead of methohexital.[15,16]

Acute confusion and delirium can pose a risk to patients and staff members in the recovery unit. Various adjuncts have been tried with varying results, in addition to avoidance of hypoxia and hypercapnia. Short-acting benzodiazepines such as midazolam, propofol boluses, haloperidol, and dexmedetomidine can be used as needed. Mechanical restraints might be necessary in some cases but should be avoided if possible.

SUMMARY

- ECT is a proven effective way of managing a variety of mood disorders refractory to medical management.
- Iatrogenic seizure induction provides uncommon challenges to anesthesiologists.
- A thorough preoperative work up geared toward addressing pre-existing cardiac diseases is essential in identifying patients at risk.
- Airway management is achieved by bag-mask ventilation.
- Methohexital is the drug of choice for induction, but propofol, ketamine, and etomidate can all be used.
- Muscle relaxation is usually achieved with succinylcholine.
- Bradycardia associated with seizure can be avoided by using anticholinergic agents in the at-risk population.
- Prompt treatment of hypertension is important, preferably with short-acting agents.
- Postprocedure delirium and cognitive impairment can be avoided by using unilateral ECT and propofol.
- Anesthesia care needs to titrated and tailored individually with every treatment.

DISCLOSURE

No financial disclosures.

REFERENCES

1. Endler NS. The origins of electroconvulsive therapy (ECT). Convuls Ther 1988; 4(1):5–23.
2. Wilkinson ST, Agbese E, Leslie DL, et al. Identifying recipients of electroconvulsive therapy: data from privately insured Americans. Psychiatr Serv 2018;69(5): 542–8.
3. Lisanby SH. Electroconvulsive therapy for depression. N Engl J Med 2007; 357(19):1939–45.
4. Kellner CH, Knapp R, Husain MM, et al. Bifrontal, bitemporal, and right unilateral electrode placement in ECT: a randomized trial. Br J Psychiatry 2010;196(3): 226–34.
5. Kolshus E, Jelovac A, McLoughlin DM. Bitemporal v. high-dose right unilateral electroconvulsive therapy for depression: a systematic review and meta-analysis of randomized controlled trials. Psychol Med 2017;47(3):518–30.
6. Rasmussen K. The practice of electroconvulsive therapy: recommendations for treatment, training, and privileging. J ECT 2002;18(1):58–9.
7. Derikx RL, van Waarde JA, Verwey B, et al. Effects on intracranial pressure of electroconvulsive therapy. J ECT 2012;28(2):e23–4.
8. Azuma I I, Fujita A, Sato K, et al. Postictal suppression correlates with therapeutic efficacy for depression in bilateral sine and pulse wave electroconvulsive therapy. Psychiatry Clin Neurosci 2007;61(2):168–73.
9. van Herck E, Sienaert P, Hagon A. Electroconvulsive therapy for patients with intracranial aneurysms: a case study and literature review. Tijdschr Psychiatr 2009;51(1):43–51 [in Dutch].
10. Gugger JJ, Dunn LE. Subarachnoid hemorrhage in the setting of electroconvulsive therapy in a patient with an unsecured cerebral aneurysm: a case report and review of the literature. J ECT 2019;35(3):212–4.
11. Anderson EL, Reti IM. ECT in pregnancy: a review of the literature from 1941 to 2007. Psychosom Med 2009;71(2):235–42.
12. Miller LJ. Use of electroconvulsive therapy during pregnancy. Hosp Community Psychiatry 1994;45(5):444–50.
13. Kellner CH, Knapp RG, Petrides G, et al. Continuation electroconvulsive therapy vs pharmacotherapy for relapse prevention in major depression: a multisite study from the Consortium for Research in Electroconvulsive Therapy (CORE). Arch Gen Psychiatry 2006;63(12):1337–44.
14. Guaranha MS, Garzon E, Buchpiguel CA, et al. Hyperventilation revisited: physiological effects and efficacy on focal seizure activation in the era of video-EEG monitoring. Epilepsia 2005;46(1):69–75.
15. Fredman B, d'Etienne J, Smith I, et al. Anesthesia for electroconvulsive therapy: effects of propofol and methohexital on seizure activity and recovery. Anesth Analg 1994;79(1):75–9.
16. Geretsegger C, Nickel M, Judendorfer B, et al. Propofol and methohexital as anesthetic agents for electroconvulsive therapy: a randomized, double-blind comparison of electroconvulsive therapy seizure quality, therapeutic efficacy, and cognitive performance. J ECT 2007;23(4):239–43.
17. Diazgranados N, Ibrahim L, Brutsche NE, et al. A randomized add-on trial of an N-methyl-D-aspartate antagonist in treatment-resistant bipolar depression. Arch Gen Psychiatry 2010;67(8):793–802.

18. Zarate CA Jr, Brutsche NE, Ibrahim L, et al. Replication of ketamine's antidepressant efficacy in bipolar depression: a randomized controlled add-on trial. Biol Psychiatry 2012;71(11):939–46.
19. Fond G, Loundou A, Rabu C, et al. Ketamine administration in depressive disorders: a systematic review and meta-analysis. Psychopharmacology (Berl) 2014; 231(18):3663–76.
20. Altinay M, Karne H, Anand A. Administration of sub-anesthetic dose of ketamine and electroconvulsive treatment on alternate week days in patients with treatment resistant depression: a double blind placebo controlled trial. Psychopharmacol Bull 2019;49(1):8–16.
21. Anderson IM, Blamire A, Branton T, et al. Ketamine augmentation of electroconvulsive therapy to improve neuropsychological and clinical outcomes in depression (Ketamine-ECT): a multicentre, double-blind, randomised, parallel-group, superiority trial. Lancet Psychiatry 2017;4(5):365–77.
22. Singh PM, Arora S, Borle A, et al. Evaluation of etomidate for seizure duration in electroconvulsive therapy: a systematic review and meta-analysis. J ECT 2015; 31(4):213–25.
23. Tzabazis A, Wiernik ME, Wielopolski J, et al. Intravenous theophylline is the most effective intervention to prolong EEG seizure duration in patients undergoing electroconvulsive therapy. BMC Anesthesiol 2017;17(1):114.
24. Mayur PM, Gangadhar BN, Janakiramaiah N, et al. Motor seizure monitoring during electroconvulsive therapy. Br J Psychiatry 1999;174:270–2.
25. Chen TL, Sun WZ, Cheng YJ, et al. Comparison of antihypertensive effects of nicardipine with nitroglycerin for perioperative hypertension. Acta Anaesthesiol Sin 1995;33(4):199–204.

Anesthesia for the Morbidly Obese Patient

Surangama Sharma, MD[a],*, Lovkesh Arora, MD[b]

KEYWORDS

- Obesity • Anesthesia for morbidly obese • Pathophysiology of obesity
- Preoperative evaluation in obese • Ambulatory surgery in obese patients
- Intraoperative management of obese patients • Postoperative care of obese patients

KEY POINTS

- Obesity is a serious and expensive health care issue, associated with a proinflammatory state, affecting multiple organ systems, prevalent in almost 40% of the US population.
- Body mass index (BMI), comorbidities, and metabolic health (better predicted by waist-hip ratio, waist circumference, total body fat) play a major role in risk stratification.
- Patients with clinical signs of obesity hypoventilation syndrome, undergoing moderate- to high-risk procedures, should be evaluated for global cardiac function.
- Ambulatory surgery in supermorbid obese patient with (BMI >50 kg/m^2) is not recommended as per Society of Ambulatory Anesthesia Consensus guidelines, because of potential need for overnight admission and inpatient monitoring.
- A multimodal, opioid-sparing approach to analgesia should be used for all patients, for better recovery profile, including early discharge.

INTRODUCTION

Obesity is one of the primary causes of preventable noncommunicable diseases (along with heart diseases, stroke, type 2 diabetes [T2DM], and certain cancers) in United States. Weight that is higher than what is considered a healthy weight for a given height is described as overweight or obese. Body mass index, or BMI, is used as a screening tool for overweight or obese.[1] Obesity can be classified as follows (**Table 1**).[1] It is a serious and costly problem that is prevalent in nearly 39.8% of the population in the United States. The estimated annual medical cost of obesity in the United States was $147 billion in 2008 US dollars; the medical costs for people who are obese were $1429 higher than those of normal weight.[2] Over the years, as obesity

[a] Department of Anesthesia, University of Iowa Hospitals and Clinics, 200 Hawkins Drive, 6417-JCP, Iowa City, IA 52242, USA; [b] Department of Anesthesia, University of Iowa Hospitals and Clinics, 200 Hawkins Drive, 6413-JCP, Iowa City, IA 52242, USA
* Corresponding author.
E-mail address: surangama-sharma@uiowa.edu

Anesthesiology Clin 38 (2020) 197–212
https://doi.org/10.1016/j.anclin.2019.10.008
1932-2275/20/© 2019 Elsevier Inc. All rights reserved.

anesthesiology.theclinics.com

Table 1
World Health Organization classification of obesity

BMI	Nutritional Status
<18	Underweight
18.5–24.9	Normal weight
25.0–29.9	Preobesity/overweight
30.0–34.9	Obesity class I
35–39.9	Obesity class II
40–49.9	Obesity class III/morbid obesity
50–69.9	Supermorbid obesity
>70	Ultraobesity

Adapted from World Health Organization (WHO) Regional Office for Europe. Body mass index – BMI. Available at: http://www.euro.who.int/en/health-topics/disease-prevention/nutrition/a-healthy-lifestyle/body-mass-index-bmi. Accessed May 6 2019; with permission.

is increasing, so is the BMI of the patient population that is encountered by anesthesiologists. It is therefore imperative to understand pathophysiologic and pharmacologic changes associated with obesity, be familiar with, and bring into practice any management strategies that can help anesthesiologists safely take care of this unique patient population.

PATHOPHYSIOLOGY

Central obesity can be defined as a waist circumference greater than 88 cm in a woman and 102 cm in a man; or a waist-to-height ratio greater than 0.55.[3] Obesity is a complex condition in which body fat distribution is associated with a proinflammatory state and metabolic alterations, affecting multiple organ systems as described in later discussion.[4]

Metabolic Syndrome

Accumulation of visceral fat, and the proinflammatory and immune activation state that accompanies it, is associated with insulin resistance and T2DM.[4]

In simple terms, risk factors causing cardiovascular diseases and diabetes are grouped together as metabolic syndrome. The presence of any 3 of the 5 listed risk factors constitutes a diagnosis of metabolic syndrome, and obesity is one of the major risk factors.[5] The diagnosis of metabolic syndrome is associated with a higher risk of morbidity after surgery.

Cardiovascular

Cardiovascular diseases are more prevalent in obese patients than the patient population with a normal weight in the same age group. In an attempt to adapt to the excess body mass and increasing metabolic demands, almost one-third of patients with long-standing obesity develop structural and functional changes that lead to obesity cardiomyopathy.[4,6] An increase in intravascular blood volume as well as an increase in cardiac output (mostly from an increase in stroke volume, even though heart rate remains normal) is noted. The increase in stroke volume leads to an increase in left ventricular load and dilation, compensatory left ventricular hypertrophy, and subsequent left ventricular failure.[6]

Hypertension
Obesity and hypertension are directly proportional. The cause of hypertension in the setting of obesity and metabolic syndrome is multifaceted, resulting from interaction between genetic factors, insulin resistance, sodium retention, activation of the sympathetic nervous system as well as the activation of the renin-angiotensin-aldosterone axis.[4,7]

Coronary artery disease
Risk factors for coronary artery disease in patients with obesity include T2DM, hypertension, dyslipidemia, heightened inflammation, and a prothrombotic state. Symptoms associated with coronary ischemia, like dyspnea on exertion and chest pain, occur commonly in obese patients and can mask a true cardiac event.[4]

Arrhythmias
Arrhythmias in the obese may be precipitated by hypoxemia, nodal dysfunction from left atrial and ventricular enlargement and fatty infiltration into the conduction system, electrolyte disturbances from diuretic therapy, an increase in plasma catecholamines, and hypercarbia. Multiple studies have demonstrated an increased risk of arrhythmias, especially atrial fibrillation,[3,4,8,9] which results in markedly increased risk of sudden cardiac death. Obesity also makes individuals prone to prolonged QT interval.[3,10]

Respiratory

Obesity is inversely related to respiratory function, primarily causing restrictive physiology, from decreased airway compliance, and visceral fat, causing diaphragmatic restriction.[11,12] Lung volumes decrease in obese patients, including total lung capacity, functional residual capacity (FRC) and expiratory reserve volume, forced vital capacity (FVC), and forced expiratory volume in 1 second (FEV_1); the FEV_1/FVC ratio is usually preserved.[12,13] Obesity is associated with increased work of breathing as a consequence of increased airways resistance and reduced respiratory system compliance.[13] Airway resistance is increased, from the increase in pleural pressure that results from the weight of the chest wall.[11] Chest wall compliance is reduced, possibly from the added pressure from chest wall and intraabdominal adipose tissue. Lung compliance is reduced as well, from increased pulmonary blood volume and early airways closure.[14] Breathing at low volumes increases airway resistance with expiratory flow limitation and gas trapping owing to early airway closure and subsequent generation of intrinsic positive end-expiratory pressure (PEEP), or auto-PEEP.[15] The presence of auto-PEEP further increases the work of breathing, which is already elevated because of reduced compliance. Above changes in lung mechanics, impair the capacity of obese patients to tolerate apneic episodes with early onset oxygen desaturation.[13,16] At baseline, ventilation-perfusion mismatch is present in the obese, with preserved perfusion to the bases and diminished ventilation to those areas from atelectasis. Exercise capacity is reduced in obesity because of increased work of breathing and cardiovascular compromise. The changes in lung function, including auto-PEEP, are more severe when the patient moves from the upright to the supine posture.[11]

Sleep-disordered breathing and obstructive sleep apnea
Sleep-disordered breathing describes the spectrum of conditions ranging from obstructive sleep apnea (OSA) through obesity hypoventilation syndrome (OHS).[3] OSA is estimated to affect between 40% and 90% of obese individuals.[17] Nocturnal hypoxia and hypercarbia associated with intermittent airway obstruction are characteristic of OSA. Chronic hypoxemia and hypercarbia lead to pulmonary hypertension,

right ventricular dysfunction, and eventually, failure.[4] Some patients with severe obesity develop OHS, characterized by alveolar hypoventilation ($Paco_2 > 45$ mm Hg) unexplained by other disorders.[18] Obese patients have a reduction in airway caliber leading to an increase in airway resistance with impairment of pharyngeal dilator activity and an increased risk of airway collapse.[17,19]

Asthma

Beuther and Sutherland[20] demonstrated that obesity increased the likelihood of asthma twice as much as individuals with a BMI < 25. Altered airway smooth muscle contractility leading to increased airway responsiveness and the chronic, low-grade inflammatory state associated with obesity were linked to higher incidence.[4] Obese patients are more likely to respond poorly to inhaled corticosteroids and long-acting β-agonists. Good response to bronchodilators rules it as true asthma rather than obesity related. In 50%, obesity-related asthma is reversible with weight loss.[3]

Pulmonary hypertension

Obese patients have multiple risk factors for developing pulmonary hypertension like OSA, OHS, left heart dysfunction, and chronic pulmonary thromboembolism.[4]

Endocrine

Diabetes mellitus

Individuals with a BMI $\geq$ 40 are 7 times more likely to have diabetes compared with individuals with a normal BMI.[4,21]

Liver Disease

Risk factors for metabolic syndrome (abdominal obesity, insulin resistance) are also risk factors for nonalcoholic fatty liver disease and nonalcoholic steatohepatitis (NASH). Fatty infiltration can progress to NASH once inflammatory changes are superimposed. In about one-fifth of these patients, NASH can progress to cirrhosis, placing them at increased risk of developing hepatocellular cancer, portal hypertension, ascites, and liver failure.[22]

Gastroesophageal Reflux Disease

Even though gastric emptying is normal in obese patients without any coexisting comorbidities, mechanical and hormonal changes increase their risk of gastroesophageal reflux disease.[4,23]

Venous Thromboembolism

Prothrombotic state increases the risk of venous thromboembolism in obese patients.

PREOPERATIVE EVALUATION AND PREPARATION
Risk Assessment

Increasing BMI is an independent risk factor for perioperative pulmonary complications. It has also been associated with increased cardiovascular complications, including Deep Vein Thrombosis, hospital length of stay, estimated blood loss, longer surgical times, surgical site infections, renal failure, and prolonged assisted ventilation. A phenomenon called "obesity paradox" has been identified. Multiple studies have suggested that overweight and class 1 obese patients, otherwise having no other comorbidities, are associated with decreased morbidity and mortality, as compared with patients with normal BMI, although outcomes were worse for underweight or morbidly obese patients.[24,25] Therefore, other than BMI, comorbidities and metabolic health (better predicted by waist-to-hip ratio, waist circumference, total body fat) play a major role in risk stratification. To maximize patient safety, a multidisciplinary team approach is advisable for major surgeries, including consultation with an anesthesiologist preoperatively.[26]

Obstructive Sleep Apnea

All suspected patients should be screened for OSA as a part of preanesthetic evaluation. Common screening tools include an updated STOP-Bang (**Table 2**). For patients who screen positive, serum bicarbonate should be measured. An elevated serum bicarbonate level increases the specificity of OSA screening tools and may indicate carbon dioxide (CO_2) retention, which can be associated with sleep-related breathing disorders.[27] Elective surgeries on patients with well-controlled OSA, that is, asymptomatic patients who are compliant with positive airway pressure (PAP), can proceed without further evaluation. Studies suggest increased risk of cardiopulmonary complications in patients with untreated OSA.[28] Per the Society of Anesthesia and Sleep Medicine Guidelines on Preoperative Screening and Assessment of Adult Patients with Obstructive Sleep Apnea, "There is insufficient evidence in the current literature to support canceling or delaying surgery for a formal diagnosis (laboratory or home polysomnography) in patients with suspected OSA. Further evaluation and preoperative cardiopulmonary optimization should be considered in patients with diagnosed, partially treated/untreated, and suspected OSA where there is suspicion of or associated uncontrolled systemic disease or additional problems with ventilation or gas exchange such as: (i) hypoventilation syndromes, (ii) severe pulmonary hypertension, and (iii) resting hypoxemia in the absence of other cardiopulmonary disease".[29] Urgent and emergency surgery should not be postponed to make a formal diagnosis of OSA or to institute treatment. Patients who are on PAP therapy for OSA should continue treatment up to the day of surgery and should bring their PAP device with them on the day of surgery. Religious use of PAP devices benefits by reducing tongue volume and increased volume of the pharyngeal space (following 4 to 6 weeks of therapy),[30] improved cardiac parameters, and improved ventilatory drive in patients with OHS.[31]

Obesity Hypoventilation Syndrome

Patients with obesity and a strong clinical suspicion of OHS who are to undergo moderate- or high-risk surgery should be screened for CO_2 retention and hypoxemia with serum electrolytes and arterial blood gases. An echocardiogram to assess global cardiac function, pulmonary hypertension, and specifically right heart function is suggested by some experts for patients with clinical signs of OHS and CO_2 retention. Most of the patients with OHS have OSA, and up to two-thirds have pulmonary hypertension. Patients with OHS are sensitive to the respiratory-depressant effects of sedatives and opioids, and supplemental oxygen may increase hypercapnia unless administered with noninvasive PAP therapy. Because of these issues, patients with OHS are more likely to have difficulty weaning from mechanical ventilation than other patients, including during emergence from anesthesia.

Hypertension

Poorly controlled hypertension is associated with labile blood pressure (BP) (exaggerated response to noxious stimuli and severe hypotension on induction), during general anesthesia and increases in cardiac, neurologic, and renal complications. No clear guidelines exist, and a case-by-case approach is the best. Elective, high-

Table 2
Summary of the principal components analysis, varimax rotation

	Factor Loadings[a]
Snoring	
1. (STOP Q1). Do you snore loudly (louder than talking or loud enough to be heard through dosed doors)?	0.596
a. Yes	
b. No	
2. (Berlin Q1). Do you snore?	0.747
a. Yes	
b. No	
c. Don't know	
3. (Berlin Q2). Your snoring is:	0.825
a. Slightly louder than breathing	
b. As loud as talking	
c. Louder than talking	
d. Very loud–can be heard n adjacent rooms	
4. (Berlin Q3). How often do you snore?	0.795
a. Nearly every day	
b. 3–4 times a week	
c. 1–2 times a week	
d. 1–2 times a month	
e. Never or nearly never	
5. (Berlin Q4). Has your snoring ever bothered other people?	0.404
a. Yes	
b. No	
c. Don't know	
Tiredness during daytime	
6. (STOP Q2). Do you often feel tired, fatigued, or sleepy during daytime?	0.674
a. Yes	
b. No	
7. (Berlin Q6). How often do you feel tired or fatigued after your sleep?	0.805
a. Nearly every day	
b. 3–4 times a week	
c. 1–2 times a week	
d. 1–2 times a month	
e. Never or nearly never	
8. (Berlin Q7). During your waking time, do you feel tired, fatigued, or not up to par?	0.743
a. Nearly every day	
b. 3–4 times a week	
c. 1–2 times a week	
d. 1–2 times a month	
e. Never or nearly never	

(continued on next page)

	Factor Loadings[a]
Stop breathing during sleep	
11. (Berlin Q5). Has anyone noticed that you quit breathing during your sleep?	0.644
a. Nearly every day	
b. 3–4 times a week	
c. 1–2 times a week	
d. 1–2 times a month	
e. Never or nearly never	
12. (STOP Q4). Has anyone observed you stop breathing during your sleep?	0.606
a. Yes	
b. No	
High blood pressure	
13. (Berlin Q10). Do you have high blood pressure?	0.947
a. Yes	
b. No	
c. Don't know	
14. (STOP Q3). Do you have or are you being treated for high blood pressure?	0.945
a. Yes	
b. No	
Questions with low factor loading for all four factors	
9. (Berlin Q8). Have you ever nodded off or fallen asleep while driving a vehicle?	
a. Yes	
b. No	
10. (Berlin Q9). How often does nodding off or fating asleep while driving a vehicle occurs?	
a. Nearly every day	
b. 3–4 times a week	
c. 1–2 times a week	
d. 1–2 times a month	
e. Never or nearly never	

Table 2
(continued)

[a] Factor loadings are correlations between the original questions and their factors. Factor loadings greater than 0.30 in absolute value are considered to be significant.

From Chung F, Yegneswaran B, Liao P, et al. STOP questionnaire: a tool to screen patients for obstructive sleep apnea. Anesthesiology 2008;108(5):816; with permission.

risk surgery may be postponed to improve management of poorly controlled, severe hypertension given the above risks (systolic >180 mm Hg and diastolic >110 mm Hg).[32–34]

Cardiovascular Disease

The American Heart Association Scientific Advisory on Cardiovascular Evaluation and Management of Severely Obese Patients Undergoing Surgery recommends that severely obese patients with at least 1 risk factor for Coronary Heart Disease (diabetes, smoking, hypertension, or hyperlipidemia) or poor exercise tolerance should have a 12-lead electrocardiogram and chest radiograph before surgery,[35] because their cardiac symptoms can easily be masked by obesity-related issues. Preoperative cardiac evaluation and management, otherwise, are similar to patients with normal BMI.

Diabetes Mellitus

T2DM is strongly associated with obesity. Patients with poorly controlled diabetes are more likely to have wound infections, acute renal failure, and postoperative leaks.[36] A target hemoglobin A1c (HbA$_{1c}$) value of 6.5% to 7.0% or less perioperatively is recommended, although an HgbA$_{1c}$ of 7% to 8% can be considered in patients with extensive comorbid conditions or difficult to control diabetes.[37]

Airway Assessment

Airway assessment should be an integral part of preanesthetic evaluation, irrespective of the type of anesthesia. Obese patients desaturate more quickly during apnea (eg, during attempts at securing the airway). Obesity and an increase in neck circumference are risk factors for difficulty with mask ventilation, supraglottic airway (SGA) ventilation, and video laryngoscopy.[38]

Ambulatory Versus Inpatient Surgery

The decision to perform surgery on an inpatient or outpatient basis must be individualized. Comorbidities should be considered when making the decision to perform ambulatory surgery in severely obese patients, including those with OSA. Other important considerations include the type of anesthesia administered (ie, monitored anesthesia care, regional anesthesia, or general anesthesia), the risk level of the surgical procedure, and requirements for postoperative care. Supermorbid obese (BMI >50 kg/m^2) patients are poor candidates for ambulatory surgery if the procedure requires general anesthesia and postoperative opioid administration. It often warrants overnight admission and observation in an inpatients unit, because these patients may be at increased risk of perioperative complications.[39] According to the Society for Ambulatory Anesthesia consensus statement on preoperative selection of adult patients with OSA scheduled for ambulatory surgery, patients with known OSA and optimized comorbidities who are able to use PAP devices can safely undergo ambulatory procedures. Also, patients with presumptive diagnosis of OSA with optimized comorbidities, if postoperative pain can be managed primarily by nonopioid techniques, can undergo ambulatory surgeries[40]

DAY OF SURGERY: PREPARATION AND MANAGEMENT
Preoperative Preparation

Availability of appropriate weighing scale, gowns, chairs, transport beds, and monitors should be checked before arrival, and the patient should be asked to trim their beard or this should be done in preoperative holding if need be. Operating Rooms should be equipped with suitable sized operating tables and gel pads for positioning, and extra personnel should be available to help with patient positioning. An experienced surgeon and anesthesiologist are ideal for supermorbidly obese patients, to minimize operating and procedure times, respectively.

Type of Anesthetic

Whenever feasible, regional anesthesia is advocated over general anesthesia in obese, especially with patients with OSA, to avoid the potential airway and respiratory problems. Neuraxial anesthesia and peripheral nerve blocks offer the advantages of improved postoperative pain control, reduced use of opioids for postoperative analgesia, and consequently, decreased potential for drug-induced respiratory depression. Peripheral nerve blocks with ultrasound guidance appear to be safe in obese patients, with relatively high block success rates, in experienced hands. However, obesity may make peripheral nerve block more difficult to perform and may be associated with higher block failure rates.[41] Obesity may be a risk factor for catheter-related infection. In a large retrospective analysis, obesity was an independent risk factor for peripheral but not neuraxial catheter-related infections.[42] Neuraxial medication should be given incrementally whenever possible, to avoid excessively high blockade; the same dose of spinal and epidural local anesthetics can spread to higher levels in obese compared with normal weight patients. If sedation is considered in conjunction with regional anesthesia, it should be kept to a minimum.[3] General anesthesia, as a backup plan, should always be considered and consent provided for, given an unsuccessful or failed regional block. General anesthesia may be the first choice given the type of procedure (laparoscopy/thoracotomy and so forth), longer-duration prone positioning cases, or procedures whereby controlled ventilation is warranted.

Pharmacology in the Obese

Pharmacokinetics and pharmacodynamics of anesthetic agents are altered in obese patients. Drug disposition is influenced as drug distribution, clearance, and elimination, and volumes of distribution (Vd) are affected as a consequence of a larger proportion adipose tissue. Using total body weight (TBW), that is, body weight of an individual without any added adjustments for all medications, is a concern in obese patients because the fatty tissue and lean body weight (LBW), that is, TBW minus the weight of fat mass, do not increase in a directly proportional fashion, and there is a risk of overdosing. In men, LBW is approximately 80% of the TBW, whereas in women it should be represented by 75% of TBW. Ideal body weight (IBW) is the weight of both men and women for what was thought to represent a maximally healthy person. It describes a relationship between the idealized weight correlated with height. For men, IBW (in kilograms) is 50 + 2.3 kg per inch greater than 5 feet, whereas in women it is 45.5 + 2.3 kg per inch greater than 5 feet. In obese patients, LBW can be estimated by increasing the IBW by close to 20% to 30%.[43] Other factors that affect dosing that need to be taken into consideration when using anesthetics in obesity include Vd and drug elimination. Factors that affect Vd include the lipophilicity/hydrophilicity of the drug, lean body mass, fat quantity, cardiac output and circulatory blood volume, total body water, and protein binding of the drug. Increased triglycerides, cholesterol, and fatty acid levels, which are all commonly seen in overweight and obese states, can decrease drug protein binding. Elimination is the process by which the body metabolizes and removes the drug. Elimination (both phase I and II) are increased in obesity. Renal clearance is increased in obesity secondary to increased renal blood flow and glomerular filtration rate.[43] Calculations should be made to determine LBW and IBW, because most anesthetic agents are dosed accordingly. For induction agents, including propofol and etomidate, anesthesia will occur before redistribution from the central compartment, and the dose needed to produce unconsciousness equates to lean body mass. For opioids (fentanyl, remifentanil, morphine, hydromorphone), using IBW as the initial dose and titrating to effect is advisable. Neuromuscular blocking agents, including rocuronium, cisatracurium, and vecuronium, are hydrophilic and distributed primarily within the central compartment. Lean body mass is a suitable dosing scalar. For suxamethonium, administration should be based on consideration of TBW, because of both an increase in plasma pseudocholinesterase and an extracellular volume in obese patients.[44] For neostigmine, studies have shown no significant difference in recovery to a train of 4 ratio of 0.7 in obese versus nonobese patients after a standard dose. However, full recovery to a train of 4 ratio of 0.9 was prolonged in obese patients.[45] Sugammadex is a reversal agent that acts by binding steroidal nondepolarizing neuromuscular blockers to its lipophilic core. Dosing of sugammadex is based on the number of posttetanic twitches or time from administration. Dosing recommendations from the manufacturer are based on TBW.[43]

Intraoperative Management

Monitoring

Use of a noninvasive BP cuff may be challenging. Appropriately sized large adult BP cuffs and unconventional sites like the forearm might be beneficial. Invasive BP monitoring may be needed for critically ill, extensive, or longer-duration procedures. An appropriately sized angiocatheter with longer cannulas and ultrasound might be needed, because venous access is more difficult in this population, making intravenous line insertion difficult.

Positioning

Studies have demonstrated an increased risk of nerve injury in the obese surgical population.[46] Prone position and steep Trendelenburg positions are especially technically challenging, with decreased lung volume in the Trendelenburg position, and airway and face edema in dependent areas in both. Caution should be excised with adequate gel padding, keeping eyes, nose, ears, and other pressure points free, minimizing risks of complications.

Premedication

Anxiolytics can be titrated for desired effect, without causing respiratory compromise. Aspiration prevention using antacids (sodium citrate), gastric stimulants (metoclopramide), or H2 blockers may be used, if the patient is also at higher risk for aspiration related to other comorbidities.[47]

Airway management

Obese patients are more likely to require intubation rather than an SGA, because they are more likely to require controlled ventilation to prevent hypoventilation during spontaneous respiration and an SGA may not maintain a seal at the higher airway pressures needed in obese patients. No specific criteria for the use of an SGA in obese patients have been established. However, a decision should be made for individual patients taking into consideration grade and distribution of obesity, type and length of surgery, and patient position to determine when its use is appropriate. When SGAs are used, second-generation devices designed for controlled ventilation, which allow for higher seal pressures and provide a gastric port, are frequently used.[48] Intubation may be more challenging in obese patients. Awake intubation is prudent when there is concern for both difficult intubation and difficult mask ventilation. Appropriate positioning with ramping (a stack of blankets or a preformed ramp can be used to elevate the patient's upper body and head with the goal of horizontal alignment between the external auditory meatus and the sternal notch), availability of backup airway management devices, and following the American Society of Anesthesiologists difficult airway algorithm are the keys for managing the obese patient's airway.[38]

Induction

Preoxygenation in the reverse Trendelenburg position in the obese, to improve FRC by decreasing pressure from abdomen and upward shift of the diaphragm, is advisable.[49] The safe apnea time should be maximized by using 100% oxygen at a flow rate high enough to prevent rebreathing (approximately 2 times the minute ventilation), aiming for an end-tidal concentration of oxygen greater than 90%. Preoxygenation with manually applied PEEP, or the use of noninvasive ventilation (NIV), will improve oxygenation in obese patients, if tolerated.[50] Passive apneic oxygenation using nasal cannula during laryngoscopy can prolong the time to desaturation during airway management.[51] Succinylcholine can be used for standard intubation or rapid sequence induction, with availability of sugammadex; an intubating dose of rocuronium is another safe option. Mask ventilation is usually difficult, so, optimal positioning should be used, and use of an oral airway, a 2-handed approach, or a Laryngeal Mask Airway (LMA) should be considered if needed for ventilation.

Anesthetic agents

The choice of induction agent used for an obese patient is the same as for a normal weight patient, although doses may need to be modified, as discussed in the section "Pharmacology in the Obese". Anesthesia can be maintained with either an inhaled anesthetic agent or a total intravenous anesthesia.

Ventilation

When patients are managed with spontaneous respiration (with either an LMA or an endotracheal tube), minute ventilation and end-tidal CO_2 should be closely monitored to assure adequate ventilation. Continuous positive airway pressure (CPAP) during spontaneous respiration should be used to improve oxygenation. When patients are unable to maintain enough volume, ventilation should be assisted or controlled. A protective ventilation strategy is reasonable to maintain oxygenation and normocapnia, and to avoid lung damage. Lung protective strategy consists of low tidal volumes, low levels of oxygen (as tolerated), PEEP, and recruitment maneuvers.[52,53] Recruitment maneuvers should not be performed unless patients are hemodynamically stable and euvolemic, because these maneuvers may lead to a transient decrease in preload.

Fluid management

Clinical judgment based on available measures of volume status and tissue perfusion should be used to guide fluid administration. Fluid therapy guided by stroke volume variation can be used as well.[54]

Reversal of neuromuscular blockade

Neuromuscular blockade may be reversed using either sugammadex or neostigmine. Some evidence suggests that sugammadex may offer additional benefits over neostigmine in certain clinical circumstances like obesity.[55]

Extubation

The head-up position is ideal to improve oxygenation and decrease work of breathing, and standard extubation criteria should be followed. Airway swelling and edema complicate an already challenging intubation. Therefore, emergency airway equipment and personnel to assist in airway management must be available to manage potential difficulties.

Analgesia

A multimodal, opioid-sparing approach to analgesia should be used for all patients. The use of potent nonsteroidal anti-inflammatory analgesics, such as ketorolac, or acetaminophen with local anesthetic wound infiltration, is beneficial. Other agents that may be used include ketamine, alpha-2 agonists (eg, clonidine and dexmedetomidine), magnesium, systemic lidocaine, and antiepileptic drugs (pregabalin and gabapentin). A multimodal strategy reduces postoperative opioid use and gives a better recovery profile, including decreased sedation and postoperative nausea and vomiting.[56]

POSTOPERATIVE CARE

Obese patients in the postanesthesia care unit (PACU) are prone to respiratory and ventilatory compromise. Obese patients are at greater risk for hypoxia in the postoperative period, so careful attention should be paid to maintaining adequate oxygenation by administration of oxygen, titrated to keep oxygen saturation at greater than 90% (by face mask or nasal cannula) and positioning the patient in head up (sitting or semisitting). The use of incentive spirometry or chest physiotherapy postoperatively improves pulmonary function and decreases complications. Administration of CPAP or other forms of NIV in patients with preoperative use, or with hypoxia unresponsive to incentive spirometry, significantly improves ventilation. An arterial blood-gas test may be used to assess hypoventilation in patients who are unable to maintain oxygen saturation despite supplementation and with altered sensorium. Hypoventilation owing to sedative medication should be ruled out; pharmacologic reversal of benzodiazepines or opioids may be used as clinically indicated. Often simply arousing a drowsy patient with a reminder to breathe deeply is sufficient, but this may need to be repeated frequently. When upper airway obstruction occurs, an oropharyngeal airway (if the patient is sedated), a nasopharyngeal airway, or both, may open the airway and permit adequate ventilation. When these maneuvers are insufficient, it is reasonable to assist these patients with NIV, which may keep them from requiring reintubation.

Discharge

Oxygen saturation on room air should return to preoperative baseline, and patients should have continuous pulse oximetry in the PACU until they have demonstrated that they can maintain adequate oxygenation when left unstimulated. Patients who cannot maintain adequate oxygenation when left undisturbed should not be discharged from the hospital but should be sent to the floor and monitored.[57]

SUMMARY

Obese patients have a unique set of physiologic and pharmacologic changes; understanding them makes caring for this subset of patients safer. Meticulous planning and interaction between surgical and anesthetic teams increase the probability of successful and satisfactory outcomes for the patient.

DISCLOSURE

The authors have no commercial or financial disclosures.

REFERENCES

1. Europe W. 2019. Available at: http://www.euro.who.int/en/health-topics/disease-prevention/nutrition/a-healthy-lifestyle/body-mass-index-bmi. Accessed May 6, 2019.
2. Prevention CDC. Adult obesity facts 2018. Available at: https://www.cdc.gov/obesity/data/adult.html. Accessed May 6, 2019.
3. Nightingale CE, Margarson MP, Shearer E, et al. Peri-operative management of the obese surgical patient 2015: Association of Anaesthetists of Great Britain and Ireland Society for Obesity and Bariatric Anaesthesia. Anaesthesia 2015; 70(7):859–76.
4. Ortiz VE, Kwo J. Obesity: physiologic changes and implications for preoperative management. BMC Anesthesiol 2015;15:97.
5. Alberti KG, Eckel RH, Grundy SM, et al. Harmonizing the metabolic syndrome: a joint interim statement of the International Diabetes Federation Task Force on Epidemiology and Prevention; National Heart, Lung, and Blood Institute; American Heart Association; World Heart Federation; International Atherosclerosis Society; and International Association for the Study of Obesity. Circulation 2009; 120(16):1640–5.
6. Kenchaiah S, Evans JC, Levy D, et al. Obesity and the risk of heart failure. N Engl J Med 2002;347(5):305–13.
7. Shihab HM, Meoni LA, Chu AY, et al. Body mass index and risk of incident hypertension over the life course: the Johns Hopkins Precursors Study. Circulation 2012;126(25):2983–9.
8. Wanahita N, Messerli FH, Bangalore S, et al. Atrial fibrillation and obesity–results of a meta-analysis. Am Heart J 2008;155(2):310–5.
9. Magnani JW, Hylek EM, Apovian CM. Obesity begets atrial fibrillation: a contemporary summary. Circulation 2013;128(4):401–5.
10. Lavie CJ, Milani RV, Ventura HO. Obesity and cardiovascular disease: risk factor, paradox, and impact of weight loss. J Am Coll Cardiol 2009;53(21):1925–32.
11. Yap JC, Watson RA, Gilbey S, et al. Effects of posture on respiratory mechanics in obesity. J Appl Physiol (1985) 1995;79(4):1199–205.
12. Steier J, Lunt A, Hart N, et al. Observational study of the effect of obesity on lung volumes. Thorax 2014;69(8):752–9.
13. Hodgson LE, Murphy PB, Hart N. Respiratory management of the obese patient undergoing surgery. J Thorac Dis 2015;7(5):943–52.
14. Sharp JT, Henry JP, Sweany SK, et al. The total work of breathing in normal and obese men. J Clin Invest 1964;43:728–39.
15. Pankow W, Podszus T, Gutheil T, et al. Expiratory flow limitation and intrinsic positive end-expiratory pressure in obesity. J Appl Physiol (1985) 1998;85(4): 1236–43.
16. Damia G, Mascheroni D, Croci M, et al. Perioperative changes in functional residual capacity in morbidly obese patients. Br J Anaesth 1988;60(5):574–8.
17. Isono S. Obesity and obstructive sleep apnoea: mechanisms for increased collapsibility of the passive pharyngeal airway. Respirology 2012;17(1):32–42.
18. Piper AJ, Grunstein RR. Obesity hypoventilation syndrome: mechanisms and management. Am J Respir Crit Care Med 2011;183(3):292–8.
19. King GG, Brown NJ, Diba C, et al. The effects of body weight on airway calibre. Eur Respir J 2005;25(5):896–901.

20. Beuther DA, Sutherland ER. Overweight, obesity, and incident asthma: a meta-analysis of prospective epidemiologic studies. Am J Respir Crit Care Med 2007;175(7):661–6.
21. Mokdad AH, Ford ES, Bowman BA, et al. Prevalence of obesity, diabetes, and obesity-related health risk factors, 2001. JAMA 2003;289(1):76–9.
22. Pais R, Charlotte F, Fedchuk L, et al. A systematic review of follow-up biopsies reveals disease progression in patients with non-alcoholic fatty liver. J Hepatol 2013;59(3):550–6.
23. Glasbrenner B, Pieramico O, Brecht-Krauss D, et al. Gastric emptying of solids and liquids in obesity. Clin Investig 1993;71(7):542–6.
24. Mullen JT, Moorman DW, Davenport DL. The obesity paradox: body mass index and outcomes in patients undergoing nonbariatric general surgery. Ann Surg 2009;250(1):166–72.
25. Thornqvist C, Gislason GH, Kober L, et al. Body mass index and risk of periop-erative cardiovascular adverse events and mortality in 34,744 Danish patients un-dergoing hip or knee replacement. Acta Orthop 2014;85(5):456–62.
26. Schumann R, Jones SB, Cooper B, et al. Update on best practice recommenda-tions for anesthetic perioperative care and pain management in weight loss sur-gery, 2004-2007. Obesity (Silver Spring) 2009;17(5):889–94.
27. Chung F, Yang Y, Brown R, et al. Alternative scoring models of STOP-bang ques-tionnaire improve specificity to detect undiagnosed obstructive sleep apnea. J Clin Sleep Med 2014;10(9):951–8.
28. Abdelsattar ZM, Hendren S, Wong SL, et al. The impact of untreated obstructive sleep apnea on cardiopulmonary complications in general and vascular surgery: a cohort study. Sleep 2015;38(8):1205–10.
29. Chung F, Memtsoudis SG, Ramachandran SK, et al. Society of Anesthesia and Sleep Medicine guidelines on preoperative screening and assessment of adult patients with obstructive sleep apnea. Anesth Analg 2016;123(2):452–73.
30. Ryan CF, Lowe AA, Li D, et al. Magnetic resonance imaging of the upper airway in obstructive sleep apnea before and after chronic nasal continuous positive airway pressure therapy. Am Rev Respir Dis 1991;144(4):939–44.
31. Cartagena R. Preoperative evaluation of patients with obesity and obstructive sleep apnea. Anesthesiol Clin North Am 2005;23(3):463–78, vi.
32. Wolfsthal SD. Is blood pressure control necessary before surgery? Med Clin North Am 1993;77(2):349–63.
33. Casadei B, Abuzeid H. Is there a strong rationale for deferring elective surgery in patients with poorly controlled hypertension? J Hypertens 2005;23(1):19–22.
34. Eagle KA, Berger PB, Calkins H, et al. ACC/AHA guideline update for periop-erative cardiovascular evaluation for noncardiac surgery–executive summary. A report of the American College of Cardiology/American Heart Association Task Force on Practice Guidelines (committee to update the 1996 guidelines on peri-operative cardiovascular evaluation for noncardiac surgery). Anesth Analg 2002; 94(5):1052–64.
35. Poirier P, Alpert MA, Fleisher LA, et al. Cardiovascular evaluation and manage-ment of severely obese patients undergoing surgery: a science advisory from the American Heart Association. Circulation 2009;120(1):86–95.
36. Perna M, Romagnuolo J, Morgan K, et al. Preoperative hemoglobin A1c and postoperative glucose control in outcomes after gastric bypass for obesity. Surg Obes Relat Dis 2012;8(6):685–90.
37. Mechanick JI, Youdim A, Jones DB, et al. Clinical practice guidelines for the peri-operative nutritional, metabolic, and nonsurgical support of the bariatric surgery

patient–2013 update: cosponsored by American Association of Clinical Endocrinologists, The Obesity Society, and American Society for Metabolic & Bariatric Surgery. Obesity (Silver Spring) 2013;21(Suppl 1):S1–27.

38. Apfelbaum JL, Hagberg CA, Caplan RA, et al. Practice guidelines for management of the difficult airway: an updated report by the American Society of Anesthesiologists Task Force on Management of the Difficult Airway. Anesthesiology 2013;118(2):251–70.

39. Kakarla VR, Nandipati K, Lalla M, et al. Are laparoscopic bariatric procedures safe in superobese (BMI ≥50 kg/m2) patients? An NSQIP data analysis. Surg Obes Relat Dis 2011;7(4):452–8.

40. Joshi GP, Ankichetty SP, Gan TJ, et al. Society for Ambulatory Anesthesia consensus statement on preoperative selection of adult patients with obstructive sleep apnea scheduled for ambulatory surgery. Anesth Analg 2012;115(5): 1060–8.

41. Nielsen KC, Guller U, Steele SM, et al. Influence of obesity on surgical regional anesthesia in the ambulatory setting: an analysis of 9,038 blocks. Anesthesiology 2005;102(1):181–7.

42. Bomberg H, Albert N, Schmitt K, et al. Obesity in regional anesthesia–a risk factor for peripheral catheter-related infections. Acta Anaesthesiol Scand 2015;59(8): 1038–48.

43. Willis S, Bordelon GJ, Rana MV. Perioperative pharmacologic considerations in obesity. Anesthesiol Clin 2017;35(2):247–57.

44. Skues MA. Perioperative management of the obese ambulatory patient. Curr Opin Anaesthesiol 2018;31(6):693–9.

45. Suzuki T, Masaki G, Ogawa S. Neostigmine-induced reversal of vecuronium in normal weight, overweight and obese female patients. Br J Anaesth 2006; 97(2):160–3.

46. Al-Temimi MH, Chandrasekaran B, Phelan MJ, et al. Incidence, risk factors, and trends of motor peripheral nerve injury after colorectal surgery: analysis of the National Surgical Quality Improvement Program Database. Dis Colon Rectum 2017; 60(3):318–25.

47. Practice guidelines for preoperative fasting and the use of pharmacologic agents to reduce the risk of pulmonary aspiration: application to healthy patients undergoing elective procedures: an updated report by the American Society of Anesthesiologists Task Force on preoperative fasting and the use of pharmacologic agents to reduce the risk of pulmonary aspiration. Anesthesiology 2017;126(3): 376–93.

48. Timmermann A, Bergner UA, Russo SG. Laryngeal mask airway indications: new frontiers for second-generation supraglottic airways. Curr Opin Anaesthesiol 2015;28(6):717–26.

49. Dixon BJ, Dixon JB, Carden JR, et al. Preoxygenation is more effective in the 25 degrees head-up position than in the supine position in severely obese patients: a randomized controlled study. Anesthesiology 2005;102(6):1110–5 [discussion: 1115A].

50. Carron M, Zarantonello F, Tellaroli P, et al. Perioperative noninvasive ventilation in obese patients: a qualitative review and meta-analysis. Surg Obes Relat Dis 2016;12(3):681–91.

51. Ramachandran SK, Cosnowski A, Shanks A, et al. Apneic oxygenation during prolonged laryngoscopy in obese patients: a randomized, controlled trial of nasal oxygen administration. J Clin Anesth 2010;22(3):164–8.

52. Aldenkortt M, Lysakowski C, Elia N, et al. Ventilation strategies in obese patients undergoing surgery: a quantitative systematic review and meta-analysis. Br J Anaesth 2012;109(4):493–502.
53. Talab HF, Zabani IA, Abdelrahman HS, et al. Intraoperative ventilatory strategies for prevention of pulmonary atelectasis in obese patients undergoing laparoscopic bariatric surgery. Anesth Analg 2009;109(5):1511–6.
54. Jain AK, Dutta A. Stroke volume variation as a guide to fluid administration in morbidly obese patients undergoing laparoscopic bariatric surgery. Obes Surg 2010;20(6):709–15.
55. Gaszynski T, Szewczyk T, Gaszynski W. Randomized comparison of sugammadex and neostigmine for reversal of rocuronium-induced muscle relaxation in morbidly obese undergoing general anaesthesia. Br J Anaesth 2012;108(2): 236–9.
56. Feld JM, Laurito CE, Beckerman M, et al. Non-opioid analgesia improves pain relief and decreases sedation after gastric bypass surgery. Can J Anaesth 2003; 50(4):336–41.
57. Gross JB, Bachenberg KL, Benumof JL, et al. Practice guidelines for the perioperative management of patients with obstructive sleep apnea: a report by the American Society of Anesthesiologists Task Force on Perioperative Management of patients with obstructive sleep apnea. Anesthesiology 2006;104(5):1081–93 [quiz: 1117–88].

Emergency Anesthesia in Resource-Limited Areas

Seung Lee, MD[a], Azuka Onye, MD[b], Asad Latif, MD, MPH[c],*

KEYWORDS

- Emergency anesthesia • Global anesthesia • Global surgery
- Resource-limited settings • Disaster settings

KEY POINTS

- Anesthesia providers often need to play central roles in the provision of care across the perioperative spectrum in resource-limited areas.
- Safe and efficient anesthesia delivery in resource-limited areas requires proper preparation based on a needs assessment coupled with a realistic understanding of locally available resources.
- Anesthetic approach and technique can depend on a variety of factors, such as training and skill of providers, availability of equipment and supplies, type of surgery, and resources for postoperative care.
- Local, spinal, and general intravenous (mainly with ketamine) anesthesia is widely used; paralysis and airway instrumentation should be avoided if possible.
- Anesthesia services need to remain in line with local resources and skills. Whenever possible, focus should be given toward training and education of local providers.

INTRODUCTION

High-quality anesthesia care can help prevent substantial death and disability in the world's poorest regions. Emergent and urgent medical conditions contribute to 90% of deaths and 84% of disability-adjusted life years worldwide, with many of these conditions requiring surgical intervention.[1] However, more than 90% of the population in low-income and middle-income countries (LMICs) lack access to emergency or essential surgical care.[2] In a 2015 report, The Lancet Commission on Global Surgery (LCoGS) estimated that 5 billion people lack access to affordable and timely surgical care and that almost 33% of all deaths worldwide are caused by

[a] Department of Anesthesiology and Critical Care Medicine, Johns Hopkins University School of Medicine, 1800 Orleans Street, 6222 Charlotte R. Bloomberg, Baltimore, MD 21287, USA;
[b] Department of Anesthesiology and Critical Care Medicine, Johns Hopkins University School of Medicine, 1800 Orleans Street, 9137 Sheikh Zayed Building, Baltimore, MD 21287, USA;
[c] Department of Anesthesiology and Critical Care Medicine, Johns Hopkins University School of Medicine, Armstrong Institute for Patient Safety and Quality, Johns Hopkins Medicine, 600 North Wolfe Street, Meyer 297A, Baltimore, MD 21287, USA
* Corresponding author.
E-mail address: alatif1@jhmi.edu

Anesthesiology Clin 38 (2020) 213–230
https://doi.org/10.1016/j.anclin.2019.10.011
1932-2275/20/© 2019 Elsevier Inc. All rights reserved.

anesthesiology.theclinics.com

untreated surgical conditions.[3] Inadequate anesthesia services are arguably a primary limitation to meeting global surgical need. In 2017, the World Federation of Societies of Anaesthesiologists (WFSA) identified 77 LMICs that do not meet the minimum anesthesia workforce density (5 per 100,000 population), with an average of 1.6 anesthetists per 100,000 people across sub-Saharan Africa.[4] The anesthesia gap results in absent or delayed care and high mortalities for many easily treatable conditions, such as obstructed labor, appendicitis, fractures, and cancer. Millions more receive unsafe anesthesia from providers with limited to no training. Anesthesia-related mortalities reflect these grim statistics and are 100 to 1000 times higher than in high-income countries (HICs), especially in obstetric and pediatric populations.[5]

Anesthesiologists from HICs often play a crucial role in providing and improving capacity for essential surgery in LMICs and frequently provide emergency care during a disaster response. Although academic partnerships with local hospitals and governments to improve education and training are important for sustainable anesthesia capacity building, many LMICs devastated by crisis, conflict, or disaster need immediate support while they develop. In these situations, volunteer anesthesia teams can offer lifesaving care with adequate training and preparation. Providing effective and safe anesthesia requires familiarity with the local infrastructure, resources, and surgical need, as well as insight into how they will affect patient care and anesthetic management. Although exceptionally trained and knowledgeable, many are unfamiliar with the resources and infrastructure available in resource-limited areas (RLAs), putting many of them outside their comfort zones and unprepared to handle the obstacles encountered.

This article categorizes and reviews some of the unique considerations and challenges to providing anesthesia care for emergency and essential surgeries in RLAs, as a first step for anesthesia providers to help organize them. It defines emergency anesthesia as anesthesia for any essential or emergency surgery in RLAs, in particular the bellwether procedures (obstetric emergencies, intra-abdominal catastrophes, and life-threatening injuries) that require immediate care to prevent death and disability.[6]

GENERAL CONSIDERATIONS FOR WORKING IN RESOURCE-LIMITED AREAS
Overall Considerations and Constraints in Resource-Limited Areas

Providing emergency anesthesia care in an RLA presents many challenges that require flexibility, resilience, and the ability to adapt to changing circumstances. Anesthesia providers often must deal with unreliable access to power, water, drugs, and equipment, as well as limited options for postoperative care and pain management. Despite these constraints, minimum standards for patient care must be followed as best as possible. The WFSA and World Health Organization (WHO) have developed international guidelines regarding essential monitoring, equipment, and medications for patient safety that are largely unobtainable in many resource-limited settings (**Table 1**).[7] In many of these settings, it is recommended that operations be restricted to emergency surgeries, and anesthesia providers must rely on clinical acumen, vigilance, and serial examinations such as visual cues, auscultation, and continuous/intermittent pulse palpation to provide safe care.

Human resource constraints
A shortage of trained anesthesia providers is one of the largest barriers to provision of safe anesthesia care in RLAs, with fewer than 1 physician anesthesiologist per million population in many countries, and some with no physician anesthesiologist at all.[4] In contrast,

Table 1
World Health Organization and World Federation of Societies of Anaesthesiologists international standards for the safe practice of anesthesia

	Level 1 Facility Small Hospital/Health Center	Level 2 Facility District/Provincial Hospital
Typical Infrastructure	Small number of beds, sparsely equipped procedure room or OR	100–300 beds, adequately equipped major and minor ORs
Treatment Capability	Small surgical procedures and emergency treatment of 90%–95% of trauma and obstetrics cases (excluding cesarean section)	Bellwether procedures[a] and short-term treatment of 95%–99% of major life-threatening conditions
Equipment[b]	Adequate lighting Tilting operating table Oropharyngeal airways Facemasks Laryngoscope and blades Endotracheal tubes Suction device and suction catheters Self-inflating bags Equipment for IV infusions and injection of medications Equipment for spinal anesthesia or regional blocks Sterile gloves Access to a defibrillator Stethoscope Pulse oximeter Carbon dioxide detector Noninvasive blood pressure monitor Electrocardiogram	System for delivering inhalational anesthesia Automated ventilator with disconnect alarm IV pressure infuser bag Device for warming IV fluids, blood Examination (nonsterile) gloves Continuous waveform capnography Temperature monitor (intermittent) Nerve stimulator Dedicated space for recovering patients
Essential Medicines[c]	Ketamine Diazepam or midazolam Morphine Local anesthetic (eg, lidocaine or bupivacaine) Dextrose (for neonates) Oxygen Epinephrine (adrenaline) Atropine Morphine Acetaminophen (paracetamol) Ibuprofen Magnesium	Thiopental or propofol Appropriate inhalational anesthetic Succinylcholine Nondepolarizing muscle relaxant Neostigmine Amiodarone Ephedrine, metaraminol, norepinephrine, or phenylephrine Hydrocortisone Salbutamol Calcium gluconate (or chloride) Hydralazine Furosemide

Abbreviations: IV, intravenous; OR, operating room.
[a] Bellwether procedures refer to cesarean delivery, laparotomy, and treatment of open fracture.
[b] The equipment listed for the level 2 facility is recommended in addition to the equipment highly recommended for the level 1 facility.
[c] The medicines listed for the level 2 facility are recommended in addition to the medicines highly recommended for the level 1 facility.
Adapted from World Health Organization (WHO). Surgical Care at the District Hospital. Anaesthetic infrastructure and supplies. Available at: https://www.who.int/surgery/publications/en/SCDH.pdf. Accessed Oct 18 2019; with permission.

the United States has an estimated 25 anesthesia providers for every 100,000 patients.[8] These shortages are compounded in rural areas owing to inequitable distribution of the existing workforce, because most health professionals are centered in urban areas. Nurses lacking specialized training are often responsible for several patients simultaneously during the patients' recovery from anesthesia, a critical period for many patients when inadequate observation and monitoring can lead to severe morbidity or mortality. Brouillette and colleagues[9] emphasized the importance of physician involvement at a teaching hospital in Ghana where 99% of perioperative deaths occurred in the postanesthesia care unit. Patients transferred to the wards are rarely better off because limited nurse staffing is associated with poor patient safety.[10]

Addressing such human resource constraints in RLAs requires novel approaches. The LCoGS suggests task sharing as a method to help fill gaps. In such scenarios, tasks are transferred to nontraditional health workers who have received focused shorter training.[11] This approach can be applied to the entire perioperative workforce, from anesthesia providers, to surgeons, to technicians and nurses. Regardless of the workforce level in RLAs, it is generally important as a principle to use the local providers as much as possible to facilitate capacity development and eventual handover of activities. To this end, anesthesia techniques during times such as surgical missions should remain in line with local capacity and knowledge, and training of local health professionals should be an integral component whenever possible. Furthermore, patients' family members are frequently deputized as care providers, especially in the perioperative period when they might be required to function as nurses during postanesthesia recovery, or medication procurers and administrators on the wards, and even physical therapists during postsurgical recovery.

Patient considerations

Many patients in RLAs present without any past medical history, given that many do not (or are unable to) seek out formal health care. The lack of history is a particular problem when patients require emergency surgery. When they do present for medical treatment, it is frequently delayed, resulting in an illness that is more severe, more difficult to treat, and complicated by resistant infection, anemia, and malnutrition.[12] Furthermore, the ability to perform a preoperative assessment may be limited by language barriers, even for safety considerations such as verifying fasting status or drug allergies. Ultimately, it can be essential to use local volunteers as a component of the perioperative team. They can act as interpreters and provide valuable insight into habits and cultural and ethical norms, among other functions.

Infrastructure, equipment, and supply constraints

In 2015, the WFSA recommended minimum standards for the safe practice of anesthesia.[5] However, most LMIC settings are unable to achieve them. A survey of 590 facilities in 22 LMICs showed that 40% of hospitals had no anesthesia machines and 35% had no access to oxygen.[13] Safe anesthesia for emergency and critically ill patients in many LMICs is made even more challenging by limited access to essential medications, support services such as laboratory and blood bank, and technologies such as advanced airway devices and invasive monitors.[14] Another study investigated the operative capacity of 78 government district hospitals in 4 sub-Saharan nations, estimating 1 operating room per 100,000 people.[15] Available equipment, often donated from HICs, is frequently outdated, broken, or inappropriate for local needs. Almost two-thirds of theaters in rural areas of LMICs did not even have pulse oximetry.[16] Anesthesia providers need to exercise flexibility in their practice, and acquaint themselves with the existing technology and equipment at their destinations.

Maintaining a steady and reliable supply of critical anesthesia drugs is frequently challenging in RLAs owing to issues with transport, storage, and regulation. A lack of ketamine may mean no anesthesia at all, and a lack of vasopressors could result in the inability to support patients hemodynamically in an emergency. At many institutions where the authors have worked, blood work and diagnostic imaging can be obtained only if family members are present to carry samples or transport the patient to an outside facility. For example, in Sierra Leone, patients can receive surgery only if family members donate a specified amount of blood based on the type of surgery. When practicing in an area without a blood bank, it may be necessary to set up a similar system for blood donation by family members. When blood products are available, the risk for transfusion-transmitted infections is much higher than in HICs.[17] Ultimately, sustainability after the departure of external aid must be planned in advance by using drugs and supplies available in the local context.

Disaster Relief Efforts in Resource-Limited Areas

The WHO defines a disaster as a situation or event that causes significant damage and overwhelms the local resources and capacity to cope.[18] Disasters can be associated with both natural hazards (eg, earthquakes, floods, hurricanes) and man-made, or complex, disasters (eg, conflict situations, oil spills, terrorist attacks). Although disasters can occur in both HICs and LMICs, countries with poor economic development are more vulnerable, and they often require outside resources and international assistance.[19] Moreover, lessons from prior disasters such as the 2010 Haiti earthquake have shown that not all help is good help. Poor planning, organization, and communication by the influx of well-intentioned volunteers can result in inefficient and unethical practices, such as duplication of services, patients lost to follow-up, and neglect for standards of patient care.

Health systems in RLAs are strained even more by the disruption to human and material resources and infrastructure intrinsic to disasters. If infrastructure is destroyed, non–purpose-built buildings such as schools and churches are often used as makeshift clinics and even operating theaters, posing challenges of maintaining sterility and infection control. Disaster and conflict zones drive many people to migrate, leaving even fewer trained professionals and health care providers to assist with perioperative care.[12] Existing poor medical record keeping becomes more unreliable, making it difficult to identify and keep track of patients. Broken transportation systems and long-distance travel to functional health facilities often worsen patients' conditions by exacerbating secondary issues such as electrolyte disturbances and intravascular depletion caused by dehydration and bleeding. Such problems must be addressed before operative management is initiated. Specific medical needs and the overall disaster assistance required vary according to the size, scope, and location of the disaster and depend on existing local capacity. Earthquakes are especially devastating because they cause extensive damage to medical infrastructure, transportation, communication lines, and energy supplies. Injuries that require urgent surgical intervention include bone fractures, soft tissue lacerations, and crush injuries, with a high prevalence of secondary issues such as soft-tissue infections and renal failure.[20,21] With tsunamis, patients typically present with near drowning, pneumonia, hypothermia, and wound infections.[22] A frequently underappreciated area is pain management. The aftermath of the 2008 Wenchuan earthquake revealed a disturbing under-recognition and undertreatment of patient pain, as well as a need for more effective pain management and awareness of the humane treatment of all patients.[21] In addition, medical, surgical, and obstetric emergencies unrelated to the disaster, as well as neglected elective surgeries, continue to accumulate and add to the burden of an already strained health care system. The number of patients presenting with chronic health conditions, burns, and infectious diseases often increases gradually as a result of overcrowding and poor water supply and sanitation.[23–25] An effective emergency medical response requires anticipation and planning for these different public health problems before they arise.

Role of the Anesthesia Provider Outside the Operating Room

Prehospital and emergency department care

In most RLAs, the responsibilities of anesthesia providers extend outside the operating room, and can range from triage and prehospital care, to management of critically ill patients in the emergency department and hospital floors. Despite having an extremely high burden of emergency conditions, many LMICs lack formal prehospital and emergency care systems. For example, prehospital care in Uganda is delivered by police and taxi drivers.[26] Systems such as this (or the lack thereof) lead to poor outcomes, such as 80% of injury deaths occurring in the prehospital setting.[27] The anesthesiologist is often the most experienced person available to provide emergency care not only for traumas and disasters but also for stabilizing patients in the emergency department. Emergency care can involve familiar procedures, such as airway management, intravenous line placement, bleeding control, cardiopulmonary resuscitation, and safe transportation. However, it can also involve unfamiliar practices such as acute medical management and triage of patients and resources. These practices are essential to maximizing the resources needed to quickly identify and treat ill patients. Throughout this process, cultural sensitivity and clear communication are critical to maintaining a good relationship with local leaders.[28]

Perioperative care

Anesthesia providers arguably play the most critical role in managing perioperative care, particularly in RLAs. They need to work closely with nursing staff, surgeons, and technicians to determine surgical capacity, ensure availability of essential equipment, and confirm that supplies are restocked. They also need to coordinate postoperative care, whether in the postanesthesia care unit or the general floors, where nurses are frequently understaffed. In addition, responsible and ethical provision of medical services necessitates reliable data collection for coordination of patient care and quality improvement.[29] Frequent roles that must be undertaken in RLAs outside the scope of normal HIC practice include managing the pharmacy, providing basic laboratory services, ensuring infection control, and collecting data. As always, local anesthesia providers should be trained whenever possible.

Care for critically ill patients

Responsibilities of anesthesia providers in RLAs not only include recognizing and treating perioperative complications but frequently extend to management of critically ill medical patients.[30] Given the severe shortage of trained workforce in RLAs, and limited number of intensive care unit beds (if any), they are called to help manage critically ill medical patients regardless of location and specialty, with complications such as acute renal failure, diabetic ketoacidosis, sepsis, and respiratory failure.[30]

ANESTHETIC TECHNIQUE AND PERIOPERATIVE CARE
Preoperative Considerations in Emergency Anesthesia

Assessment and documentation

The preoperative assessment is a standard of care set forth by the WHO and the WFSA and needs to be used to develop a safe anesthetic plan. An effective preoperative plan needs accurate knowledge about the patient's diagnosis, medical conditions, medications, and allergies; a focused physical examination; any available laboratory data; airway examination; and nil-by-mouth status. Experiences from disaster areas such as the 2008 Wenchuan earthquake revealed that anesthetic risk was increased, in part because of inadequate preoperative assessment.[31] Even in nondisaster settings, cultural and language barriers can make assessing prior medical history and status challenging, especially in emergency situations. Record keeping is an established norm in anesthesia care, and it is adopted as a standard by the recent WHO-WFSA guidelines to be filed with the patient's medical records.[7] The documentation should include details of the preoperative assessment, anesthetic management, and any complications. Record keeping is vital for the safe transfer of patient care between providers and locations. More importantly, documentation of procedures and outcomes provides a valuable metric to influence future quality-improvement programs.

Imaging

Imaging can be an important component of the preoperative anesthesia evaluation, especially during emergencies when other sources of information might be sparse. However, the tools required for formal imaging are often unavailable in RLAs, and, if they are available, patients cannot afford them.[32] Providers are forced to work without imaging modalities when patients cannot afford them, which can complicate both surgical and anesthetic management of these patients.

Point-of-care ultrasonography (POCUS) offers some interesting possibilities in this regard, because of its utility as an effective diagnostic tool in the hands of trained physicians, even in RLAs.[33] After initial acquisition costs, POCUS can provide tremendous value because of its mobility, reusability, and ability to provide imaging at minimal cost compared with tradition radiologic studies. With advancements in technology, portable handheld ultrasonography machines have become more affordable and reliable. Numerous case reports have shown that handheld devices are effective when used for patient-management decisions in RLAs. Shorter and Macias[34] described how, during the 2010 Haiti earthquake, handheld ultrasonography changed the clinical management in 70% of patients with regard to decisions for emergent surgery, transfer to a higher level of care, or use of certain medications. Bedside POCUS can be used to triage and identify potentially critical issues such as pericardial effusion, pleural effusion, pneumothorax, and intra-abdominal and pelvic disorders. Therapeutic interventions such as thoracentesis and paracentesis are safer under ultrasonography guidance.[32] POCUS can also be used to characterize cardiac function and guide fluid management and resuscitation.[35]

Resuscitation

Emergency surgical patients may present to the hospital in shock secondary to distributive, obstructive, cardiogenic, or neurogenic causes. Preoperative evaluation reveals many patients who are dehydrated or under-resuscitated and who will benefit from preoperative fluid therapy to ensure safety and stability before and during anesthesia. The choice of fluids is often limited in RLAs, as can be their availability as well. The patient's family members may need to purchase supplies and medication before any possible intervention, so appropriate anticipation by anesthesia providers can help minimize delays in care. Blood products should be administered when indicated, especially in unstable, hemorrhaging patients. Patients, or more commonly their family members, often must pay for the blood before it is administered. Furthermore, family members may need to donate their own blood if supply is inadequate.

Intraoperative Considerations in Emergency Anesthesia

Checklists

To help improve perioperative outcomes, the WHO developed both the Surgical Safety Checklist and the Anesthesia Safety Checklist, which should be used for every surgical procedure. The surgical version has been shown to reduce patient complications and deaths in a variety of settings globally.[36,37] Although less known and studied, the newer Anesthesia Safety Checklist is intended to serve the same purpose, including items to ensure verification of fasting status, working intravenous access, equipment checks, and the presence of adequate personnel for induction (**Box 1**).

Monitoring

Multiple standards for intraoperative monitoring have been developed. WFSA and WHO include monitoring oxygenation, ventilation, circulation, urine output, temperature, neuromuscular function, and depth of anesthesia. Where resources are limited, clinical acumen, physical examination, and the support of anesthesia assistants can be critical to provide safe patient care. Using physical examination alone to look for cyanosis during anesthesia can lead to catastrophic outcomes because it is often a late finding. In addition, many patients in RLAs are anemic and do not show specific signs of poor perfusion.[38] It is highly recommended that all patients receiving any type of anesthetic be monitored with a pulse oximeter along with clinical observation.[7] Patients who are intubated should be monitored by capnography to ensure adequate gas exchange. Where pulse oximetry or capnography is unavailable, other techniques

---

Box 1
Anesthesia safety checklist

Before induction of anesthesia

Is an experienced and trained assistant available to help you with induction?
☐ Yes
☐ Not applicable

Has the patient had no food or drink for the appropriate time period?
☐ Yes
☐ Not applicable

Is there intravenous access that is functional?
☐ Yes

Is the patient on a table that can be rapidly tilted into a head-down position in case of sudden hypotension or vomiting?
☐ Yes

Equipment check
☐ If compressed gas will be used, is there enough gas and a reserve oxygen cylinder?
☐ Anesthetic vaporizers are connected?
☐ Breathing system that delivers gas to the patient is securely and correctly assembled?
☐ Breathing circuits are clean?
☐ Resuscitation equipment is present and working?
☐ Laryngoscope, tracheal tubes, and suction apparatus are ready and clean?
☐ Needles and syringes are sterile?
☐ Drugs are drawn up into labeled syringes?
☐ Emergency drugs are present in the room, in case they are needed?

From World Health Organization Integrated Management for Emergency and Essential Surgical Care toolkit – Quality and Safety Tools. Available at: https://www.who.int/surgery/publications/s15980e.pdf?ua=1. Accessed May 2019; with permission.

need to be used, including clinical observation of chest rise, intermittent chest auscultation for bilateral breath sounds, use of a precordial stethoscope, and/or continuous palpation of the radial or carotid pulse.[39]

Equipment

Per the WHO-WFSA guidelines, facilities that provide emergency surgical interventions, and hence emergency anesthesia services, should be equipped with an oxygen supply, oropharyngeal airways, facemasks, appropriately sized laryngoscopes and endotracheal tubes, intubation aids such as forceps and a bougie, and suctioning equipment.[7] Again, this is not always the case in many RLAs.

An oxygen delivery system (eg, oxygen cylinder, oxygen concentrator) should be available for all procedures in which anesthesia is being provided. It is recommended that the inspired-oxygen concentration be monitored with a low-oxygen concentration alarm, as well as an oxygen fail-safe alarm and interlocking systems to prevent hypoxic gas mixtures. These measures are often unavailable owing to the absence of batteries, fuel cells, or even pressure gauges.[7] The development of small, portable oxygen concentrators has made access to oxygen delivery much easier in RLAs. Oxygen concentrators work by passing atmospheric air through zeolite, which absorbs the nitrogen, leaving behind 95% oxygen.[39] Both the Universal Anesthesia Machine (UAM) by Gradian Health Systems and the Glostavent by Diamedica are anesthesia machines that incorporate an oxygen concentrator and can be used in draw-over or continuous mode.[39,40]

Anesthetic Plan

The anesthetic plan needs to be tailored to the local context with consideration for patient characteristics, surgical procedure, and available resources. Given the inherent constraints of emergency anesthesia added to working in RLAs, such as delayed presentation, limited oxygen supply, and variable perioperative care, anesthetic techniques that avoid unstable hemodynamics and muscular relaxation while facilitating earlier recovery and discharge from the facility are preferred. Spinal, regional, and intravenous anesthesia (mainly ketamine with or without benzodiazepines) are well suited for these purposes. **Table 2** summarizes common anesthetic techniques, including ketamine dosing regimen for RLAs. An analysis of Medicines Sans Frontier anesthesia practices revealed significantly lower odds of perioperative death when spinal, regional, or general anesthesia without intubation was used than when general anesthesia with intubation was used.[41] In a meta-analysis of maternal mortality in LMICs, 54% of all anesthesia-related deaths were caused by airway complications.[42] In RLAs, less is often more, but providing quality anesthesia requires a thorough assessment of patient risk balanced with resources.

Inhalational anesthesia

Halothane and ether are widely used in many LMICs because they are inexpensive. Ether does not cause respiratory depression, provides analgesia, and is useful in patients with shock because it does not cause myocardial depression, whereas halothane can cause significant myocardial depression. Ether has a more stable hemodynamic profile, but can lead to significant postoperative nausea and vomiting, has a pungent smell, and is highly soluble in blood, leading to a slow onset. All of these disadvantages make ether a poor induction agent when providing emergency anesthesia, especially when the risk of aspiration of gastric content is high.[39]

Inhaled anesthetics such as halothane can be delivered via continuous flow or the draw-over technique. Continuous flow is used in most HICs. Its advantages include

Table 2
Anesthesia techniques for resource-limited areas

Technique	Strategy and Considerations
Ketamine[46,55,56]	
Advantages and disadvantages	Advantages: • Excellent analgesia with preservation of airway reflexes • Hemodynamic stability • Wide therapeutic range, rapid onset, and short half-life Disadvantages: • Hallucinations, delirium, nausea, and excessive salivation
Induction and Bolus maintenance	
IV ketamine	Dose: 1–2 mg/kg IV; given over 60 s, followed by 25%–50% of induction dose every 10–15 min. Coadministered with midazolam 2–5 mg IV or diazepam 2–5 mg IV to reduce emergence delirium Onset, 60 s; duration, 10–15 min
IM ketamine	Dose: 4–5 mg/kg IM; total of 10 mg/kg given over 5–10 min for short procedures Onset, 5–10 min; duration, 20–30 min
Infusion	Dose: 1–6 mg/kg/h; place 500 mg of ketamine in 500 mL of saline. Via standard 20 drop/mL chamber, start infusion at 2 drops/kg/min until adequate level of anesthesia then decrease rate to 1 drop/kg/min
Analgesia	IV ketamine, <1 mg/kg; IM ketamine, 0.5 mg/kg Infusion: 60–180 μg/kg/h; 500 mg ketamine in 500 mL of saline and administer at 40–80 mL/h
Regional Anesthesia	
Spinal[57]	Advantages: • Excellent operating conditions with superior analgesia • Avoids airway and hemodynamic complications of deep sedation or general anesthesia • Does not rely on availability of oxygen • Simple and portable equipment • Rapid recovery from anesthesia Disadvantages: • Significant hypotension • Risk of high spinal anesthesia leading to respiratory distress and possibly cardiac arrest
Intrathecal lidocaine	Dose for block to T10 dermatome: 50–75 mg Dose for block to T4 dermatome: 75–100 mg Onset, 3–5 min; duration: 60–90 min
Intrathecal bupivacaine	Dose for block to T10 dermatome: 8–12 mg Dose for block to T4 dermatome: 14–20 mg Onset, 5–8 min; duration, 90–120 min Pediatric dose: infants, 0.5–1.0 mg/kg; 1–7 y old, 0.3–0.5 mg/kg; >7 y old, 0.2–0.3 mg/kg

(continued on next page)

Table 2 (continued)	
Technique	**Strategy and Considerations**
Inhalational Anesthesia	
Volatile gas[55]	Advantages: • Predictable surgical anesthesia and amnesia • Fast induction in emergency situations Disadvantages: • Relies on availability of oxygen, medical gases, anesthesia circuits, and power • Relies on availability of narcotic drugs for analgesia • Longer recovery period
Halothane	MAC% (0.75) Side effects: myocardial and respiratory depression

Abbreviations: IM, intramuscular; MAC%, minimum alveolar concentration percentage.

a reservoir bag, easier inhalational induction, use of a T piece, and the ability to give continuous positive airway pressure. However, continuous flow requires a steady supply of compressed gas, such as with liquid oxygen and oxygen cylinders, which can be scarce in LMICs.[39] The draw-over technique is more commonly used in austere environments because the system is portable, easy to piece together, and requires little to no maintenance. Draw-over vaporizers include the EMO (Esptein, Macintosh, Oxford) and the OMV (Oxford Miniature Vaporizer). Such vaporizers have a low internal resistance and provide a constant output over a range of tidal volumes and temperatures. They are also designed to be easy to clean, dismantle, and reassemble.[39]

The best anesthetic machine for delivering volatile gases depends on the availability of reliable electrical supply and access to compressible gases, both of which can be highly variable in RLAs. Anesthesia providers in RLAs need to be mindful that patients who require endotracheal intubation and ventilation during an emergency may need to be bag masked for prolonged periods unless a mechanical ventilator is available. Patients intubated for airway protection can often be allowed to breathe spontaneously via a bag as long as ventilation, oxygenation, and perfusion are adequately monitored.[43] It is crucial to have help available to assist in such scenarios.

Intravenous anesthesia

Ketamine is considered the anesthetic of choice for major surgery in RLAs because of its favorable safety profile, ease of administration, preservation of airway reflexes, and provision of both anesthesia and analgesia.[44–46] Ketamine is especially useful in emergency situations for its cardiovascular effects, which include an increase in blood pressure and heart rate. For these reasons, ketamine is listed as a WHO essential medication for level 1 facilities (see **Table 1**). Ketamine can be used alone or in combination with other intravenous agents to provide total intravenous anesthesia. Most commonly, ketamine is used in conjunction with a benzodiazepine such as midazolam or diazepam to help minimize agitation and/or hallucinations.

Other medications that can be used for the induction of anesthesia include thiopental and propofol, which are WHO essential medications for a level 2 facility (see **Table 1**). Although not common in HICs, thiopental is still widely available in LMICs. It is a short-acting anesthetic that has a quick onset. However, it can cause hemodynamic instability by reducing left ventricular outflow and inducing hypotension. If available, propofol can also be given in a bolus dose to induce anesthesia. However, like thiopental, propofol can cause profound hypotension and respiratory depression, which can be detrimental in emergency surgical procedures.

The shortage of anesthesia providers and essential medications can make it challenging to provide a safe anesthetic to patients in need of emergency surgery.[47] The Every Second Matters–Ketamine (ESM-Ketamine) package was developed by Massachusetts General Hospital to support emergency surgery, essential surgery, and sedation at facilities in RLAs that may not have a trained anesthesia provider. The package includes a checklist with ordered instructions for using the kit (**Box 2**).[44] Evidence suggests that minimalist protocolized approaches such as this can be used successfully by both anesthesia and nonanesthesia providers to provide safe anesthesia care.[44–46]

Regional anesthesia

Regional anesthesia has been widely used in RLAs and has been shown to be an effective tool during times of crisis.[48–50] Regional anesthesia can be the sole anesthetic to avoid risks associated with general anesthesia, which is far more resource intensive in terms of equipment, labor, and monitoring requirements. Alternatively, regional technique can supplement other forms of anesthesia to provide excellent surgical conditions and postoperative pain relief. Spinal blocks are far more common than peripheral nerve blocks despite being more invasive and associated with more complications such as hypotension, partly because of the relative ease with which the correct technique can be taught, as well as the wide variety of surgeries that can be performed under neuraxial anesthesia as the sole anesthetic modality. Spinal anesthesia can be used for surgical interventions in the upper abdomen, lower abdomen, perineum, and lower

---

Box 2
ESM-Ketamine checklist

Emergency, essential surgery, and procedural sedation

☐ Completed ESM-Ketamine clinical record

☐ Confirmation of ketamine concentration

☐ Equipment check

☐ Intravenous (IV) line placement with confirmation of fluids freely flowing (normal saline, lactated Ringer solution)

☐ Pulse oximeter placement on side of IV line

☐ Confirm blood pressure cuff on opposite arm of IV and pulse oximeter

☐ Place oxygen on patient via nasal cannula or face mask

☐ Titrate IV ketamine to appropriate patient effect depending on the procedure
  1. Emergency/essential surgery
     • 2 mg/kg over 30 to 60 seconds (initial dose)
     • 1 to 2 mg/kg every 10 to 15 minutes
  2. Procedural sedation
     • 1 mg/kg over 30 to 60 seconds (initial dose)
     • 0.25 to 1 mg/kg thereafter as needed

☐ Complete ESM-Ketamine Clinical Record

Adapted from Burke TF, Suarez S, Sessler DI, et al. Safety and Feasibility of a Ketamine Package to Support Emergency and Essential Surgery in Kenya when No Anesthetist is Available: An Analysis of 1216 Consecutive Operative Procedures. World J Surg 2017;41:2992; with permission.

extremities.[49] As portable ultrasonography becomes more accessible, there is a growing role for peripheral nerve blocks in emergency and low-resource settings. Epidural or peripheral nerve catheter placement is generally avoided because of logistical and safety constraints. Despite its benefits and prevalence in some regions, many anesthesia providers in LMICs do not have the experience or education necessary to perform neuraxial anesthesia procedures.[49] Moreover, even when a neuraxial block is used as the sole anesthetic, emergency airway equipment must be available, including oxygen and a bag mask, in case general anesthesia must be induced.

Postoperative Considerations in Emergency Anesthesia

Postoperative monitoring

Emergence from anesthesia is a period during which a patient can experience significant harm. Patients are at increased risk for aspiration and acute respiratory failure. Before emergence from general anesthesia and extubation, patients should have their gastric contents suctioned. Patients should also be spontaneously breathing and following commands unless a deep extubation is warranted.

All patients should be observed in a postanesthesia care unit before they are considered recovered from anesthesia. The level of training of staff and the nurse/patient ratio can be significantly different than those found in HICs. Communication is

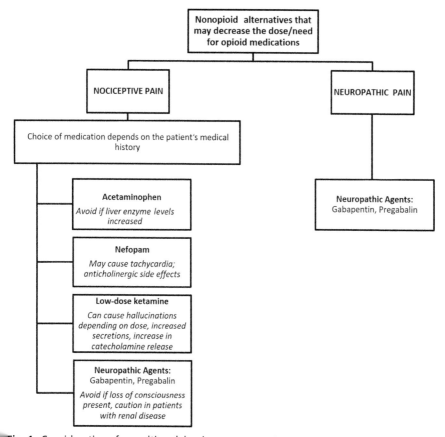

Fig. 1. Considerations for multimodal pain management.

crucial, with a need for clear orders for vital sign parameters and pain management to the managing providers in the recovery unit, as well as who to contact and how.[51]

Pain control

Inadequate pain control in the postoperative period can lead to many complications besides discomfort for the patient, including splinting, suboptimal ventilation, and immobility, which delays patient recovery and increases length of stay and risk for infections. Furthermore, poor pain control can lead to the development of postsurgical chronic pain. Although the WHO identifies analgesia as a crucial part of the postoperative period, about 80% of the global population lives in areas where access to pain medication is inadequate.[51,52]

Anesthesia providers can offer unique skills and approaches to postoperative pain control, particularly in the acute period. Pain management can be achieved with local anesthetics via peripheral nerve blocks or neuraxial analgesia, opioid medications, and multimodal analgesics, such as acetaminophen and ketamine. In 2018, the Society of Critical Care Medicine revised the clinical practice guidelines for pain management to include a multimodal algorithm for pain management that can be used to avoid or minimize the use of opioid medications. Recommended analgesics to consider include acetaminophen, nefopam, ketamine, and gabapentinoids. No matter the choice of analgesic medication, patients should be monitored frequently and examined to ensure adequate pain coverage (**Fig. 1**).[53,54]

SUMMARY

As the burden of surgical disease continues to outpace growth of anesthesia capacity in many LMICs, volunteers from HICs can offer critical support to regions overwhelmed by poverty and disaster. Safe, high-quality anesthesia is possible even in the most austere environments but requires recognition of the unique challenges likely to be encountered and preparation in line with local context. Anesthesiologists need to be flexible and adapt to settings with unreliable power supply, airway and monitoring equipment, medications, and even staff. Infrastructure, resources, and needs may vary depending on the circumstances and location, but the guiding principles for providing safe and responsible anesthesia in RLAs remain the same. First, do no harm. Professionals based or trained in HICs should only engage in activities with which they are familiar and well trained. Second, international standards should be adhered to as closely as possible. Bare minimum standards include the use of informed consent, surgical safety checklists, and adequate postoperative monitoring and pain management. In the absence of standard monitors, volunteers should practice extreme vigilance by using auscultation, pulse oximetry, and clinical signs to keep patients safe. In addition, anesthetic technique should be kept simple with the goal of altering the patient's own physiology as little as possible. Although all types of anesthesia have been shown to be safe and effective in RLAs, the choice likely depends on provider experience, availability of assistants and equipment, and circumstances in which anesthesia is delivered. Clear communication is important for good outcomes in difficult environments. Anesthesiologists play a critical role in facilitating effective teamwork and ensuring the safety and well-being of patients.

DISCLOSURE

The authors have no real or potential commercial or financial conflicts of interest to report.

REFERENCES

1. Chang CY, Abujaber S, Reynolds TA, et al. Burden of emergency conditions and emergency care usage: new estimates from 40 countries. Emerg Med J 2016; 33(11):794–800.

2. Ozgediz D, Jamison D, Cherian M, et al. The burden of surgical conditions and access to surgical care in low- and middle-income countries. Bull World Health Organ 2008;86(8):646–7.

3. Shrime MG, Bickler SW, Alkire BC, et al. Global burden of surgical disease: an estimation from the provider perspective. Lancet Glob Health 2015;3(Suppl 2):S8–9.

4. Kempthorne P, Morriss WW, Mellin-Olsen J, et al. The WFSA global anesthesia workforce survey. Anesth Analg 2017;125(3):981–90.

5. McQueen K, Coonan T, Ottaway A, et al. Anesthesia and perioperative care. In: Debas HT, Donkor P, Gawande A, et al, editors. Essential surgery: disease control priorities, vol. 1, 3rd edition. Washington, DC: The International Bank for Reconstruction and Development/The World Bank; 2015. p. 263–78.

6. Bickler SN, Weiser TG, Kassebaum N, et al. Global burden of surgical conditions. In: Debas HT, Donkor P, Gawande A, et al, editors. Essential surgery: disease control priorities, vol. 1, 3rd edition. Washington, DC: The International Bank for Reconstruction and Development/The World Bank; 2015. p. 19–40.

7. Gelb AW, Morriss WW, Johnson W, et al. World Health Organization-World Federation of Societies of Anaesthesiologists (WHO-WFSA) International Standards for a Safe Practice of Anesthesia. Anesth Analg 2018;126(6):2047–55.

8. Dubowitz G, Detlefs S, McQueen KAK. Global anesthesia workforce crisis: a preliminary survey revealing shortages contributing to undesirable outcomes and unsafe practices. World J Surg 2010;34(3):438–44.

9. Brouillette MA, Aidoo AJ, Hondras MA, et al. Anesthesia capacity in ghana: a teaching hospital's resources, and the national workforce and education. Anesth Analg 2017;125(6):2063–71.

10. Ogbolu Y, Johantgen ME, Zhu S, et al. Nurse reported patient safety in low-resource settings: a cross-sectional study of MNCH nurses in Nigeria. Appl Nurs Res 2015;28(4):341–6.

11. Meara JG, Hagander L, Leather AJM. Surgery and global health: a Lancet Commission. Lancet 2014;383(9911):12–3.

12. Paix BR, Capps R, Neumeister G, et al. Anaesthesia in a disaster zone: a report on the experience of an Australian medical team in Banda Aceh following the "Boxing Day Tsunami". Anaesth Intensive Care 2005;33(5):629–34.

13. Daniel Vo, Cherian MN, Bianchi S, et al. Anesthesia capacity in 22 low and middle income countries J Anesth Clin Res 2012;3:207.

14. Hadler RA, Chawla S, Stewart BT, et al. Anesthesia care capacity at health facilities in 22 low- and middle-income countries. World J Surg 2016;40(5):1025–33.

15. LeBrun DG, Chackungal S, Chao TE, et al. Prioritizing essential surgery and safe anesthesia for the Post-2015 Development Agenda: operative capacities of 78 district hospitals in 7 low- and middle-income countries. Surgery 2014;155(3): 365–73.

16. Funk LM, Weiser TG, Berry WR, et al. Global operating theatre distribution and pulse oximetry supply: an estimation from reported data. Lancet 2010; 376(9746):1055–61.

17. Jayaraman S, Mabweijano JR, Lipnick MS, et al. First things first: effectiveness and scalability of a basic prehospital trauma care program for lay first-responders in Kampala, Uganda. PLoS One 2009;4(9):e6955.

18. World Health Organization. Humanitarian Health Action. Glossary of humanitarian terms. 2018. Available at: http://www.who.int/hac/about/definitions/en/. Accessed April 10, 2019.

19. Wallemacq P, House R. Economic losses, poverty and disasters 1998-2017. Geneva (Switzerland): United Nations Office for Disaster Risk Reduction (UNISDR); 2018. p. 31.

20. Missair A, Pretto EA, Visan A, et al. A matter of life or limb? A review of traumatic injury patterns and anesthesia techniques for disaster relief after major earthquakes. Anesth Analg 2013;117(4):934–41.

21. Chen G, Lai W, Liu F, et al. The dragon strikes: lessons from the Wenchuan earthquake. Anesth Analg 2010;110(3):908–15.

22. Kongsaengdao S, Bunnag S, Siriwiwattnakul N. Treatment of survivors after the tsunami. N Engl J Med 2005;352(25):2654–5.

23. Noji EK. Public health issues in disasters. Crit Care Med 2005;33(1 Suppl): S29–33.

24. Chu K, Trelles M, Ford N. Rethinking surgical care in conflict. Lancet 2010; 375(9711):262–3.

25. von Schreeb J, Riddez L, Samnegård H, et al. Foreign field hospitals in the recent sudden-onset disasters in Iran, Haiti, Indonesia, and Pakistan. Prehosp Disaster Med 2008;23(2):144–51 [discussion: 152].

26. Kobusingye OC, Guwatudde D, Owor G, et al. Citywide trauma experience in Kampala, Uganda: a call for intervention. Inj Prev 2002;8(2):133–6.

27. Mock CN, Donkor P, Gawande A, et al. Essential surgery: key messages from Disease Control Priorities, 3rd edition. Lancet 2015;385(9983):2209–19.

28. Morey TE, Rice MJ. Anesthesia in an austere setting: lessons learned from the haiti relief operation. Anesthesiol Clin 2013;31(1):107–15.

29. Craven RM. Managing anaesthetic provision for global disasters. Br J Anaesth 2017;119(suppl_1):i126–34.

30. Kuza CM, McIsaac JH. Emergency preparedness and mass casualty considerations for anesthesiologists. Adv Anesth 2018;36(1):39–66.

31. Wang Z, Sun Y, Wang Z, et al. Anesthetic management of injuries following the 2008 Wenchuan, China earthquake. Eur J Trauma Emerg Surg 2011;37(1):9–12.

32. Stachura M, Landes M, Aklilu F, et al. Evaluation of a point-of-care ultrasound scan list in a resource-limited emergency centre in Addis Ababa Ethiopia. Afr J Emerg Med 2017;7(3):118–23.

33. Wydo SM, Seamon MJ, Melanson SW, et al. Portable ultrasound in disaster triage: a focused review. Eur J Trauma Emerg Surg 2016;42(2):151–9.

34. Shorter M, Macias DJ. Portable handheld ultrasound in austere environments: use in the Haiti disaster. Prehosp Disaster Med 2012;27(2):172–7.

35. Becker DM, Tafoya CA, Becker SL, et al. The use of portable ultrasound devices in low- and middle-income countries: a systematic review of the literature. Trop Med Int Health 2016;21(3):294–311.

36. Kwok AC, Funk LM, Baltaga R, et al. Implementation of the World Health Organization surgical safety checklist, including introduction of pulse oximetry, in a resource-limited setting. Ann Surg 2013;257(4):633–9.

37. Haynes AB, Weiser TG, Berry WR, et al. A surgical safety checklist to reduce morbidity and mortality in a global population. N Engl J Med 2009;360(5):491–9.

38. Herbert LJ, Wilson IH. Pulse oximetry in low-resource settings. Breathe 2012; 9(2):90–8.

39. McCormick BA, Eltringham RJ. Anaesthesia equipment for resource-poor environments. Anaesthesia 2007;62(Suppl 1):54–60.

40. Gradian Health Systems. Universal Anaesthesia Machine (UAM). Anaesthesia Workstation 2019. Available at: https://www.gradianhealth.org/our-products/uam/. Accessed May 10, 2019.

41. Ariyo P, Trelles M, Helmand R, et al. Providing anesthesia care in resource-limited settings: a 6-year analysis of anesthesia services provided at Médecins Sans Frontières Facilities. Anesthesiology 2016;124(3):561–9.

42. Sobhy S, Zamora J, Dharmarajah K, et al. Anaesthesia-related maternal mortality in low-income and middle-income countries: a systematic review and meta-analysis. Lancet Glob Health 2016;4(5):e320–7.

43. Krishnamoorthy V, Vavilala MS, Mock CN. The need for ventilators in the developing world: An opportunity to improve care and save lives. J Glob Health 2014;4(1):010303.

44. Burke TF, Suarez S, Sessler DI, et al. Safety and feasibility of a ketamine package to support emergency and essential surgery in kenya when no anesthetist is available: an analysis of 1216 consecutive operative procedures. World J Surg 2017;41(12):2990–7.

45. Tran KP, Nguyen Q, Truong XN, et al. A comparison of ketamine and morphine analgesia in prehospital trauma care: a cluster randomized clinical trial in rural Quang Tri province, Vietnam. Prehosp Emerg Care 2014;18(2):257–64.

46. Villegas S, Suarez S, Owuor J, et al. Intraoperative awareness and experience with a ketamine-based anaesthesia package to support emergency and essential surgery when no anaesthetist is available. Afr J Emerg Med 2019;9(Suppl): S56–60.

47. Notrica MR, Evans FM, Knowlton LM, et al. Rwandan surgical and anesthesia infrastructure: a survey of district hospitals. World J Surg 2011;35(8):1770–80.

48. Missair A, Gebhard R, Pierre E, et al. Surgery under extreme conditions in the aftermath of the 2010 Haiti earthquake: the importance of regional anesthesia. Prehosp Disaster Med 2010;25(6):487–93.

49. Schnittger T. Regional anaesthesia in developing countries. Anaesthesia 2007; 62(Suppl 1):44–7.

50. Lehavi A, Meroz Y, Maryanovsky M, et al. Role of regional anaesthesia in disaster medicine: field hospital experience after the 2015 Nepal Earthquake. Eur J Anaesthesiol 2016;33(5):312–3.

51. World Health Organization (WHO). Postoperative Care. 2003. Available at: https://www.who.int/surgery/publications/Postoperativecare.pdf. Accessed May 8, 2019.

52. Goucke CR, Chaudakshetrin P. Pain: a neglected problem in the low-resource setting. Anesth Analg 2018;126(4):1283–6.

53. Wampole CR, Smith KE. Beyond opioids for pain management in adult critically ill patients. J Pharm Pract 2019;32(3):256–70.

54. Devlin JW, Skrobik Y, Gélinas C, et al. Clinical practice guidelines for the prevention and management of pain, agitation/sedation, delirium, immobility, and sleep disruption in adult patients in the ICU. Crit Care Med 2018;46(9):e825–73.

55. Mellor AJ. Anaesthesia in austere environments. J R Army Med Corps 2005; 151(4):272–6.

56. Mahoney PF, editor. Anaesthesia handbook. International Committee of the Red Cross (ICRC); 2017. Available at: https://www.icrc.org/en/publication/anaesthesia-handbook. Accessed May 10, 2019.

57. Chin A, van Zundert A. Chapter 13. Spinal anesthesia. In: Hadzic A, editor. NY-SORA textbook of regional anesthesia and acute pain management. New York: The McGraw-Hill Companies; 2017. p. 328–69.

Ethical Issues in Organ Transplantation at End of Life: Defining Death

Wendy Suhre, MD[a], Gail A. Van Norman, MD[b,c],*

KEYWORDS

- Ethics • Brain death • Vital organ transplantation • Donation after cardiac death
- Religion

KEY POINTS

- Vital organ transplantation has special ethical considerations, including defining death of the donor before organ procurement.
- More than 50 years after the Harvard committee described brain death (BD), definitions of medical aspects of death and permanent loss of consciousness remain elusive, and the concept of BD is poorly accepted among many cultural groups.
- Death involves physical, spiritual, and social aspects that, out of respect for donors and families, should not be overlooked by physicians.
- Legislative treatment of the concept of BD is likely to undergo significant change in the future.

INTRODUCTION

In 2013, 13-year-old Jahi McMath had a cardiac arrest caused by massive bleeding following tonsillectomy. She was declared brain dead by her doctors, because of iso-electric electroencephalogram (EEG), lack of brain blood flow, and apnea on medical testing. Her family sued, disputing the diagnosis of brain death (BD) and claiming that they had also been pressured to donate her organs. The court declared her legally dead, and the family appealed on constitutional privacy and religious grounds. Jahi's case was complicated by concerns of possible malpractice and racism, and witness reports that she moved to commands. The hospital refused to place a tracheostomy or

Commercial Affiliations: Dr W. Suhre has no competing commercial affiliations; Dr G.A. Van Norman has funding from the American College of Cardiology for medical writing not related to this work.

[a] Department of Anesthesiology and Pain Medicine, University of Washington School of Medicine, Box 356540, 1959 Northeast Pacific Street, Seattle, WA 98195, USA; [b] Anesthesiology and Pain Medicine, University of Washington, Seattle, WA, USA; [c] Bioethics, University of Washington, Seattle, WA, USA
* Corresponding author. 2601 West Boston Street, Seattle, WA 98199.
E-mail address: gvn@uw.edu

Anesthesiology Clin 38 (2020) 231–246
https://doi.org/10.1016/j.anclin.2019.10.009
1932-2275/20/© 2019 Elsevier Inc. All rights reserved.

feeding tube to stabilize potential future care, claiming it would be grotesque to do so on a dead body, but released Jahi to the Alameda County coroner with her intravenous lines and ventilator intact. The coroner issued an official death certificate and released Jahi to her mother. A tracheostomy and feeding tube were placed at an undisclosed facility in New Jersey, currently the only state that recognizes a religious exception regarding BD.[1,2] In October 2014, the family sued to reverse the death certificate, claiming that Jahi no longer met BD criteria because medical tests now showed brain blood flow and electrical activity, and videos seemed to show her moving her fingers on command. Jahi succumbed to internal bleeding and kidney failure on June 22, 2018. Her brain was donated to science, and her family continues to pursue a malpractice action and a civil rights lawsuit to amend the date of her death.[3–5]

The moral terrain of end-of-life vital organ donation is populated with complicated questions of beneficence and nonmaleficence, donor desires and recipient needs, hastening death versus double effects. However, woven through all of them are 2 of the most fundamental questions of all: what it means to be alive, and when are people actually dead?

Transplant of vital organs presents singular ethical issues. Survival of the donor is impossible, and the viability of organs depends on minimizing ischemic time, from removal of the organ from circulation in the donor to reconnection to circulation in the recipient body. Ethical medical principles require equal consideration for living persons regardless of individual differences, such as sex, ethnicity, religion, nationality, age, disabilities, and whether they are approaching end of life. Furthermore, taking a life or hastening death for the purpose of procuring organs constitutes homicide. Ethics of vital organ transplantation have thus long relied on the so-called dead-donor rule: a vital organ donor must be dead before the organs are removed.

FIFTY YEARS OF BRAIN DEATH

Historically, death of an individual was considered to occur when the heart stopped beating and breathing ceased. However, by the mid twentieth century, Claude Beck had performed the first successful cardiac defibrillation (1947)[6]; the first positive pressure ventilators were deployed (1955)[7]; and, in response to concerns of the World Congress of Anesthesiologists, Pope Pius the XII proclaimed that withdrawal or withholding of life-sustaining measures in futile cases was neither homicide nor suicide (1957).[8,9] In an era when physicians could sustain a human life far beyond its natural limits, when was it appropriate to simply stop?

In 1968, the Ad Hoc Committee of the Harvard Medical School was convened under the leadership of Henry Beecher, Chair of Anesthesiology, to redefine death.[10] Much has been debated about whether the true goal of the committee was to facilitate organ transplants. The committee itself offered only a utilitarian rationale for redefining death: to free up beds occupied by permanently comatose patients, and to allow the procurement of organs for transplant.[10] However, it is clear that its leaders had other complex ethical and philosophic concerns. Beecher[11] had long decried perpetuating futile medical care to permanently unconscious patients as intruding on the rights of individuals, and amounting to human experimentation.[11,12] Joseph Murray, who performed the first successful kidney transplant in 1954, stated, "When to declare death is a problem to be solved, whether or not organ transplantation follows."[13]

Eventually, the committee settled on 2 kinds of death: irreversible cardiopulmonary death and irreversible whole-brain BD. Using neurologic criteria on bedside examination, including unresponsiveness to noxious stimuli, complete absence of movement and breathing, no presence of reflexes, and electrically silent EEG, the patient was defined to have irreversible cerebral damage, and therefore could be declared dead. Testing had to be completed by a physician in the absence of central nervous depressants and hypothermia.

On the day of publication of the Harvard Criteria, the World Medical Association also declared that death, "is a gradual biological process at the cellular level with tissues varying in their ability to withstand deprivation of oxygen," stating that "clinical interest lies not in the state of preservation of isolated cells, but in the fate of a person."[14,15] However, BD was met with a reticence on the part of many physicians, philosophers, and the lay public that continues to this day.[16]

By 1980, nearly half of the United States legally recognized BD,[17] although the language of statutes varied from state to state. A President's Commission (PC) was convened to provide guidelines for determination of death, including model legislation to bring conformity to the language adopted by each state: the Uniform Determination of Death Act (UDDA). It also stated that determination of BD must be made using accepted medical standards that were not then specifically defined.

Brain Death Criteria

Globally, the developing BD criteria varied, and are not uniform to this day (**Tables 1** and **2**).[18–22] For example, in the United Kingdom, BD was determined only by the absence of brainstem function. No testing of cortical function, such as EEG, auditory evoked potentials, or angiography, was performed, although some such tests were required in other parts of Europe.[23] These differences led to the paradox that a person who was legally dead in the United Kingdom, for example, can be simultaneously legally alive in the United States,[15] although some have questioned whether any relevant clinical distinction exists between whole-brain BD and brainstem death.[24]

In 1981, the PC issued another report to justify BD, this time finding that an essential characteristic of a living organism was organismal integration, without which the individual ceased to exist. The brain was the master integrator; therefore, when the whole brain ceased to function, the person was dead.[25,26] This was further clarified in a 2008 report in which the President's Council on Bioethics defined death as the point at which an organism is no longer able to undertake its "vital work," through its "need driven commerce with the surrounding world."[27]

By 1995, the American Academy of Neurology (AAN) published guidelines for determining BD based on 3 clinical findings: coma, apnea, and absence of brainstem reflexes (**Box 1**). Although silent EEG and absence of brain blood flow are missing from the criteria, the AAN did state that such ancillary testing should be used if there is uncertainty in the clinical examination findings or apnea test.[28] In 2010, the AAN further declared that a literature search did not find any legitimate "reports of patients recovering brain function when the criteria for brain death determination was used appropriately."[29]

These criteria were challenged in Nevada in 2015 in the case of Aden Hailu, who had been declared brain dead using the AAN criteria, despite activity present on 3 separate EEGs before a positive apnea test and absent brainstem reflexes.[30] The Nevada Supreme Court declared that, under Nevada's UDDA law, AAN guidelines do not meet accepted medical standards for BD, notably in part because they do not require EEG and brain blood flow tests.[31]

Table 1
Brain death certification in Europe and United Kingdom

Country	AAN Guidelines (Concordant or Discordant)[a]	Ancillary Tests Required[b] (Yes/No)	BD Designated by Law or Practice[c]
Austria	Discordant	Yes	Law
Belgium	Concordant	No	Law
Czech Republic	Discordant	No	Law
Denmark	Concordant	No	Law
Finland	Discordant	No	Law
France	Concordant	Yes	Law
Germany	Concordant	No	Law
Greece	Discordant	No	Law
Hungary	Concordant	No	Law
Ireland	Discordant	No	Law
Italy	Discordant	Yes	Law
Norway	Concordant	Yes	Law
Poland	Discordant	No	Law
Portugal	Concordant	No	Law
Spain	Concordant	No	Law
Sweden	Concordant	No	Law
Switzerland	Discordant	Yes	Uncertain
Turkey	Concordant	No	Law
United Kingdom	Discordant	No	Law

Abbreviation: AAN, American Academy of Neurology.

[a] Country's practice or law differs from AAN guidelines; for example, in 1 study 23% of institutions did not check spinal reflexes.

[b] Ancillary tests include EEG and somatosensory evoked potentials (SSEPs) to evaluate electrophysiology of the brain, and intracranial blood flow tests such as angiography, radionuclide scan, and transcranial Doppler.

[c] The country may have practical guidelines established to determine BD, but if they have not been enacted into law, BD is designated by physician practice, even if the country has enacted an organ donation law.

Data from Refs.[19–22]

Concerns Regarding Validity of the Concept of Brain Death

The brain as the great integrator

Are currently accepted medical standards, whether set by the AAN or state courts, sufficient to guarantee that a person is dead? It is now known that some so-called integrative brain functions continue in patients in whom medical testing is consistent with BD, such as elimination of waste from the body, energy balance, maintenance of body temperature and ability to develop fever and fight infection, cardiovascular and hormonal stress responses to unanesthetized incision, successful gestation of a fetus, and sexual maturation in a child.[32] If loss of integration is the defining feature of BD, such cases seem to challenge the validity of BD as a diagnosis.

Timing of examination and the global ischemic penumbra

Even if current BD criteria can withstand scientific challenges, the timing of the clinical examination is of extreme importance; sufficient time must be allowed before medical testing for brain recovery from acute injury, but how much time is appropriate? In 1

Table 2
Brain death certification in Asia

Country	Whole Brain or Brainstem	Ancillary Tests Required[a] (Yes/No)	BD Designated by Law or Practice[b]
China	Whole brain	Yes	Practice
Hong Kong	Brainstem	No	Practice
India	Brainstem	No	Practice
Indonesia	Whole brain	No	Practice
Japan	Whole brain	Yes	Law
Malaysia	Whole brain	2 EEG for <1 y old	Practice
Myanmar	Whole brain	No	Law
Philippines	Whole brain	No	Law
Singapore	Brainstem	No	Law
South Korea	Whole brain	Yes	Law
Sri Lanka	Whole brain	No	Law
Taiwan	Brainstem	No	Practice
Thailand	Whole brain	No	Practice
Vietnam	Whole brain	No	Practice

Country's practice or law differs from AAN guidelines; for example, in 1 study 23% of institutions did not check spinal reflexes.

[a] Ancillary tests include EEG and SSEPs to evaluate electrophysiology of the brain, and intracranial blood flow tests such as angiography, radionuclide scan, and transcranial Doppler.

[b] The country may have practical guidelines established to determine BD, but if they have not been enacted into law, BD is designated by physician practice, even if the country has enacted an organ donation law.

Data from Refs.[19–22]

study, 10% of patients that clinically met criteria for BD had normal brain at autopsy,[33] and histopathologic examination identifies normal or very little ischemic change in all regions of the brain in approximately 40% of patients.[34] Some investigators hypothesize that a global ischemic penumbra may account for this finding: reduction in blood flow throughout the brain suppresses transmission in the cerebral cortex, but without apparent permanent ischemic neuronal damage.[35] Neurogenesis and neuroplasticity in the adult brain does occur. Would the clinical neurologic deficits signaling BD have been reversible in these patients, if they had been given enough time to recover? In a recent study, researchers were able to reestablish neuronal communication in the brains of pigs that had been dead for 4 hours.[36] They did not detect any EEG activity, although this could have been caused by neuronal blockers in the perfusate used to bathe the cells. Although the researchers did not believe there was organized neuronal function that could produce consciousness, the experiment lasted only 6 hours and it is unknown what would have been seen in the absence of neuronal blocking agents if the experiment were allowed to continue. The potential to reestablish brain activity after BD conflicts with a critical requirement of irreversibility in defining BD.

Defining unconsciousness

The Harvard committee discussed BD in the context of a state of irreversible unconsciousness.[10] Can current neurologic testing determine the presence or absence of consciousness? One significant problem with a consciousness-driven definition of death is that there is no clear definition of what consciousness is. Unresponsiveness does not equate to unconsciousness. Disorders of consciousness can include absent

---

Box 1
American Academy of Neurology 1995 criteria for diagnosing brain death

A. Baseline criteria
  • Clinical or neuroimaging evidence of acute central nervous system catastrophe compatible with a clinical diagnosis of BD, plus
  • Exclusion of complicating medical conditions that might confound clinical assessment (eg, severe electrolyte, acid-base, or endocrine disturbance)
  • No drug intoxication or poisoning
  • Core temperature greater than or equal to 32°C (90°F)

B. Three cardinal findings with clinical testing
  • Coma or unresponsiveness: no cerebral motor responses to pain in all extremities (eg, nail bed pressure and supraorbital pressure)
  • Absence of brainstem reflexes
    ○ Pupils: no pupillary response to bright light and pupils midposition (4 mm) to dilated (9 mm)
    ○ Ocular movement: no oculocephalic reflex (do not test in the presence of cervical spine fracture or instability); no deviation of the eyes to irrigation in each ear with 50 mL of cold water (allow 1 minute after injection and greater than or equal to 5 minutes between testing on each side)
    ○ Facial sensation and facial motor response: no corneal reflex to touch; no jaw reflex; no grimacing to deep pressure on nail bed, supraorbital ridge, or temporomandibular joint
    ○ Pharyngeal and tracheal reflexes: no response after stimulation of the posterior pharynx with a tongue blade, no cough response to bronchial suctioning
    ○ Positive apnea test (ie, no respiratory response): testing described in AAN statement

C. Confirmatory tests
  • Optional, but highly recommended
    ○ Repeat clinical testing: 6 hours after first testing is recommended, time interval is arbitrary
  • Desirable in patients in whom specific components of the clinical testing cannot be reliably performed or evaluated
    ○ Conventional cerebral angiography showing no intracerebral filling at the level of the carotid bifurcation or circle of Willis
    ○ Electroencephalography showing absent electrical activity for greater than or equal to 30 minutes of recording
    ○ Transcranial Doppler showing small systolic peaks in early systole without diastolic flow or reverberating flow
    ○ Technetium-99m hexamethylpropylene-amineoxime brain scan showing no uptake of isotope in brain parenchyma
    ○ Somatosensory evoked potentials: bilateral absence of N20-P22 response with median nerve stimulation

Adapted from Report of the Quality Standards Subcommittee of the American Academy of Neurology. Practice parameters for determining brain death in adults (summary statement). Neurology 1995;45:1012-1014; with permission.

(not present and unrecoverable), latent (not present but can reemerge in the future), and covert (present but cannot be discerned from a third party) brain function, all of which are on a continuum of variable degrees of conscious awareness.[37] Individuals that had severe brain injuries and have been deemed to lack consciousness based on neurologic testing have later been found to have latent or covert consciousness using functional MRI studies.[38] In 1996, a startling study revealed that 43% of patients thought to be in a persistent vegetative state were conscious of their environments and could communicate under certain circumstances.[39] Consciousness can be present even if the EEG is silent; the surface EEG is unreliable in detecting electrical activity in the deep cortical structures[40] and may even be present in the dying brain after circulatory arrest.[41] Moreover, regions of the human brain have been shown to retain the capacity for electrophysiologic responsiveness postmortem.[42]

If cognition/consciousness is functionally dissociated from the behavioral motor response, the absence of movement on clinical examination may lead to misdiagnosis of BD.[43] Movement or motor reflexes may be absent if there is a disconnection of communication between the cortex and the brainstem, leading to a false diagnosis of unconsciousness, and therefore should not be used to determine whether or not higher integrative functions are present in the cerebral cortex.[43] Such disconnections are known to occur, for example, in certain types of thalamic injury. It is also thought that such disconnections are accentuated by certain drugs such as GABAergic drugs, potentially explaining why patients who appear unconscious under general anesthesia using an isolated forearm technique do not move despite potentially being aware.[44]

The apnea test, used to rule out the presence of brainstem function, is also unreliable in certain circumstances. Disconnection of the medulla from supraspinal centers; infarction of the spinal cord at the junction of the medulla[33]; and injury to the spinal cord, spinal nerves, or respiratory muscles can result in a positive apnea test in the presence of normal respiratory centers in the medulla.[45] In the words of Karakatsanis,[43] "a compelling argument against even the notion of absence of cerebral functions is that, in the context of brain stem infarction/destruction—which is always part of 'brain death'—it is impossible to test for any cerebral function by clinical bedside exam, because the tracts of passage to and from the cerebrum through the brain stem are destroyed or nonfunctional."[43]

Inability of brain monitors to detect consciousness

It is now known that a large proportion of patients (in some studies using the isolated forearm technique, more than 72%) who were previously thought to be unconscious under general anesthesia are both conscious and aware.[46,47] Recent studies also suggest that consciousness survives for a time after circulatory death.[41]

At present, no technological means exist by which consciousness can be reliably confirmed or ruled out.[48] For example, processed EEG and other neurologic monitors developed to detect awareness under anesthesia do not reliably detect awareness even when it is clearly demonstrable using an isolated forearm technique.[49–51] Human patients given muscle paralytic agents using isolated forearm techniques, but without any sedation, register as unconscious on neuromonitors, despite showing awareness through trained signaling, the ability to solve complex mathematics problems, and the ability to recount stories told to them[52] while paralyzed. In the absence of a solid definition of consciousness, and without any means by which to reliably rule it out, a determination of death that relies on consciousness criteria becomes extremely problematic.

Neurologically disabled persons

The Ad Hoc Committee grappled with a consciousness-driven definition of death, and/or death of personhood, and found it too disquieting to provide clear guidance on the ethical treatment of living human beings.[10] A part of the problem is the issue of degree: how much personhood can someone lose and still remain a living, human being? On a spectrum of neurologic disabilities, how disabled must people be in order to lose their living human rights? Although all lives may be equally valuable, they are not all equally enabled and independent, and part of an ethical society and a core function of the practice of medicine is to try to either restore health and independence to patients or to promote the ability of those who cannot be restored to health to enjoy autonomy and as much "ableness" as is possible within their individual limitations. Trying to decide what constitutes untenable disability is fraught. In whose judgment is what degree of disability sufficiently dehumanizing to call an individual no longer alive? History has shown that social systems are prone to make adverse judgments about the abilities of people who do not sufficiently resemble the norms in wealth, race, gender identification, abilities, and other characteristics. Surveys clearly show that physicians and other health care workers not only have these prejudices but also are notoriously willing to act on them and deny lifesaving care to disabled patients.[53,54]

The Fiction of Brain Death Acceptance

Is BD the equivalent of biological death? Legally, BD is an accepted equivalent of death; however, philosophically, this may not be so. To believe that BD is the death of the organism, it must be believed that the human being is the brain and that functioning of the body is not another feature of the human essence. Examination of various cultural and theological norms shows that this assertion is not as widely accepted as many physicians would like to believe, and that an assertion of global BD acceptance is simply false.

Eastern and Western beliefs about death

Western religions from the Abrahamic tradition (Jewish, Christian, Muslim) tend to rely on the cessation of function of various organs to define death, but Eastern religions (eg, Hinduism, Buddhism, Jainism) are more likely to see the cessation of organ function as merely a beginning of death, and rely more on concepts of consciousness and the soul to define completion of the dying process. A particular example of this dichotomy can be found between Western (Catholic) Christianity and Eastern (Orthodox) Christianity. Western Catholicism supports the concept of BD,[55] whereas the Orthodox Christian Church carefully avoids any clear-cut statements that define death related to cessation of the function of the brain or any other organ.[9]

Protestant Christian groups do not generally prohibit the concept of BD, but many do not have official statements on BD (eg, American Baptists, Jehovah's Witnesses, Seventh-day Adventists, Southern Baptists, and Unitarians), instead defaulting to the beliefs of the individual. Some conservative Jewish sects insist that persons are alive for as long as the heart is beating.[9,56] In 1 survey of Islamic jurists, more than 90% disagreed that BD equaled death.[9,57] Although India passed BD legislation in 1994, many Hindus are uncomfortable with the concept.[58] Buddhism generally disagrees with defining death by neurologic criteria[1] and defines death by the absence of 3 things: vitality, heat, and consciousness. However, in this context, consciousness is not specifically a neurologic state of awareness but is more akin to the soul. Some contemporary Buddhist scholars assert that consciousness continues to exist in a person whose heart and respirations have stopped,[59] a belief that is also reflected in Taoism. Although Japan legislated BD criteria in 1997, BD is not well accepted in Japan because a predominant religion, Shintoism, generally does not recognize death in the presence of a heartbeat.[9,60] In addition, many indigenous beliefs and practices oppose declarations of death and do not accept BD.[9,60]

Cultural beliefs in collision

Western countries increasingly are "melting pots" of populations of both Western and Eastern origin, with diverse philosophic and theological beliefs and cultural practices that defy the uniformity demanded by legislation. As a result, families are increasingly pressing for a religious exemption to the declaration of BD. Lawsuits have been filed in California, Massachusetts, Michigan, and Washington DC.[31,60] Prolife groups are also beginning to argue against BD in their advocacy platforms.[61,62] Laws requiring religious or other exemption or accommodation now exist in 4 of the United States **(Table 3)**.[60,63–66] As this trend continues, even if BD could be said to have a solid foundation in medical theory and practice, it is unlikely that its legal foundation will continue in its current form.

CARDIOPULMONARY DEATH AND ORGAN DONORS
Is Cardiopulmonary Death Really Brain Death in Disguise?

Ironically, in the debate over BD, reliability of cardiopulmonary death criteria has also been questioned. As Siminoff[67] stated, "Even cardiopulmonary death can be considered a fiction, as it is certainly the case that electrical activity in the brain can continue for a span of time after the heart and lungs cease to function."[67] In the past, cessation of heartbeat was thought to be associated with loss of consciousness and brain function within seconds to minutes. However, it is now known the brain can survive loss of circulation for variable periods of time, and partial brain survival occurs for prolonged intervals after cessation of heartbeat occurs in animals.[36] It is presumed that eventually the master integrator will inevitably die if deprived of blood and oxygen, but there is significant controversy about how long that process takes, and the point at which integration is irreversibly lost is not known.

This question becomes particularly important in organ donation after cardiac death (DCD), in which withdrawal/withholding of life-sustaining treatments is discontinued, and vital organ procurement commences after cardiopulmonary arrest. How long does an organ procurement team have to wait to ensure that the donor is permanently unconscious and/or indisputably dead?

Table 3	
Religious or other exemption/accommodation legislation regarding brain death in the United States	
State	**Details**
New Jersey, 1991	Exemption: the law provides exemption for those objecting to BD on religious grounds, and requires that cardiopulmonary death be the standard applied to declare death
New York, 2011	Accommodation: the law requires that hospitals "establish written procedures for the reasonable accommodation of the individual's religious or oral objections to the use of the brain death standard"[65] Such accommodation may include continuation of ventilator support, and hospital policies should specify the duration of the accommodation. In 2 cases in New York, both involving children, courts constrained the hospital from discontinuing physiologic support for 7 d, in order that the family could find an alternative facility
California, 2009	Accommodation: law requires accommodation of all objections to BD, whether or not they are based on moral or religious objections. The hospital is required to continue only previously ordered cardiopulmonary support, and the time period of accommodation is "an amount of time afforded to gather family or next of kin at the patient's bedside," usually 24–36 h
Illinois, 2007	Accommodation: the physician is allowed to take into account the patient's religion and continue life support after BD, but the period of accommodation is left to the physician's discretion

Data from Refs.[60,63–66]

Timing of declaration of death and organ donation after cardiac arrest

The timing of determination of death following cessation of heart beat in DCD organ donation has been left largely to institutional, state, or international policies, which is a significant problem, as the Institute of Medicine expressed in a report in 2000.[68,69] Waiting times vary significantly, from as short as 75 seconds in Colorado to 5 minutes in the United Kingdom to 20 minutes in Italy.[70,71] Shorter wait times are more likely to provide higher-quality organs for transplant, and this clearly presents a conflict of interest in DCD donation; there is concern that transplant teams who are dedicated to the cause of lifesaving organ transplantation may justify premature declaration of death, or administration of medications that hasten death, to benefit the recipient, thus encroaching on the dead-donor rule and devaluing the last minutes of the donor's life. Such accusations have indeed been levied, as in the case against Dr Hootan Roozrokh, a transplant surgeon who was accused of administering high doses of morphine and lorazepam to hasten a donor's death in order to procure kidneys and liver for transplant. Dr Roozrokh stated that the medications were ordered only to relieve the donor's suffering, and not to hasten death, and the donor ultimately did not die quickly after withdrawal of ventilator support. Dr Roozrokh was ultimately acquitted of charges, but the perception of conflict of interest persists.[72]

Increasingly, concerns have been raised about short wait times in DCD organ transplantation. In the first place, autoresuscitation (the spontaneous return of circulation) in continuously monitored patients has been clearly shown to occur at least as late as 10 minutes following cardiac arrest, and some investigators have reported cases as long as 33 minutes after arrest; therefore, the criterion of irreversible cessation of cardiopulmonary function for declaration of death has not been met after 75 seconds or even 5 minutes. In the second, the brain has almost certainly not irreversibly lost function after only 10 minutes of loss of circulation, and therefore irreversibility of loss of whole-brain function as a condition of death has not been met.[73] These problems have led to debate about whether the statements "irreversible," "permanent," and "will not be reversed" are ethically, biologically, and legally equivalent, a conversation that is too lengthy to detail here.

SOCIAL DEATH

A significant problem with defining death in solely medical terms is that it fails to recognize that death is a profoundly social event and not merely a biological one. Japanese journalist Kunio Yanagida described what he called "death in the second-person point of view" in his book *Sacrifice*, the story of his own son's BD diagnosis. He posited that, even in the state of "BD," the patient's life continues to exist, in the midst of human relationships among the patient and family members.[74] Death moves families from caring for the sick to mourning the loss of a loved one. There are essential cultural, ceremonial, and emotional transitions to make, and for which societies have developed important, specific processes. Any definition of death that only recognizes its physical aspects ignores this reality. Perhaps the most glaring of shortcomings of the Harvard criteria is that they attempted to create a social construct for death using medical terms; although the body is still living, it could be treated as though it were dead.

More than 50 years after the Harvard declaration, defining death remains elusive scientifically, sociologically, theologically, and ethically. In addition, as recent cases show, enforcement of the concept of BD contributes to suffering for some dying patients and their families. More importantly, the debate has distracted clinicians at times from a critical core value in medicine: compassion. It is telling that in many reports following the McMath case, concern was expressed over the devastating impact the case might have on organ transplantation, rather than on the devastating effect an entrenched, purely medical approach to death can have on patients and families who, for religious or personal reasons, do not accept BD as a concept, or have reasons to mistrust the health care system as a whole.[75]

Concerns About Premature Declaration of Death for Organ Donation

The McMath case is one of many cases in which organ procurement has been alleged to be at the root of potentially premature declarations of death[76–78] (**Table 4**). This concern, as well as religious and other objections to BD as a legitimate definition of death, has led families and others to take action.[72–74] In addition to lawsuits, legislative efforts have been designed to prevent declaration of death by BD criteria in several states. In Kansas and Montana, the law now requires informed consent for the medical

Table 4
Sample judicial cases regarding brain death determination and organ donation

Case	Summary of Issues, Findings, and Implications
Jahi McMath (Oakland Children's Hospital, CA) 2013	Summarized in case description leading this article. Mother disagreed with BD determination, and alleged that the hospital pressured her into donating Jahi's organs. Some neurologists believe that she regained sufficient brain function to not meet BD criteria
Gregory Jacobs v CORE, Erie, PA; 2007	Parents alleged that their teenage son, who had sustained traumatic brain injury on a ski trip, had been declared brain dead by doctors prematurely for the purpose of obtaining his organs. This case was settled out of court for >$1 million. No criminal charges were filed against physicians
Colleen Burns (St Joseph's Hospital, Syracuse, NY) 2009	Colleen Burns was declared brain dead after a drug overdose despite showing signs of responsiveness. She was taken to the operating room for organ retrieval, where she opened her eyes. Burns was released from the hospital 2 wk later. Hospital was fined $6000 by New York Department of Health and sanctioned by the Centers for Medicare and Medicaid Services. No lawsuit was filed and Burn committed suicide 2 y later
Morgan Westhoff (Oakland Children's Hospital, CA) 2013	21-month-old girl died after alleged malpractice during vascular surgery. Parents did not dispute BD diagnosis. However, the lawsuit alleged that the hospital lied about performing an autopsy and subjected the parents to "multiple aggressive attempts" to get them to donate Morgan's organs
McMahon v NY Organ Donor Network, 2012	A former transplant coordinator for the New York Organ Donor Network alleged that the network pressured hospital staffers to declare patients brain dead so that organs could be obtained. He alleged that 1 in 5 patients declared brain dead still showed brain activity. He cited a 2011 case in which a 19-year-old man was still making respiratory efforts and had brain activity, but was nevertheless declared brain dead. McMahon was fired for disclosing violations

Abbreviation: CORE, Center for Organ Recovery & Education.
Data from Refs.[75–78]

tests necessary to declare BD. Without that consent, physicians cannot test for BD, and are therefore be unable to declare death based on neurologic criteria.[60] Although 2 states, Virginia and Nevada, have explicitly legislated that doctors do not need such consent,[60] the issue is not going away. In 2017, the mother of Israel Stinson brought forth a complaint in the state of California alleging that doctors had performed an apnea test without her permission on her 2-year-old son in order to declare him brain dead, and in Illinois Lydia Cassaro has filed a similar lawsuit on behalf of her son, Randall Bianchi.[31]

SUMMARY

Can there ever be a single definition of death? As Zink[79] points out, "Multiple and sometimes competing definitions are permitted, because we do exist in a world where individual understanding creates different (and sometimes competing) world views." BD may be acceptable for some families, and not others. In a paradigm in which different definitions of death are allowed to coexist, BD is merely 1 of many possible concepts of death. It is a concept that is legally permissive of vital organ transplant, but only when it aligns with the beliefs and wishes of the donors and their families. A BD diagnosis could not in that model be used to "shoehorn" a family into terminating treatments for persons who, in their social and cultural concepts of death, are still alive.

Defining either the physical or spiritual aspects of death remains elusive. For physicians, rather than focusing on creating rules and definitions that define death in purely medical terms for the purpose of legislative convenience, to facilitate organ transplant, or to manage medical resource deployment, the primary ethical emphasis should be on the question of how clinicians can and should act in a way that maintains and shows respect for dying persons (the donors and their loved ones) during the end-of-life transition,[80] even if this sometimes leads to fewer transplantable organs. What do the donors value about their existence? What are they willing to accept? As Nabi and Wilson[3,81] have said, greater emotional and cultural intelligence and sensitivity in the McMath case, for example, might have left the family feeling more respected, and perhaps avoided a protracted legal contest, regardless of the eventual outcome.

REFERENCES

1. Son RG, Setta SM. Frequency of use of the religious exemption in New Jersey cases of determination of brain death. BMC Med Ethics 2018;19:76.
2. Olick RS. Brain death, religious freedom, and public policy: New Jersey's landmark legislative initiative. Kennedy Inst Ethics J 1991;1:275–88.
3. Wilson Y. Hastings Center Bioethics Forum. 2018. Available at: https://www.thehastingscenter.org/jahi-mcmath-race-bioethics/. Accessed May 30, 2019.
4. Schmidt S. Jahi McMath, the Calif. Girl in life-support controversy, is now dead. The Washington Post. 2018. Available at: https://www.washingtonpost.com/news/morning-mix/wp/2018/06/29/jahi-mcmath-the-calif-girl-declared-brain-dead-4-years-ago-is-taken-off-life-support/?utm_term=.17fe8496c8b4. Accessed May 30, 2019.
5. Aviv R. What does it mean to die? The New Yorker. 2018. Available at: https://www.newyorker.com/magazine/2018/02/05/what-does-it-mean-to-dieM. Accessed May 30, 2019.
6. Beck CS, Prochard WH, Feil HS. Ventricular fibrillation of long duration abolished by electric shock. JAMA 1947;135:985.

7. Puri N, Puri V, Dellinger RP. History of technology in the intensive care unit. Crit Care Clin 2009;15:185–200.
8. Pope Pius XII. The Prolongation of Life. 1957.
9. Setta SM, Shemie SD. An explanation and analysis of how world religions formulate their ethical decisions on withdrawing treatment and determining death. Philos Ethics Humanit Med 2015;10:6.
10. A definition of irreversible coma. Report of the Ad Hoc Committee of the Harvard Medical School to examine the definition of brain death. JAMA 1968;205:337–40.
11. Beecher HK. Ethics and clinical research. N Engl J Med 1966;274:1354–60.
12. Belkin GS. Death before dying: history, medicine and brain death. New York: Oxford University Press; 2014.
13. Wijdicks EF. The neurologist and Harvard criteria for brain death. Neurology 2003;61:970–6.
14. Machado C, Korein J, Portel L, et al. The Declaration of Sydney on human death. J Med Ethics 2007;33:699–703.
15. De Georgia MA. History of brain death as death: 1968 to the present. J Crit Care 2014;29:673–8.
16. Silverman D. Irreversible coma associated with electrocerebral silence. Neurology 1970;20:525–33.
17. The President's Commission. Special Communication: guidelines for the determination of death. JAMA 1981;246:2184–7.
18. Citerio G, Crippa KA, Bronco A, et al. Variability in brain death determination in Europe: looking for a solution. Neurocrit Care 2014;21:376–82.
19. Wijdicks EFM. Brain death worldwide. Accepted fact but no global consensus in the diagnostic criteria. Neurology 2002;58:20–5.
20. Chua HC, Kwek TK, Morihara H, et al. Brain death: the Asian perspective. Semin Neurol 2015;35:152–61.
21. Wahlster S, Wijdicks EFM, Patel PV, et al. Brain death declaration. Practices and perceptions worldwide. Neurology 2015;84:18870–9.
22. Smith M. Brain death: the United Kingdom perspective. Semin Neurol 2015;35:145–51.
23. Young PJ, Matta BF. Anesthesia for organ donation in the brainstem dead—why bother? Anaesthesia 2000;54:105–6.
24. Varelas PM. Brainstem or entire brain-based declaration of death: is there a difference? Pract Neurol 2016;16:85–6.
25. President's Commission for the Study of Ethical Problems in Medicine and Biomedical and Behavioral Research. Defining death: medical, legal and ethical issue in the determination of brain death. 1981. Available at: https://repository.library.georgetown.edu/bitstream/handle/10822/559345/defining_death.pdf?sequence=1. Accessed May 29, 2019.
26. Nguyen D. A holistic understanding of death: ontological and medical considerations. Diametros 2018;55:44–62.
27. President's Council on Bioethics. Controversies in the determination of death: a white paper by the President's Council on Bioethics. 2008. Available at: https://bioethicsarchive.georgetown.edu/pcbe/reports/death/. Accessed May 29, 2019.
28. The Quality Standards Subcommittee of the American Academy of Neurology. Practice parameters for determining brain death in adults (summary statement). Neurology 1995;45:1012–4.
29. The Quality Standards Subcommittee of the American Academy of Neurology. Evidence-based guideline update: determining brain death in adults. Neurology 2010;74:1911–8.

30. Yanke G, Rady MY, Verhijde JL. In re guardianship of Hailu: the Nevada Supreme Court casts doubt on the standard for brain death diagnosis. Med Sci Law 2017; 57:100–2.
31. Pope TM. Brain death forsaken: growing conflict and new legal challenges. J Leg Med 2017;37:265–324.
32. Shewmon DA. The brain and somatic integration: insight into the standard biological rationale for equating "brain death" with death. J Med Philos 2001;26:457–78.
33. Walker E. Pathology of brain death. Ann N Y Acad Sci 1978;315:272–80.
34. Wijdicks EF, Pfeiffer EA. Neuropathology of brain death in the modern transplant era. Neurology 2008;70:1234–7.
35. Coimbra CG. Implications of ischemic penumbra for the diagnosis of brain death. Braz J Med Biol Res 1999;32:1479–87.
36. Vrselja Z, Daniele SG, Silbereis J, et al. Restoration of brain circulation and cellular functions hour post-mortem. Nature 2019;568:336–43.
37. Verhijde JL, Rady MY, Potts M. Neuroscience and brain death controversies: the elephant in the room. J Relig Health 2018;57:1745–63.
38. Naci L, Graham M, Owen AM, et al. Covert narrative capacity: mental life in patients thought to lack consciousness. Ann Clin Transl Neurol 2016;4:61–70.
39. Andrews K, Murphy L, Munday R, et al. Misdiagnosis of the vegetative state: Retrospective study in a rehabilitation unit. BMJ 1996;313:13–6.
40. Kroeger D, Florea B, Amzica F. Human brain activity patterns beyond the isoelectric line of extreme deep coma. PLoS One 2013;8:e75257.
41. Parnia S, Spearpoint K, de Vos G, et al. AWARE—AWAreness during resuscitation. A prospective study. Resuscitation 2014;85:1799–805.
42. Rouleau N, Murugan NJ, Tessaro LWE, et al. When is the brain dead? Living-like electrophysiological responses and photo emissions from applications of neurotransmitter in fixed post-mortem human brains. PLoS One 2016;11:e0167231.
43. Karakatsanis KG. "Brain death": should it be reconsidered? Spinal Cord 2008;46: 396–401.
44. Sanders RD, Tononi G, Lureys S, et al. Unresponsiveness ≠ Unconsciousness. Anesthesiology 2012;116:946–59.
45. Joffe AR, Anton NR, Duff JP. The apnea test: rationale, confounders, and criticism. J Child Neurol 2010;25:1435–43.
46. Russell IF. Midazolam-alfentanil: an anaesthetic? An investigation using the isolated forearm technique. Br J Anaesth 1993;70:42–6.
47. Sanders 2012 Linassi F, Zanatta P, Tellarli P, et al. Isolated forearm technique: a meta-analysis of connected consciousness during different general anaesthesia regimens. Br J Anaesth 2018;121:198–209.
48. Karatkatsanis KG. Brain dead patients: critically ill or dead? A potential answer to the problem. J Intensive Crit Care 2016;2:2.
49. Kerssens C, Gaither JR, Sebel PS. Preserved memory function during bispectral index-guided anesthesia with sevoflurane for major orthopedic surgery. Anesthesiology 2009;111:18–24.
50. Russell IF. The ability of bispectral index to detect intraoperative wakefulness during total intravenous anaesthesia compared with the isolated forearm technique. Anaesthesia 2013;68:502–11.
51. Russell IF. The ability of bispectral index to detect intraoperative wakefulness during isoflurane/air anaesthesia, compared with the isolated forearm technique. Anaesthesia 2013;68:1010–20.
52. Schuller PJ, Newell S, Strickland PA, et al. Response of bispectral index to neuromuscular block in awake volunteers. Br J Anaesth 2015;115(Suppl 1):i95–103.

53. Gerhart K, Koziol-McLain J, Lowenstein S, et al. Quality of life following spinal cord injury: knowledge and attitudes of emergency care providers. Ann Emerg Med 1994;23:807–12.
54. Madorsky J. Is the slippery slope steeper for people with disabilities? West J Med 1997;166:410–1.
55. Why brain death is valid as a definition of death. The signs of death. Statement by the Pontifical Academy of Sciences and responses to objections. Vatican City, 2008. pp54. Available at: http://www.casinapioiv.va/content/accademia/en/publications/extraseries/braindeath.html. Accessed June 12, 2019.
56. Zohar NJ. The end of humanity: does circumventing "death" help the cause? Am J Bioeth 2003;3:12–3.
57. Haque OS. Brain death and its entanglements: a redefinition of personhood for Islamic ethics. J Relig Ethics 2008;36:13–36.
58. Nagal S. Ethics of organ transplantation. Indian J Med Ethics 1995;3:19–22.
59. Tsomo KL. Into the jaws of Yama, Lord of death: Buddhism, bioethics and death. New York: Albany State University Press of New York; 2005.
60. Pope TM. Brain death and the law: hard cases and legal challenges. Hastings Center Special Report: Defining Death: organ transplantation and the fifty-year legacy of the Harvard report on brain death. Hastings Ctr Rep 2018;46:S46–8.
61. Dubois JM. Brain death and organ donation: some pro-life groups are questioning the criteria for organ transplants. Pope John Paul II would have disagreed. America; the Jesuit Review. 2009. Available at: https://www.americamagazine.org/politics-society/2009/02/02/brain-death-and-organ-donation-some-pro-life-groups-are-questioning. Accessed June 1, 2019.
62. Devine DJ. Oakland girl's brain death divides pro-life camp. World: Health. 2014. Available at: https://world.wng.org/2014/01/oakland_girls_brain_death_divides_pro_life_camp. Accessed June 1, 2019.
63. N.J Rev. Stat. §26:6A-3.
64. New York State Department of Health and New York State Task Force on Life and the Law. Guidelines for determining brain death. 2011. Available at: https://www.health.ny.gov/professionals/hospital_administrator/letters/2011/brain_death_guidelines.pdf. Accessed June 9, 2019.
65. Calif Health and Safety Code §1254.4(b)(2012).
66. 210 Ill. Comp. Statt. 85/6.23 (2012).
67. Siminoff LA. The dead donor rule: not dead yet. Am J Bioeth 2003;3:30.
68. Herdman R, Beauchamp TL, Potts JT Jr. The Institute of Medicine's report on non-heart-beating organ transplantation. Kennedy Inst Ethics J 1998;8:83–90.
69. Cassel C, Allee M, Beasley C, et al. Non-heart beating organ transplantation: practice and protocols. a report of the Committee on Non-Heart Beating Transplantation II, Institute of Medicine. Washington (DC): National Academy; 2000.
70. Page A, Messer S, Large SR. Heart transplantation from donation after circulatory determined death. Ann Cardiothorac Surg 2018;7:75–81.
71. Ortega-Deballon I, Horby L, Shemie SD. Protocols for uncontrolled donation after circulatory death: a systematic review of international guidelines, practices and transplant outcomes. Crit Care 2015;19:268–83.
72. McKinley J. Doctor cleared of harming man to obtain organs. The New York Times. 2008. Available at: https://www.nytimes.com/2008/12/19/health/12doctor.html. Accessed June 9, 2019.
73. Joffe AR, Carcillo J, Anton N, et al. Donation after cardiocirculatory death: a call for a moratorium pending full public disclosure and fully informed consent. Philos Ethics Hum Med 2011;6:17–35.

74. Morioka M. Feminism, disability, and brain death. Alternative voices from Japanese bioethics. J Philos Life 2015;5:19–41.
75. Eachempati Soumitra R. A tragedy compounded: the heart-wrenching case of Jahi McMath may have devastating consequence to organ donation. The Daily Beast. 2014. Available at: https://www.thedailybeast.com/a-tragedy-compounded-the-heart-wrenching-case-of-jahi-mcmath-may-have-devastating-consequences-to-organ-donation. Accessed May 30, 2019.
76. Lupkin S. Patient wakes up as doctors get ready to remove organs. ABC news. 2013. Available at: https://abcnews.go.com/Health/patient-wakes-doctors-remove-organs/story?id=19609438. Accessed June 12, 2019.
77. Pope TM. Legal briefing: brain death and total brain failure. J Clin Ethics 2014;25: 245–57.
78. Birkle C, Pope T. Brain death: legal obligations and the courts. Semin Neurol 2015;35:174–9.
79. Zink S. Death and donation: a reply to Koppelman. Am J Bioeth 2003;3:29–30.
80. Hester DM. "Dead donor" versus "respect for donor" rule: putting the cart before the horse. Am J Bioeth 2003;3:24–6.
81. Nabi J. "No one was listening to us." Lessons from the Jahi McMath Case. Hastings Ctr Bioethics Forum. 2018. Available at: https://www.thehastingscenterorg/no-one-listening-us-lessons-jahi-mcmat-case/. Accessed June 9, 2019.

Moving?

Make sure your subscription moves with you!

To notify us of your new address, find your **Clinics Account Number** (located on your mailing label above your name), and contact customer service at:

Email: journalscustomerservice-usa@elsevier.com

800-654-2452 (subscribers in the U.S. & Canada)
314-447-8871 (subscribers outside of the U.S. & Canada)

Fax number: 314-447-8029

Elsevier Health Sciences Division
Subscription Customer Service
3251 Riverport Lane
Maryland Heights, MO 63043

*To ensure uninterrupted delivery of your subscription, please notify us at least 4 weeks in advance of move.

Printed and bound by CPI Group (UK) Ltd, Croydon, CR0 4YY

08/05/2025

01864746-0004